GERIATRIC SECRETS
Second Edition

MARY ANN FORCIEA, MD
Clinical Associate Professor of Medicine
Division of Geriatric Medicine
University of Pennsylvania School of Medicine
Hospital of the University of Pennsylvania
Presbyterian Medical Center
Pennswood Life Care Community
Philadelphia, Pennsylvania

RISA LAVIZZO-MOUREY, MD, MBA
Professor of Medicine
Director, Institute on Aging
Chief, Division of Geriatric Medicine
University of Pennsylvania School of Medicine
Hospital of the University of Pennsylvania
Presbyterian Medical Center
Veterans Administration Medical Center
Philadelphia, Pennsylvania

EDNA P. SCHWAB, MD
Assistant Professor of Medicine
Division of Geriatric Medicine
University of Pennsylvania School of Medicine
Hospital of the University of Pennsylvania
Veterans Administration Medical Center
Presbyterian Medical Center
Philadelphia, Pennsylvania

HANLEY & BELFUS, INC./ Philadelphia

Publisher: HANLEY & BELFUS, INC.
                   Medical Publishers
                   210 South 13th Street
                   Philadelphia, PA 19107
                   (215) 546-7293; 800-962-1892
                   FAX (215) 790-9330
                   Web site: http://www.hanleyandbelfus.com

Note to the reader: Although the information in this book has been carefully reviewed for correctness of dosage and indications, neither the authors nor the editors nor the publisher can accept any legal responsibility for any errors or omissions that may be made. Neither the publisher nor the editors make any warranty, expressed or implied, with respect to the material contained herein. Before prescribing any drug, the reader must review the manufacturer's current product information (package inserts) for accepted indications, absolute dosage recommendations, and other information pertinent to the safe and effective use of the product described. This is especially important when drugs are given in combination or as an adjunct to other forms of therapy.

Library of Congress Cataloging-in-Publication Data

Geriatric secrets / edited by Mary Ann Forciea, Risa J. Lavizzo-Mourey,
   Edna P. Schwab.—2nd ed.
        p. ; cm.—(The Secrets Series®)
   Includes bibliographical references and index.
   ISBN 1-56053-417-6 (alk. paper)
   1. Geriatrics—Miscellanea.   I. Forciea, Mary Ann, 1949–
II. Lavizzo-Mourey, Risa.   III. Schwab, Edna.   IV. Series.
   [DNLM: 1. Geriatrics—Examination Questions.   2. Aging—Examination
Questions.   WT 18.2 G369 2000]
   RC952.5 .G44346 2000
   618.97—dc21
                                                        00-022109

GERIATRIC SECRETS, 2nd Edition   ISBN 1-56053-417-6

Last digit is the print number: 9   8   7   6   5   4   3   2   1

CONTENTS

CONTRIBUTORS

Janet L. Abrahm, M.D.
Associate Professor, Division of Hematology and Oncology, Department of Medicine, University of Pennsylvania School of Medicine; Hospital of the University of Pennsylvania; Presbyterian Medical Center; Pennsylvania Hospital, Philadelphia, Pennsylvania

Steven E. Arnold, M.D.
Assistant Professor, Departments of Psychiatry and Neurology, University of Pennsylvania School of Medicine; Hospital of the University of Pennsylvania, Philadelphia, Pennsylvania

Michelle Battistini, M.D.
Associate Professor, Department of Obstetrics and Gynecology, University of Pennsylvania School of Medicine; Hospital of the University of Pennsylvania, Philadelphia, Pennsylvania

Marie A. Bernard, M.D.
Professor and Chairman, Donald W. Reynolds Department of Geriatric Medicine, University of Oklahoma College of Medicine, Oklahoma City, Oklahoma

John Bruza, M.D.
Division of Geriatric Medicine, Department of Medicine, University of Pennsylvania Health System, Philadelphia, Pennsylvania

John D. Cacciamani, M.D.
Geriatric Fellow, Division of Geriatric Medicine, Department of Medicine, University of Pennsylvania School of Medicine, Philadelphia, Pennsylvania

Elizabeth Capezuti, Ph.D., R.N., FAAN
Research Assistant Professor, University of Pennsylvania School of Nursing, Philadelphia, Pennsylvania

Lesley Carson, M.D.
Assistant Professor, Division of Geriatric Medicine, Department of Medicine, University of Pennsylvania School of Medicine; Staff Physician, Hospital of the University of Pennsylvania; Presbyterian Medical Center, Philadelphia, Pennsylvania

Stephen I. Chavin, M.D.
Professor, Department of Medicine, MCP Hahnemann School of Medicine; Albert Einstein Medical Center, Philadelphia, Pennsylvania

Christopher M. Clark, M.D.
Associate Professor, Department of Neurology, University of Pennsylvania School of Medicine; Hospital of the University of Pennsylvania, Philadelphia, Pennsylvania

Grace A. Cordts, M.D., M.S., M.P.H.
Faculty, Internal Medicine, York Health System, York Hospital, York, Pennsylvania

Hollis Day, M.D., M.S.
Clinician Educator Fellow, Division of Geriatric Medicine, Department of Medicine, University of Pennsylvania School of Medicine, Philadelphia, Pennsylvania

Susan C. Day, M.D., M.P.H.
Adjunct Associate Professor, Department of Medicine, University of Pennsylvania School of Medicine, Philadelphia, Pennsylvania; Chestnut Hill Hospital, Chestnut Hill, Pennsylvania

Angela DeMichele, M.D.
Instructor in Medicine, Division of Hematology and Oncology, Department of Medicine, University of Pennsylvania School of Medicine, Philadelphia, Pennsylvania

William F. Edwards, M.S.N., R.N., C.S., CRNP
Geriatric Nurse Practitioner and Research Project Manager, University of Pennsylvania Hospital, Philadelphia, Pennsylvania

Roy S. Feldman, D.D.S., DMSc
Adjunct Professor of Periodontics, University of Pennsylvania School of Dental Medicine; Chief, Dental Service, Veterans Administration Medical Center, Philadelphia, Pennsylvania

Mary Ann Forciea, M.D.
Clinical Associate Professor, Division of Geriatric Medicine, Department of Medicine, University of Pennsylvania School of Medicine; Hospital of the University of Pennsylvania; Presbyterian Medical Center; Pennswood Life Care Community, Philadelphia, Pennsylvania

Robert Goldman, M.D.
Assistant Professor, Department of Rehabilitation Medicine, University of Pennsylvania School of Medicine; Hospital of the University of Pennsylvania; Presbyterian Medical Center, Philadelphia, Pennsylvania

Nalaka S. Gooneratne, M.D.
Fellow, Division of Pulmonary and Critical Care, Department of Medicine, University of Pennsylvania School of Medicine; Hospital of the University of Pennsylvania, Philadelphia, Pennsylvania

Richard H. Greenberg, M.D.
Department of Hematology and Oncology, Hospital of the University of Pennsylvania, Philadelphia, Pennsylvania

David Guha, M.D.
Division of Internal Medicine, Department of Medicine, Brooklyn Hospital Center, Brooklyn, New York

Raquel E. Gur, M.D., Ph.D.
Professor, Department of Psychiatry, University of Pennsylvania School of Medicine; Director, Neuropsychiatry, Hospital of the University of Pennsylvania, Philadelphia, Pennsylvania

Ruben C. Gur, Ph.D.
Professor, Department of Psychiatry, University of Pennsylvania School of Medicine; Director, Brain Behavior Laboratory, Hospital of the University of Pennsylvania, Philadelphia, Pennsylvania

Diane Hershock, M.D., Ph.D.
Clinical Instructor of Medicine, Division of Hematology and Oncology, Department of Medicine, University of Pennsylvania School of Medicine; Hospital of the University of Pennsylvania, Philadelphia, Pennsylvania

Dennis S. Hsieh, M.D.
Division of Geriatric Medicine, Department of Medicine, University of Pennsylvania Health System, Philadelphia, Pennsylvania

Howard Hurtig, M.D.
Professor and Interim Chair, Department of Neurology, University of Pennsylvania School of Medicine; Hospital of the University of Pennsylvania; Pennsylvania Hospital, Philadelphia, Pennsylvania

Jerry C. Johnson, M.D.
Associate Professor, Department of Medicine, University of Pennsylvania School of Medicine; Attending Staff Physician, Hospital of the University of Pennsylvania; Presbyterian Medical Center, Philadelphia, Pennsylvania

Fran E. Kaiser, M.D.
Adjunct Professor of Medicine, Department of Geriatric Medicine, St. Louis University School of Medicine, St. Louis, Missouri

Jason H. T. Karlawish, M.D.
Assistant Professor, Department of Medicine, University of Pennsylvania School of Medicine; Hospital of the University of Pennsylvania, Philadelphia, Pennsylvania

Bruce Kinosian, M.D.
Division of Geriatric Medicine, Department of Medicine, University of Pennsylvania Health System, Philadelphia, Pennsylvania

Glenn W. Knox, M.D.
Courtesy Clinical Associate Professor, Department of Surgery, University of Florida Health Science Center; Baptist-St. Vincent's Medical Center, Jacksonville, Florida

Joyann A. Kroser, M.D.
Assistant Professor of Medicine, Division of Gastroenterology, Department of Medicine, University of Pennsylvania School of Medicine; Hospital of the University of Pennsylvania; Presbyterian Medical Center, Philadelphia, Pennsylvania

Matthew M. Kurtz, Ph.D.
Postdoctoral Fellow, Neuropsychiatry Program, Department of Psychiatry, University of Pennsylvania Health System, Philadelphia, Pennsylvania

Risa Lavizzo-Mourey, M.D., M.B.A.
Professor of Medicine; Director, Institute on Aging; Chief, Division of Geriatric Medicine, Department of Medicine, University of Pennsylvania School of Medicine; Hospital of the University of Pennsylvania; Presbyterian Medical Center; Veterans Administration Medical Center, Philadelphia, Pennsylvania

Thomas E. Lawrence, M.D.
Clinical Assistant Professor, Institute on Aging, Division of Geriatric Medicine, Department of Medicine, University of Pennsylvania School of Medicine; Hospital of the University of Pennsylvania; Presbyterian Medical Center, Philadelphia, Pennsylvania

Bruce T. Liang, M.D.
Associate Professor, Departments of Medicine and Cardiology, University of Pennsylvania School of Medicine; Cardiology Staff, Hospital of the University of Pennsylvania, Philadelphia, Pennsylvania

Elizabeth R. Mackenzie, Ph.D.
Research Assistant Professor, Division of Geriatric Medicine, Department of Medicine, University of Pennsylvania Health System, Philadelphia, Pennsylvania

Cheng-An Mao, M.D., M.P.H.
Clinical Assistant Professor, Department of Family Medicine, University of Medicine and Dentistry of New Jersey; St. Joseph's Hospital and Medical Center; Medical Director, St. Vincent's Nursing Home, Paterson, New Jersey

David J. Margolis, M.D., MSCE
Associate Professor, Departments of Dermatology and Biostatistics and Epidemiology, University of Pennsylvania School of Medicine; Attending Physician and Director, Cutaneous Ulcer Center, Department of Dermatology, Hospital of the University of Pennsylvania, Philadelphia, Pennsylvania

Joseph R. McClellan, M.D., FACC, FACP
Assistant Professor, Department of Medicine, University of Pennsylvania School of Medicine; Associate Director, Cardiovascular Medicine Program, Hospital of the University of Pennsylvania; Chief of Cardiovascular Medicine, Presbyterian Medical Center, Philadelphia, Pennsylvania

Paula McCrae-Patton, M.D.
Primary Care Provider, Living Independently for Elders Program, University of Pennsylvania School of Nursing; Clinical Associate, Temple University Hospital; Presbyterian Medical Center, Philadelphia, Pennsylvania

Harold Mignott, M.D.
Assistant Professor, Department of Medicine, University of Pennsylvania School of Medicine; Hospital of the University of Pennsylvania, Philadelphia, Pennsylvania

David S. Miller, M.D.
Associate Professor, Department of Psychiatry, University of Medicine and Dentistry of New Jersey Robert Wood Johnson Medical School, Piscataway, New Jersey; Director of Geriatric Psychiatry, Carrier Clinic, Belle Mead, New Jersey

Jeffrey Miller, M.D.
Department of Dermatology, University of Pennsylvania School of Medicine, Philadelphia, Pennsylvania

Paul J. Moberg, Ph.D.
Assistant Professor of Neuropsychology, Department of Psychiatry, University of Pennsylvania School of Medicine; Clinical Director of Neuropsychology, Hospital of the University of Pennsylvania, Philadelphia, Pennsylvania

David W. Oslin, M.D.
Assistant Professor, Department of Psychiatry, University of Pennsylvania School of Medicine, Philadelphia, Pennsylvania

Sheila Pasupathy, B.A.
Program Manager, Geriatrics Education, Institute on Aging, University of Pennsylvania Health System, Philadelphia, Pennsylvania

Michael Pazianas, M.D.
Associate Professor, Division of Geriatric Medicine, Department of Medicine, University of Pennsylvania Health System, Philadelphia, Pennsylvania

Daniel J. Rader, M.D.
Assistant Professor, Department of Medicine, University of Pennsylvania School of Medicine; Director, Preventive Cardiology, University of Pennsylvania Medical Center, Philadelphia, Pennsylvania

Iris M. Reyes, M.D.
Assistant Professor, Department of Emergency Medicine, University of Pennsylvania School of Medicine; Hospital of the University of Pennsylvania, Philadelphia, Pennsylvania

Keith M. Robinson, M.D.
Associate Professor, Department of Rehabilitation Medicine, University of Pennsylvania School of Medicine; Pennsylvania Hospital, Philadelphia, Pennsylvania

Madhurika Samakur
Division of Geriatric Medicine, Department of Medicine, University of Pennsylvania Health System, Philadelphia, Pennsylvania

Edna P. Schwab, M.D.
Assistant Professor of Medicine, Division of Geriatric Medicine, Department of Medicine, University of Pennsylvania School of Medicine; Hospital of the University of Pennsylvania; Veterans Administration Medical Center; Presbyterian Medical Center, Philadelphia, Pennsylvania

Eugenia L. Siegler, M.D.
Associate Professor of Clinical Medicine, Department of Medicine, New York University School of Medicine, New York, New York; Chief of Geriatrics, Brooklyn Hospital Center, Brooklyn, New York

Charles L. Spencer, M.D., Ph.D., C.M.D.
Assistant Clinical Professor, Division of Geriatric Medicine, Department of Medicine, University of Pennsylvania School of Medicine; Hospital of the University of Pennsylvania, Philadelphia, Pennsylvania

Joel E. Streim, M.D.
Associate Professor, Department of Psychiatry, University of Pennsylvania School of Medicine, Philadelphia, Pennsylvania

Dana L. Suskind-Liu, M.D.
Assistant Professor, Department of Pediatric Otolaryngology, Louisiana State University Medical Center, New Orleans, Louisiana

Areena Swarup, M.D.
Geriatric Fellow, Division of Geriatric Medicine, Department of Medicine, University of Pennsylvania School of Medicine, Philadelphia, Pennsylvania

Raymond R. Townsend, M.D.
Associate Professor, Department of Medicine, University of Pennsylvania School of Medicine; Faculty, Hospital of the University of Pennsylvania, Philadelphia, Pennsylvania

David J. Vaughn, M.D.
Associate Professor, Division of Hematology and Oncology, Department of Medicine, University of Pennsylvania School of Medicine; Attending Physician, Hospital of the University of Pennsylvania, Philadelphia, Pennsylvania

Christopher L. Vojta, M.D., M.B.A.
Fellow, Division of Geriatric Medicine, Department of Medicine, University of Pennsylvania School of Medicine, Philadelphia, Pennsylvania

Sandeep Wadhwa, M.D., M.B.A.
Adjunct Assistant Professor, Division of Geriatric Medicine, Department of Medicine, University of Pennsylvania School of Medicine; Hospital of the University of Pennsylvania, Philadelphia, Pennsylvania

Katherine E. Waltman, PharmD
Clinical Assistant Professor of Pharmacy Practice, University of the Sciences, Philadelphia College of Pharmacy; Clinical Pharmacy Specialist, Division of Geriatric Medicine, Presbyterian Medical Center, Philadelphia, Pennsylvania

Joan Weinryb, M.D., C.M.D.
Clinical Assistant Professor, Division of Geriatric Medicine, Department of Medicine, University of Pennsylvania School of Medicine; Hospital of the University of Pennsylvania; Presbyterian Medical Center, Philadelphia, Pennsylvania

Susan E. Wiegers, M.D.
Director, HUP Cardiac Clinic; Associate Director, Noninvasive Imaging, Cardiovascular Division, Hospital of the University of Pennsylvania, Philadelphia, Pennsylvania

Jean Yudin, M.S.N., R.N, C.S.
Division of Geriatric Medicine, Department of Medicine, University of Pennsylvania School of Medicine, Philadelphia, Pennsylvania

PREFACE

Geriatric Secrets is designed for medical students and other health care professionals who are learning the principles of geriatric practice. We use a direct approach familiar to students, the question-answer format, because of its ability to cut to the chase. Now more than ever, students must assimilate large amounts of information quickly and effectively. The Socratic method, whether applied on rounds or in board review books, is an effective, efficient method of imparting information. We attempted to make the book reader-friendly. Where possible, we encouraged the use of summary tables and bullets rather than long passages of text.

This second edition has been expanded to include a new section that deals with health systems and alternative sites of care, such as nursing homes and patients' homes. We have also included a chapter on osteoporosis and its complications as well as chapters on anticoagulation, dehydration, and incontinence.

Consider this book a handbook, not a textbook. It provides an overview of the salient issues in the practice of geriatrics, rather than a comprehensive or exhaustive discussion. Within these constraints, we have tried to emphasize the art of geriatrics—the personal touch, the team approach, the clinical challenges, and the tremendous satisfaction of improving the quality of someone's life, however briefly. Chapter 1 focuses on the art of practicing geriatrics and introduces some of the patients who have taught us the real "secrets" of geriatrics.

Next to the satisfaction of practicing geriatrics, our greatest pleasure comes from teaching it. For many reasons, too few students are exposed to geriatric medicine early enough and often enough to experience its rewards. We take pleasure in the fact that the impact of this book will be felt not only by the students who learn directly from its pages, but also by the clinicians of tomorrow who will benefit from the educational programs of the Institute on Aging at the University of Pennsylvania, to which the royalties from the sale of the book will be donated.

Finally, we gratefully acknowledge those whose contributions helped us turn a concept into a book, the authors for providing content and the project team, Sheila Pasupathy and Robert Stein, for making it happen.

Mary Ann Forciea, M.D.
Risa Lavizzo-Mourey, M.D., M.B.A.
Edna P. Schwab, M.D.

I. Overview

1. THE ART AND PRACTICE OF GERIATRICS

Risa Lavizzo-Mourey, M.D., M.B.A., and Mary Ann Forciea, M.D.

Most of this book focuses on the practice of geriatrics. It strives to impart the basics of geriatric medicine by using a direct approach—questions and answers. However, the art of caring for older patients is as important as the clinical facts, albeit less appreciated. The principles that underlie the art and inherent satisfaction of practicing geriatrics are the "Geriatric Secrets" revealed in this chapter. As with all health care, the real secrets reside in the patients. Although every patient is unique, the commonality among them often defines the approach and direction of a specialty or a discipline. Sometimes the commonality is as simple as a particular disease. In the case of geriatrics, the commonalities are more complex, going beyond age, specific diseases, or particular organ systems. This chapter introduces a few of our patients who, over the years, defined the art and practice of geriatrics for us.

Complex Medicine—Mrs. M.

Geriatric patients have multiple chronic diseases, along with all the sequelae and treatments that chronic conditions entail. Chronic disease, coupled with a vulnerability to acute illness and disability, means that geriatric clinical situations are rarely simple. As clinicians, mostly we are taught to make the diagnosis, to find the malady, and to cure it. In geriatrics there rarely is one diagnosis; the average is four. The diagnoses may be related, sharing organ systems or pathophysiology, but just as often coexisting conditions merely fulfill the dictum that common diseases occur commonly together. Whichever the case, multiple chronic diseases interact, adding ambiguity and complications. As a result, geriatric clinical situations are almost always challenging, requiring knowledge, judgment, and good problem-solving skills.

Mrs. M. illustrates this point. At 75 years of age, Mrs. M. has coronary artery disease and a history of two myocardial infarctions (MIs) despite a series of angioplasties and a coronary artery bypass graft. Mrs. M. is a slight woman with limited bone mass and has been on hormonal replacement therapy (HRT) since menopause. We did not question estrogen replacement until she developed stage I breast cancer. The tumor was quickly and effectively treated with lumpectomy and radiation. Then came the complicated question of whether to continue the HRT. Estrogen could stimulate tumor growth, but without it she was at greater risk for another MI and osteoporosis. Moreover, Mrs. M. suffered from debilitating hot flushes whenever the HRT was discontinued. Ultimately we continued the HRT, following closely for signs of cancer recurrence. Knowledge, judgment, and active consideration of Mrs. M.'s preference led us to the best "solution" for her. Another patient, less compliant or with more advanced cancer, might warrant a different approach.

As challenging as juggling the management of half a dozen chronic diseases—such as diabetes, hypertension, polymyalgia rheumatica, coronary artery disease, nephrosclerosis, and cataracts—can be, it is the superimposed acute disease that often tests one's clinical acumen.

Mr. H.

A 92-year-old retired engineer, Mr. H. moved in with his son and daughter-in-law after the death of his wife. Mr. H. is limited in mobility by coronary artery disease and severe osteoarthritis of both knees. Despite his mobility limitations, Mr. H. leads an active intellectual and social life through telephone conversations and visits from neighbors.

One winter, Mr. H. developed a severe respiratory tract infection. A chest x-ray revealed multiple smooth pulmonary nodules, which almost certainly represented multiple metastases. His respiratory tract infection resolved. Mr. H. and his family discussed diagnostic and therapeutic options with the geriatrics team. Mr. H. decided not to pursue further evaluation of the metastases.

Eighteen months later, Mr. H. continues to be pain-free. He is unable to leave his room due to his dyspnea but still plays a vital role in his family and neighborhood.

In caring for patients with multiple illnesses, the key is to facilitate patients or their surrogates in determining which symptoms are the most burdensome. The impact of treatment on "critical" symptoms must be evaluated, both in terms of efficacy and potential side effects. To Mr. H., dyspnea was familiar and tolerable. He had adjusted his lifestyle to this limitation and was not frightened by the thought of progression of breathlessness. He was terrified by the prospect of pain or nausea. In his family meetings, he finally concluded that he wished no disruption of his life unless pain intervened. The geriatrics team and Mr. H.'s family were able to focus on Mr. H.'s view of his life and to design a program of care that responded to his wishes.

Differentiating Aging from Disease—Mr. I.

Shakespeare characterized old age as a second childhood: "sans eyes, sans teeth, sans everything."

The body changes with aging, and many organs and organ systems become more limited in their capacity to carry out prescribed functions. However, the losses conjured by Shakespeare's words generally result from disease, not normal aging. Differentiating the consequences of normal aging from disease so that disease can be treated or managed is a fundamental principle of geriatrics. For example, the ratio of type I to type II muscle fibers changes with age, but does not cause debilitating muscle atrophy. Sleep patterns change—less deep sleep and increased ratios of REM to non-REM sleep. Yet daytime somnolence, insomnia, and early awaking, while common complaints among the elderly, are not a part of normal aging. Part of the art of geriatrics is not only knowing the difference between normal aging and disease, but also being able to convince patients of the difference.

Mr. I. could not hear as well as he did as a young man. He saw it as an inevitable consequence of aging and was prepared to accept the attendant inconveniences. It was his wife who insisted that he "look into it." She complained about the blaring television and was growing tired of repeating herself or arguing about what had been said. Mr. I.'s hearing loss was severe and asymmetric, involving low- as well as high-frequency ranges. Presbycusis, commonly seen in elders (see Chapter 11), typically involves high frequencies. Mr. I.'s problem was not normal aging and was treatable with a hearing aid.

Convincing Mr. I. that he had a treatable problem meant correcting a lot of misconceptions without creating unrealistically high expectations. After he got a hearing aid, his hearing improved but was not perfect. He admits to being more comfortable in social situations and is amazed at how isolated he had become. In accepting the treatment, he improved his quality of life and taught his physicians the value of pursuing treatable diseases in old age.

Limited Physiologic Reserve—Miss O.

Conceptually, older people often tolerate illness and other threats to homeostasis poorly, because they have limited "physiologic reserve." An 80-year-old's minute ventilation may be adequate at rest, but he or she does not have the reserve necessary to handle two flights of stairs in the setting of a viral upper respiratory infection. Physiologic changes in most organ systems contribute to the diminished reserve observed in the elderly. For example, lean body mass decreases with age, as does muscle strength. Cardiac output with exertion decreases with age. Cognitive functioning, with the exception of executive functions, attenuates. All of these examples can have clinical consequences, particularly when older adults are stressed with an acute illness. Anticipating the consequences of limited physiologic reserves is fundamental to practicing high-quality geriatrics. For example, decreased muscle strength is associated with rapid deconditioning and necessitates attention to ambulation and physical therapy, even during relatively brief ill-nesses. Miss O. was the patient who first peaked our interest in this aspect of geriatrics. She was in her 80s, mildly demented, but still independent in all activities of daily living. Her sister, with whom she shared an apartment, brought her to the emergency department because of her ob-tunded state. According to the sister, Miss O. had been "fine" two days earlier save for a slight fever and foul-smelling urine. Over 48 hours the patient's oral intake progressively worsened, and lethargy developed. On admission to the hospital her serum sodium was 178 mg/dl. That such severe hypernatremia could develop so rapidly seemed improbable at the time, yet we now appreciate that the patient had virtually no reserve and was severely stressed physiologically. Her total body water at baseline was compromised by several factors, including her small size and age-related decreases. Her acute illness, pyelonephritis, exacerbated the dehydration by causing mild diabetes insipidus. Although one cannot be sure that she did not have the infection for longer than two days (but was afebrile), the severity of the dehydration, the devastating effect on her mental status, and the complete reversal of symptoms with hydration left an indelible impres-sion of the need to anticipate the clinical consequences of limited physiologic reserve.

The Interdisciplinary Team Approach—Mrs. W.

All too often the uninitiated believe geriatrics to be overwhelming and depressing. Many pa-tients are frail and often have social problems in addition to complex illnesses. To be sure, pro-viding care to such patients in the context of a busy, single-discipline office practice is daunting. Geriatrics is inherently interdisciplinary. To provide comprehensive care (see later section), a well-functioning, interdisciplinary team is critical.

An interdisciplinary team usually has members with defined but fluid roles that, to some degree, frequently overlap. For example, both nurse practitioner and physician may provide pri-mary care, with the nurse taking responsibility for assessment of functional status or other fac-tors, depending on the availability of physical or occupational therapy. Similarly, case management may fall to nursing, social work, or, in complicated situations, medicine. The hall-marks of a well-functioning cooperative team are flexibility, mutual respect, and the ability to stay focused on the patient's needs and goals.

Mrs. W. is a 68-year-old woman with insulin-dependent diabetes mellitus of 30 years' dura-tion; complications involve almost every organ system. She requires chronic intermittent bladder catheterization because of autonomic nervous system dysfunction. She cannot perform this task for herself because of peripheral neuropathy involving her fingers. She requires help in drawing up her insulin because of the neuropathy and decreased vision. At a routine office visit, review of her diabetic diary revealed marked deterioration in glucose control. Careful questioning made clear that Mrs. W. is no longer certain about guidelines for adjusting her insulin doses to changes in blood sugar level.

A team meeting is followed by a meeting of the team with the patient and her family. The family meeting includes an update of Mrs. W.'s current complications and their impact on her daily life. The medical team members develop new medication schedules and guidelines. Mrs. W. agrees to allow her family to assist in her care and in the adjustment of her insulin doses. Family members volunteer to be trained in insulin administration and in bladder catheterization; team nurses conduct the training sessions. Home health aides are recruited by the team social worker to assist the patient in personal hygiene while the family members are at work.

One month later, the patient and family are much more satisfied with Mrs. W.'s daily life. Her diary reveals much improved glycemic control. The entire team as well as the patient and her family participated in a series of changes in Mrs. W.'s daily routine. A crisis that would have re-quired hospitalization for serious hyper- or hypoglycemia was almost certainly averted; the qual-ity of Mrs. W.'s daily life improved.

Care Across the Continuum—Mrs. Z.

Geriatricians and the teams of care to which those geriatricians belong care for patients in a variety of sites: the office, the hospital, the long-term care facility, and the patient's home. The constancy of the relationship between the patient, family, and geriatric team can be a powerful asset during diagnosis and treatment of an illness.

Mrs. Z. is an 88-year-old retired bookkeeper who lives with her daughter. She has been "shy" all her life: she has little social contact outside her family and dislikes crowds. Her daughter convinced her to seek medical care for long-term arthritis of both knees. She established an ongoing relationship with the geriatrician and the practice nurse. One Sunday morning, Mrs. Z. trips on a bathroom rug, falls to the floor, and is unable to rise. Mrs. Z. is taken to the ER, where a hip fracture is diagnosed. Despite severe pain, she refuses surgery and becomes increasingly agitated with efforts to obtain consent for surgery. Her geriatrician arrives, is able to calm her (draws the curtains to create privacy, sits down next to her, and speaks quietly), and she agrees to surgery. She tolerates hip replacement well, but has postoperative problems with anticoagulation and heart failure. The geriatrician and orthopedist work together to manage these problems and speak daily with the family. The patient is transferred to a skilled nursing facility for rehabilitation after reassurance that "her" doctor will continue to see her during rehabilitation. The geriatrician continues to provide medical care for the patient; the home care nurse practitioner meets the patient in the nursing home. After 1 month, the patient is discharged to home. She can stand but cannot leave the house. The home care team oversees home physical therapy and therapy for her congestive failure. After 3 months, the patient is able to travel by car and returns to the office for ongoing care.

The continuing presence of a familiar physician and other team members allowed Mrs. Z. to accept necessary care. That continuity also facilitates management of new problems and medications (such as anticoagulation) in a safer fashion.

Family Involvement—Miss K.

Geriatrics is a family-oriented specialty. The geriatrician frequently relies on an older person's family to implement the care plan, to be a surrogate decision-maker, and in many ways to function as a member of the team. Yet the family member's unique role and perspective must be preserved. Similarly, geriatricians are faced with the challenge of keeping the patient's interests paramount when day-to-day interactions frequently involve communication only with family members. The rewards of becoming closely involved not only with a patient but also with his or her family are among the most significant in geriatric practice—particularly when the "family" extends beyond the usual definition. Although a geriatrician's interactions with family members are complex, four dimensions seem universal: emotional support, decision making, provision of care, and education.

Education is the foundation on which a sound relationship with the family is built. The willingness to take the time to explain the cause of a clinical event, the next stage of the illness, alternative treatment, and the contents of articles that appear in the newspapers or other lay publications is consistently mentioned by both patients and families as key determinants of their satisfaction or dissatisfaction with physicians. A family that is attempting to cope with a frail elder who may be deteriorating functionally and cognitively is filled with anxiety because they do not know what to expect or when. By educating the family, the clinician not only builds rapport but also gains a critical member of the care team. Family members and other caregivers are the first-line decision-makers in any changing clinical situation. The family decides when to call the physician as well as whether to carry out the physician's suggestion, seek an alternative healer, or do nothing at all. Moreover, the geriatrician frequently must make a medical judgment based on the information provided by family members. Confidence in the accuracy and reliability of this information makes decision making easier.

In their roles as caregivers, family members interact with geriatricians in two other ways: as surrogate decision-makers and as potential patients. When an elderly person is cognitively impaired, it is often the family who participates in medical decision making rather than the patient. The challenge of keeping the patient's interests paramount while meeting the family's needs can be accomplished only through open communication between the family and geriatric team. When effective, such communication produces gratifying rapport, respect, and closeness. Moreover, it forms the basis for providing ongoing emotional support to the family and offers insight into when more intensive intervention is needed to preserve the caregiver's health and well-being.

The Role of Culture in the Picture of Geriatrics—Mr. M.

Culture is the set of shared beliefs, values, and morals that guide individual behaviors. Culture plays an important role in the way every individual interacts with the health care system. With the elderly, it is often a critical element in the physician-patient relationship. The unprecedented advances in technology and medicine that have shaped much of present-day American culture contrast starkly with the environment that influenced many of our elders' values. Moreover, many of America's present-day elders are immigrants or first-generation descendants of immigrants, making them much closer to a set of values that may be quite different from the dominant values of the U.S. today. Most elderly patients were teenagers during the late 1930s and early 1940s, and many immigrated to the United States under political or economic duress. African-American elders endured the humiliation of segregation. Although we take antibiotics, chemotherapy, and sophisticated diagnostic procedures, such as magnetic resonance imaging (MRI), for granted, rest and good air were the predominant treatment for almost every ailment when most elderly patients were growing up. They were adults when the first antibiotics became available and are all too familiar with the devastation that diseases such as polio can cause. Now most Americans receive more than 13 years of formal education, whereas most elderly people had on average only eight years of formal education. Seventy years ago, health education classes were not a standard part of the curriculum. The basic concepts of biology and human physiology that we take for granted in explaining medical conditions to our patients are not necessarily a part of our older patients' fund of knowledge. An elder's understanding of disease and illness may be rooted in religion rather than biology. Every effort should be made to learn the elderly patient's perspectives and values and to give them careful consideration in explanations, conversations, and care planning.

Mr. M. is an 86-year-old African-American man who grew up in the rural southeastern part of the United States. Despite little formal education, he is articulate and extremely skilled in social interactions. He is quite vocal about his major regrets in life, the most prominent being the missed opportunity to go to college. Mr. M.'s two clinical problems were hypertension and hearing loss. The hypertension was easily controlled, but over several years the hearing loss became more disabling. Audiometry revealed classic presbycusis, yet Mr. M. adamantly refused a hearing aid. As his disability from the hearing loss progressed and attempts to persuade him to use a hearing aid were repeatedly spurned, an exploration of his health beliefs was initiated. Surprisingly, this worldly gentleman believed that all illness was punishment from God. Once the hearing loss was discussed in the context of a disease caused by God's wrath rather than neuronal loss, we were able to identify the ways in which a hearing aid could be useful. Mr. M. illustrates a vital lesson: the sharing of many values, such as love of education, does not necessarily mean that one shares all values, including a belief in the biomedical model.

Bioethics

Unlike clinical situations with younger populations, in which ethical issues arise infrequently, geriatricians often grapple with thorny ethical dilemmas. The difficult decision-making surrounding end-of-life choices often gets media attention. However, other decisions—such as the timing of nursing home placement, whether to proceed with a surgical therapy, or whether to place a feeding tube when an elderly person seems unwilling or unable to eat—are equally difficult. The geriatrician's role is complex. The tasks may shift from educator to advisor to sounding board. However, the critical and unwavering role always must be as patient advocate. Older patients can find themselves particularly vulnerable and therefore need the security of knowing that someone always will be their advocate.

Because ethical issues surrounding treatment choices are likely to touch most older people, geriatricians must be comfortable in discussing such issues with their patients. Discussions should occur in the context of the patient's cultural values. Some patients who come from family-centered cultures may prefer to involve family members in the decision-making process, whereas patients from Western cultures are generally comfortable making decisions autonomously. In short, the ethical issues call on all of the other principles of the art and practice of geriatrics. The geriatrician must be knowledgeable about the complexity of medical care in older patients; be able to base prognostications on a clear differentiation between disease and aging; know when to use the other members of an interdisciplinary team; and, above all, discuss such complex issues in the context of the patient's culture and family. Failure to do so can be devastating to the therapeutic relationship and to compliance with recommendations.

2. BIOLOGY OF AGING

Mary Ann Forciea, M.D.

1. Are the changes we associate with aging under any control?

The question underlying all aging research is whether aging changes are due to random (stochastic) processes or whether alterations are under the control of a regulated program. Although no two people age in exactly the same way, most people display similar changes with increasing years. We do not often confuse a 20-year-old patient with one of 80, for example, although we often may mistake a patient of 70-years for one of 80. We postulate that programmed change is responsible for predictable change in a population, whereas random changes may influence changes in an individual within a population.

Another way to address this question is to ask where in the level of complexity of organisms we first begin to see aging in populations. For instance, we do not recognize aging changes in populations of most single-celled organisms such as yeast. Even some multicellular organisms do not display any time-associated changes, such as loss of replicative vigor, biochemical marker changes, or anatomic alterations. We first begin to see "aging" changes in organisms that develop differentiated cell functions. The relationship between differentiation and aging is central not only to aging research, but also to research in oncology and developmental biology.

2. What is the difference between gerontology and geriatrics?

Gerontology is the study of aging itself, as well as of any processes or phenomena that develop around aging change. Gerontology is a research discipline that employs methods and paradigms from biology, sociology, epidemiology, political science, and economics, to name only a few fields. Scientists who study aging are called **gerontologists**.

Geriatrics is the clinical practice of a professional who works with older people in areas such as geriatric medicine, geriatric psychiatry, geriatric nursing, and geriatric social work. Any of these professionals may be called a **geriatrician**, although the term *geriatrician* has currently come to refer to a physician.

3. What are the major theories of aging?

Aging theories fall into two major groups: random change theories and programmed change theories.

Theories of Aging

RANDOM CHANGE	PROGRAMMED CHANGE
Errors	Genetic
Chance	Developmental
Environmental toxins	Metabolic
Chemicals	Autoimmune
Radiation	
Bacteria	
Free radicals	
Wear and tear	

4. Describe the major random change theories of aging.

Error theories hold that aging changes are produced by mistakes in the replication of DNA, in transcription into RNA, in protein translation, and in enzymatic biochemistry.

These mistakes produce mutations and/or dysfunctional processes, such as cross-linking of proteins and other macromolecules. Mistakes are expected to increase in the presence of radiation or certain toxins. As individuals age, the opportunity for such errors to occur and accumulate increases. Older individuals have had more opportunity to experience errors and experience declines as a result of these errors.

The increasing understanding of the independence of mitochondrial DNA within the cell and the relationship of mitochondrial DNA to energy metabolism within the cell has given another dimension to potential sites for errors. Mitochondrial DNA may be injured without affecting nuclear DNA. Techniques in cell biology that allow independent analysis of mitochondrial and nuclear DNA are essential in these studies.

Free radicals are small molecules generated by biochemical reactions at the cellular level. Free radicals are highly toxic because of their instability: they rapidly combine with nearby compounds and produce molecular changes that inactivate many compounds or cause mutation in nucleic acids. Although the generation of these molecules and the changes that the free radicals produce clearly fall into the category of error theories, the area of free radical speculation is so prominent in the lay press and in the marketing of antiaging products that free radicals deserve special mention. A variety of compounds have been discovered that can, in the laboratory, capture (or "scavenge") free radicals as the radicals are generated. These include "antioxidants" such as vitamin E, vitamin C, and beta-carotene. Other naturally occurring antioxidants, such as the enzyme superoxide dismutase, also have been isolated.

Exposure to **environmental toxins** is another theory of aging, which holds that aging changes accumulate because of contact with harmful influences in the environment as we grow older. The categories of outside influences are wide ranging and include such diverse elements as trauma (e.g., auto accidents), radiation, air and chemical pollutants, occupational hazards, and infectious organisms. Exposure to many of these influences can produce an illness or chronic disease; repeated encounters may produce some of the declines in vitality that we associate with aging.

Wear and tear theories hold that individuals are born with a finite capacity in many systems. As the years proceed, these systems become exhausted or damaged and loss of vigor results. The increase in degenerative arthritis due to cartilage damage is an example of a disease process caused by wear and tear.

5. What are the major programmed change theories of aging?

Genetic theories postulate that individuals inherit their life-span; longevity is encoded in the genome. Species have a characteristic life-span. Studies from several species have demonstrated that selectively breeding the longest-lived individuals can extend the life-span of that species by a modest amount. The vitality of these longer-lived individuals is usually extended in such populations.

Developmental theories are invoked by scientists who believe that aging changes are a natural developmental stage in the individual (just as puberty is a developmental stage), with its own endocrinology and anatomic characteristics, and that aging changes are the manifestations of that developmental program. Because the logical place for this program to be encoded is in the genome, many include these theories in the genetic family of aging theories. Support for the existence of a program is provided by the existence of at least one "mutation": children with progeria have been described. Such children appear normal until the age of 2 years and then begin to experience "accelerated aging," in which they develop atherosclerotic cardiovascular disease, graying of hair, thinning of skin, and non–insulin-dependent diabetes mellitus. They often succumb to these illnesses in their 20s. At the other extreme, researchers are now describing families in which large numbers of individuals reach the age of 90 years or older. Careful genetic studies of both these "early aging" and "late aging" clusters will be of great interest.

The discovery of **telomeres**, terminal fragments of chromosomes that are lost during cell division, has generated excitement in the fields of developmental biology, cellular biology of aging, and oncology. Long telomeres occur not only in germ cells but also in pluripotential cells (e.g., bone marrow stem cells) and cells isolated from tumors. With divisions associated with differentiation, the telomeres shorten. Better understanding of how the loss of terminal DNA material may affect cell function (and serve as a "biologic clock") is of central interest to gerontologists and oncologists.

Metabolic theories state that the "rate of living" influences length of life. These theories are sometimes called "pacemaker" theories, because it is postulated that the individual organism can keep track of biologic events and that vigor is reduced as vital substances are consumed. Evidence to support metabolic theories has been cited from studies that have shown that caloric restriction can prolong vigor and life-span in various species, and that modest environmental hypothermia can prolong life-span in some species. Another avenue of support for these theories has come from the observation that body size is generally linked to species longevity: larger species tend to have longer life-spans.

Autoimmune theories hold that aging changes are produced by the accumulation of antibodies that react to proteins in the self; these antibody/antigen complexes then produce disease, which decreases function. The prevalence of many autoantibodies does increase during aging.

6. What model systems are used to study the biology of aging?

Gerontologists use a wide range of **animal species** for study, from very simple invertebrates to insects such as fruit flies and mammals such as rodents. Smaller, simple organisms are desirable because of their short life-spans and large numbers, but more complex organisms may be used to explore more complex processes as well as those more directly linked to human pathology.

The culture of **individual cells** is widely used, especially to examine biochemical changes during aging, to study the effects of various toxic exposures, and to study the controls of lifespan. Diploid cells in culture have a limited ability to divide and reproduce themselves (the "Hayflick phenomenon"). This limitation on replicative life-span of the individual somatic cell has proven to be a fruitful area of research, not only in the field of aging but also in oncology, because cancer cells are immortal in tissue culture.

Investigations of humans throughout their life-span are being conducted through various **human longitudinal studies** in which epidemiologists follow cohorts of healthy individuals throughout their life-span.

7. What is the relationship between normal aging and disease?

Many changes that we associate with normal aging have little consequence to the individual and his or her ability to function in the world. Gray hair, for instance, does not impair physical function. Critical physiologic functions tend to have substantial reserve capacity (such as glomerular filtration rate), so age-associated declines may not be associated with decreased function for many years. On the other hand, reduction in reserve capacity may leave the individual more prone to acute illness or to the development of chronic impairment in function. Some of the physiologic changes formerly ascribed to normal aging have been shown to be reversible (such as VO_2max declines with aging that can improve with exercise). The goal of maximizing functional abilities throughout the life-span is the goal of both gerontology and geriatrics.

BIBLIOGRAPHY

1. Finch CE: Longevity, Senescence, and Genome. Chicago, University of Chicago Press, 1990.
2. Miller RA: The biology of aging and longevity. In Hazzard WR, Blass JP, Ettinger WH, et al (eds): Principles of Geriatric Medicine and Gerontology, 4th ed. New York, McGraw-Hill, 1999, pp 1–19.
3. Schneider EL, Rowe JW (eds): Handbook of the Biology of Aging. San Diego, Academic Press, 1996.
4. Smith JR, Pereira-Smith OM: Replicative senescence: Implications for in vivo aging and tumor suppression. Science 273:63, 1996.
5. Weindruch R: Caloric restriction and aging. Sci Am (January):46, 1996.

II. Symptoms

3. AGING AND NEUROCOGNITIVE FUNCTIONING

Ruben C. Gur, Ph.D., Paul J. Moberg, Ph.D., Matthew M. Kurtz, Ph.D., and Raquel E. Gur, M.D., Ph.D.

1. What is the pattern of cognitive decline in normal aging?

As you might suspect, most cognitive abilities decline with age after adulthood is reached, just like physical abilities. However, not all "mental muscles" "shrivel" at the same rate, and it is important to weigh the negative effects of reduced mental abilities against the positive impact of experience. Thus, even though psychological test performance may decline with age, for particular real-life tasks the relevant experience of an individual may be much more important than the score on a cognitive test. For example, a test may show decline in verbal fluency, but an experienced lawyer would perhaps be better able to select the more effective, if fewer, words compared with younger and likely more fluent counterparts.

Numerous specific changes in cognitive performance are exhibited by persons with dementia. Such changes differ both in magnitude and extent from those seen in the normal aging process. Abilities more commonly affected in dementia include verbal and nonverbal memory, perceptual-organizational abilities, communication skills, and psychomotor performance. The nature, extent, and rate of decline depend on the cause, the person's educational attainment, activity level, and general health status. It is important to remember that about 80% of people living into very old age never experience a significant memory loss or other symptoms of dementia. A slight forgetfulness is common as we age, but it is usually not enough to interfere with our functioning. Pablo Picasso, Margaret Mead, and Duke Ellington were productive well past their 75th birthdays, suggesting that successful aging is both possible and probable.

A long-standing body of research has documented differential patterns of age-related decline on different measures of intelligence. Based on these data, prior research has proposed a taxonomy of cognitive abilities in which cognitive skills can be grouped into one of two functional domains: *crystallized* versus *fluid* intelligence. In this context fluid intelligence represents cognitive abilities that handle novel problems and require flexible and rapid information processing skills. These skills are highly sensitive to the effects of age and are thought to be more closely linked to neurobiologic changes. In contrast, crystallized intelligence represents the repertoire of cognitive skills that are the result of the application of fluid intelligence to the environment. These skills include overlearned information, such as expressive vocabulary, or our general fund of information. These skills are highly influenced by our educational and social history and are relatively resistant to the impact of aging.

Most recent research suggests that cognitive changes associated with aging are most intimately related to a generalized slowing of "cognitive speed." This theoretical model has generated increasing attention to the cognitive processes that underlie performance on a variety of cognitive tasks. By this view, performance on tasks that "load" on, or are more dependent upon, overlearned verbal knowledge are preserved during aging, relative to tasks that require cognitive speed. This "slowing" of cognition, however, may be modified to some extent by general health, use of medications, and physical activity.

2. How is cognition assessed?

To understand which cognitive activities decline more than others, we need to divide cognition into components or domains. It is customary to evaluate the following clusters of cognitive abilities:

Executive functions: the ability to plan, to abstract principles from examples of a set, to shift sets, and to keep ongoing operations in "working memory."

Attention and vigilance: the ability to select relevant stimuli for further processing and response and to concentrate on specific tasks for extended periods.

Learning and memory: the ability to acquire new information and to retrieve it on demand. This ability seems to differ—and perhaps follow specific rules—for verbally encoded and spatial information.

Language and related functions: the ability to speak fluently, communicate effectively, to comprehend accurately and effectively, to name and identify things and people in the environment, to retrieve words in running speech, reading abilities, and writing skills.

Intellectual functions: analytic abilities, fund of information and vocabulary, and effectiveness of processing complex information. These abilities also seem to differ for verbal and spatial functions.

Sensorimotor functions: the acuity of the senses and the speed and accuracy of motor responses.

Of these domains of behavior, there is evidence for age-related decline in attentional processing, memory (both verbal and spatial), intellectual functions (primarily spatial), and the sensorimotor domain, particularly motor speed. On the other hand, executive functions seem relatively preserved. Declines in speed of response and processing are among the most characteristic changes seen with aging and can be observed in any of the above domains.

3. Can the effects of age on cognition be separated from the effects of illness?

A difficulty in answering the question of domain-specific cognitive decline is the need to separate normal aging effects from the effects of age-related disorders likely to influence cognitive dysfunction. As we age, we are more likely to experience accidents in which we lose consciousness, our arteries harden, and we may experience subclinical ischemic episodes that could nonetheless affect specific cognitive abilities. Other brain disorders also are more prevalent in older age. One way to address this methodologic problem is to screen research subjects carefully for any disorder that may affect cognition. In addition, it is helpful to examine the effects of aging within the younger age range, where it is less likely that age-related disorders have occurred. Obviously the effects of age will be smaller in this population, but the effects observed would point to the cognitive systems that are most vulnerable to the normal aging process. One should also bear in mind that some functions may show little if any decline initially and steeper decline after a certain age.

4. Are there sex-related differences in this decline?

This issue has been relatively less investigated, because for a long time such differences were ignored and frequently only men were studied. However, there seems to be evidence that the rate of decline with age is faster for men than for women. (See figure at top of opposite page.)

5. What causes age-related changes in cognitive functioning?

Most likely the cognitive decline associated with aging is linked to brain function, and indeed there is evidence for both anatomic and physiologic brain changes with normal aging. Brain volume is reduced with normal aging, and the reduction in the volume of brain tissue is accompanied by an increase in the volume of the cerebrospinal fluid (CSF). This was demonstrated initially by direct postmortem measurements of brains, using the old Archimedes method of measuring the volume of displaced liquid into which the brain is immersed. More recently, computed tomography (CT) and magnetic resonance imaging (MRI) have been used to measure brain volume. These methods are based on computerized "segmentation" of tissue into brain and CSF, which give different image intensities. Such studies confirm the results of postmortem measurements and also suggest sex differences in the rate at which tissue is lost with normal aging. Men show a steeper loss of tissue and increase in CSF than women. Indeed, the decline in the frontal

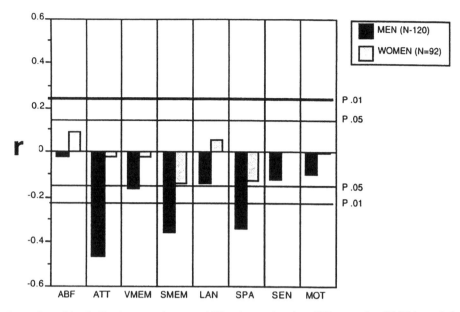

Rates of cognitive decline in men and women. ABF = abstract function; ATT = attention; VMEM = verbal memory; SMEM = spatial memory; LAN = language; SPA = spatial function; SEN = sensory perception; MOT = motor function.

and temporal regions is so pronounced in men compared with women that, whereas young men have larger volumes than young women (commensurate with their overall larger bodies), the volumes in elderly men and elderly women are identical. (See figure below.)

6. How is the pattern different in the dementias?

As noted earlier, changes in brain structure and function are inevitable with the aging process. For example, speed of response tends to slow, and mild forgetfulness is usually present

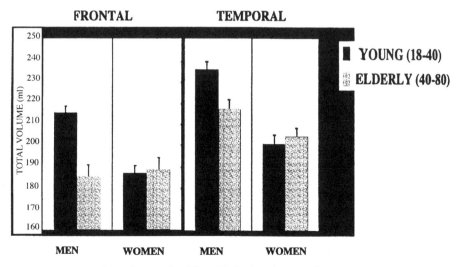

Loss of temporal and frontal brain tissue in men and women.

as a person gets older. Some level of cognitive decline is expected with age, but at what point does it become abnormal? The basic question is whether a person exhibits cognitive changes above and beyond those expected for his or her age. Research with healthy, aged individuals provides a benchmark of mental abilities for people of various ages and educational and occupational backgrounds as well as gender. Such abnormality is typically assessed against this benchmark. For example, an elderly person with a dementing illness may remember only 50% of what is said to them, whereas a healthy person matched in age, gender, and education may remember 80% or more. In addition, the person with dementia shows other deficits of a substantial scope and magnitude in addition to "forgetfulness." Deficits in problem-solving, language, and visual-perceptual abilities are often present. The stigma attached to cognitive decline is not applied to age-associated physical ailments. Older adults suffering from heart disease are not labeled as abnormal, but this term is applied to those suffering from "dementia." Yet just as the definition of aging can include heart disease, so can it include dementia. Many names have been given to the symptoms of memory loss and loss of cognitive abilities in older adults. Terms such as *senility, hardening of the arteries,* and *organic brain syndrome* have been commonly used. *Alzheimer's disease, multi-infarct disease,* and *senile dementia* are terms often used by health care professionals. The word *dementia* means a loss or impairment of mental abilities; it does not mean "crazy": It comes from two Latin words which translate into *away* and *mind*. Dementia is a term chosen by health care professionals to describe a group of symptoms expressed by various disease states. The question is whether dementia is the inevitable end-point of the normal aging process if one lives long enough. While the evidence for either outcome is not entirely clear, the prevailing thought is that the degenerative organic brain state known as dementia is not part of normal aging. Many types of illnesses are associated with dementia, including Alzheimer's disease, multi-infarct disease, Parkinson's disease, Pick's disease, and progressive supranuclear palsy. The most common causes of dementia in elderly persons are Alzheimer's disease and multi-infarct disease.

Dementia knows no social or racial lines: rich and poor, wise and simple alike can be victims. Many brilliant and famous people have suffered from dementing illnesses, and it is likely that we all know someone with such cognitive impairment. Many elderly people live in the community with mild levels of dementia. Typically they can function if environmental supports (e.g., a caring wife, husband, family members) are available. This impairment becomes clinically meaningful when it impairs the person's level of day-to-day functioning. Although we may all be irritated by occasional forgetfulness, it does not prevent us from performing our daily duties and activities.

7. How do the medicines that older people take affect cognitive function?

The concept that medicine can alter a person's cognitive processes is generally well-accepted by most investigators. Aging brings changes in the way that medicine is broken down and used by the body. For example, studies have shown that age-related changes in the gastrointestinal system, increases in body fat, cardiovascular alterations, reduction in blood flow in the brain, reductions in liver and kidney function, and changes in tissue response to hormones interact with medicines and their effect on the patient. In addition, age has a definite impact on the person's ability to adapt to internal or external stressors. For example, elderly people tend to recover more slowly from the adverse side effects of many medications. This issue becomes more complicated if the older adult is also taking more than one medicine. The disorders for which elderly people most commonly receive medication are depression, anxiety, and apprehension; cognitive and memory impairment; sleep disturbances; and behavior disorders. Drugs with anticholinergic properties (e.g., antidepressants, antihistamines, antimotion sickness medications) are the most likely to cause cognitive side effects. Whereas younger people may experience minimal cognitive effects, such effects are magnified in the elderly by physiologic changes. The cognitive effects of drugs used to treat most medical conditions have not, however, been studied systematically.

The greater sensitivity to drug effects in elderly persons also makes the ingestion of "social drugs" problematic and can clearly increase the frequency of negative drug reactions. It is a common practice for patients with diabetes to change their diet to help control the illness. In contrast, it is not unusual to see patients arrive at a precise combination of medicines and dosages through close consultation with their physician—and yet ingest 10–20 cups of coffee a day! Caffeine, nicotine, and other chemicals in common day-to-day beverages and foods can also interact with medicine (or act on their own) to produce adverse cognitive and physiologic effects. Coffee and cola drinks are not the only culprits in such "social drug" consumption. Tea, chocolate, cocoa, cigarettes, and alcohol also must be listed. In addition, seemingly harmless over-the-counter medications (e.g., cold capsules, sleep medicines, pain relievers) can interact with prescribed medications. Perhaps the claim of homeopathic physicians that they successfully treat patients with a minimal dosage of drugs can be explained by their close attention to diet and its direct relationship to the taking of prescribed drugs.

In general, many medicines can have an impact on cognitive processes, especially when the increased vulnerability of the brain and associated physical systems is considered. However, such concerns are often secondary to the cognitive effects of the illnesses for which such medications are prescribed. For example, untreated hypertension or diabetes has a greater adverse effect on cognitive function than the medicines used to treat either condition.

BIBLIOGRAPHY

1. Birren JE, Fisher LM: Aging and speed of behavior: Possible consequences for psychological functioning. Ann Rev Psychol 46:329–353, 1995.
2. Cowell PE, Turetsky BT, Gur RC, et al: Sex differences in aging of the human frontal and temporal lobe. J Neurosci 14:4748–4755, 1994.
3. Salthouse TA: Adult Cognition: An Experimental Psychology of Human Aging. New York, Springer-Verlag, 1982.
4. Salthouse TA: Pressing issues in cognitive aging. In Schwarz N, Park DE (eds): Cognition, Aging, and Self-reports. Hove, UK, Erlbaum, 1999.
5. Salthouse TA, Hambrick DE, McGuthry KE: Shared aged-related influences on cognitive and noncognitive variables. Psychol Aging 13:486–500, 1998.
6. Salzman C, Shader RI, Van Der Kolk BA: Clinical psychopharmacology and the elderly patient. N Y State J Med 76:71–77, 1976.
7. Stuart-Hamilton I: Intellectual changes in late-life. In Woods RT (ed): Clinical Psychology of Ageing. New York, Wiley, 1996.
8. Wilson RS, Bennett DA, Schwartzendruber A: Age-related change in cognitive function. In Nussbaum PD (ed): Handbook of Neuropsychology and Aging. New York, Plenum, 1997.

4. ACUTE CONFUSIONAL STATES AND THE SYNDROME OF DELIRIUM

Joel E. Streim, M.D.

1. Are confusion and disorientation part of the normal aging process?

Aging is normally associated with some decline in specific areas of cognitive performance, especially information acquisition, processing, and retrieval and some language functions. Mild forgetfulness may also be apparent.

Despite this decline in the *speed* of several cognitive functions, older adults normally retain full or nearly full *capacity* to learn and remember new information, perform problem-solving, and communicate. Confusion and disorientation, or cognitive impairment that interferes with the person's ability to function in everyday activities, are *not* normal aging phenomena. They are almost always manifestations of pathologic processes, and some may represent medical emergencies. (See also Chapter 3.)

2. Which conditions are associated with confusion in elderly patients?

Delirium and **dementia** are the two syndromes most often associated with confusional states in older adults. These syndromes, in turn, may each be caused by a wide variety of underlying illnesses and may be exacerbated by environmental factors. Delirium and dementia may also be concurrent.

3. How is delirium distinguished from dementia?

Delirium involves a disturbance of consciousness associated with impaired alertness and attention. This may be manifest clinically as waxing and waning lethargy or diminished arousability, with or without intercurrent periods of agitation. By contrast, patients with **dementia** are consistently arousable and able to remain alert without alterations in their level of consciousness, even though they too may have difficulty concentrating on a task or may become agitated at times.

The onset and clinical course of confusion also help to distinguish delirium from dementia. Confusional states with acute onset should always suggest **delirium**. Typically, the syndrome of delirium develops over a short time, becoming clinically apparent over a few minutes, hours, or days—with the level of consciousness and cognitive and perceptual disturbances tending to fluctuate. By contrast, when confusion is due to **dementia**, it usually begins insidiously and becomes apparent over weeks, months, and years. While patients with dementia may exhibit some day-to-day variability in level of confusion, their cognitive and perceptual capacities do not change dramatically over a period of hours or days, and for most patients, the clinical course tends to be stable or gradually progressive, depending on the underlying cause of the dementia syndrome.

4. What causes acute confusional states or delirium?

Almost any medical illness and many medications. The differential diagnosis includes any condition associated with:

- Cerebral hypoperfusion (e.g., due to hypotension, myocardial infarction, low cardiac output states, arrhythmias)
- Cerebral hypoxia (e.g., due to pneumonia, chronic obstructive pulmonary disease, congestive heart failure, pulmonary emboli) or hypercarbia
- Dehydration (mild dehydration as well as intravascular volume depletion)
- Electrolyte disturbances (e.g., hypo- and hypernatremia, hypo- and hypercalcemia, hypo- and hypermagnesemia, hyperammonemia)
- Hypo- and hyperglycemia and hyperosmolar states

- Infection (e.g., cystitis, urosepsis, pneumonia, peritonitis, and less common central nervous system (CNS) infections such as meningitis and encephalitis)
- Fever or hypothermia
- Pain or discomfort (including distress from urinary retention or fecal impaction)
- Intracranial processes (e.g., stroke, subdural hematoma, neoplasm, infection)
- Intoxication or withdrawal states (e.g., alcohol and other drugs)
- Other adverse drug effects (e.g., central anticholinergic, antihistaminic effects)

While this list of potential causes includes conditions that occur commonly in older patients, it is not exhaustive. In many cases of acute confusion or delirium, it is impossible to identify or confirm a single cause. More often, one identifies multiple factors that are suspected to cause, contribute to, or aggravate confusion.

5. Which classes of drugs commonly cause confusion in older adults?

Virtually all drugs that affect CNS function have the potential to cause confusion.

    Sedative/hypnotic drugs (e.g., benzodiazepines, barbiturates)
    Analgesics (e.g., opiates, nonsteroidal anti-inflammatory drugs)
    Histamine blockers (used for gastrointestinal disorders, insomnia, pruritus, allergy)
    Antisecretory agents (atropinic-like drugs)
    Antidiarrheals
    Incontinence agents
    Tricyclic antidepressants
    Antipsychotics (esp. chlorpromazine, thioridazine, mesoridazine)
    Antiarrhythmic drugs (e.g., lidocaine, procainamide)
    Some antineoplastic agents

6. Who is at risk for developing delirium?

Persons most likely to develop delirium are the very old, those with preexisting brain damage (e.g., from degenerative dementia, cerebrovascular insults, traumatic brain injury), and those with sensory loss (e.g., hearing and visual impairment). Acute confusional states are also more likely to occur in unfamiliar surroundings and environments that cause sensory overload or sensory deprivation.

7. Is sensory deprivation the cause of "sundowning"?

The term "sundowning" usually refers to acute confusional episodes that begin late in the day or at night. The temporal association with the sun's going down has suggested that sensory deprivation may be a cause. However, patients often exhibit a pattern of confusion that has its onset late in the day but before the sun sets. Also, nocturnal confusion has frequently been observed to persist even when adequate lighting and sensory stimulation are maintained after nightfall. Thus "sundowning" may be a misnomer, and some diurnal factor other than altered sensory input may explain the time of onset of confusion.

8. Why is it always important to recognize and evaluate acute confusion or delirium?

Delirium often is the only apparent clinical manifestation of a serious medical illness. For example, myocardial infarction or pulmonary embolus in older adults may present initially with confusion in the absence of chest pain or dyspnea. Urosepsis and pneumonia often occur in older adults without somatic complaints, fever, or leukocytosis, and delirium may be the sole initial clue to these and other infectious diseases. Similarly, abdominal catastrophes (e.g., bowel infarction, perforation, peritonitis) may be heralded by confusion in the very old. Thus, delirium can be an important clinical sign that leads to early recognition, diagnosis, and treatment of serious illness.

Even when delirium is caused by less serious conditions (mild dehydration, constipation, use of low-dose antihistamines), it can lead to significant, potentially reversible comorbidity and excess disability, especially in frail, older adults. When the underlying conditions are identified and are properly managed, the confusion and other cognitive disturbances associated with delirium are usually reversible. Treatment interventions can also alleviate comorbidity, reduce distress and disability, increase function, and improve quality of life. Recognition and evaluation of acute confusion or delirium is therefore essential for the identification and treatment of reversible conditions.

9. How should acute confusion be evaluated?

The work-up for acute confusion or delirium should include:
Complete history
Chart review (with close attention to medications administered, including those taken as needed [PRNs])
Physical and mental status examinations
Laboratory evaluation including:
Urinalysis
Complete blood count
Chemistry profile (with electrolytes including calcium and magnesium)
Electrocardiogram

The use of further tests, such as chest x-ray, CSF examination, electroencephalogram, or brain imaging, should be directed by the specific findings from the history, record review, and patient examination.

10. How is acute confusion or delirium treated?

Appropriate treatment of delirium begins with ensuring the patient's safety, attending to medical emergencies, and managing any other underlying medical conditions, medication effects, or environmental factors that are thought to be contributing to the delirium. Thus, the treatment of delirium and amelioration of the acute confusional state will depend on the specific etiologic factors identified.

11. When should psychotropic medications be used in the management of elders with acute confusion or delirium?

Psychotropic medications are often used in acute and long-term care settings when acute confusional states are associated with agitated or combative behaviors, psychotic symptoms (e.g., hallucinations and delusions), or severe disruption of the normal sleep-wake cycle. The medications usually used for calming these agitated patients are the high-potency neuroleptic/antipsychotics and the short half-life benzodiazepines. Benzodiazepines are the first-line treatment for delirium due to alcohol or benzodiazepine withdrawal. However, few controlled clinical trials have been conducted to determine the efficacy or safety of drugs commonly used to treat delirium due to other causes. For cases of delirium with a variety of etiologies, it is not generally known whether these drugs diminish or exacerbate agitation, combativeness, psychosis, insomnia, or confusion; whether they shorten or prolong the course of the delirium; or whether they reduce the excess disability and mortality associated with delirium.

Although clinical experience suggests that some patients' agitation and psychosis may be effectively quieted with these medications, these agents can also complicate the course of delirium. They can cause sedation and worsen lethargy. The benzodiazepines can also cause increased confusion, anterograde amnesia, disinhibition, and paradoxical excitation. The neuroleptic/antipsychotics can induce akathisia, a syndrome of motor restlessness that may worsen the agitation. When this occurs, it is usually difficult to distinguish the effects of the drugs from the symptoms and signs of delirium.

For this reason, it is usually preferable to manage agitation, sleep disruption, and psychosis by first addressing medical conditions, medication effects, and environmental factors that may be causing these symptoms, with an emphasis on proper nursing care. Pharmacologic strategies should generally be reserved for those patients who are refractory to these measures and who remain highly distressed or physically unsafe without medication to calm them down. Benzodiazepines and neuroleptics should not be used as a treatment for acute confusion when it is uncomplicated by agitation, insomnia, or psychosis. Some clinicians report benefit from the use of chloral hydrate on an empiric basis to calm agitated patients and to treat insomnia when it is thought to be associated with severe sleep deprivation that complicates treatment.

12. What safety precautions should be observed for acutely confused patients?
For many patients with delirium, acute confusion will be accompanied by lethargy or agitation. Patients whose level of responsiveness is diminished may require airway protection or aspiration precautions. For those who are agitated, there may be a need for safeguards against injury: prevention of falls; restriction of access to arterial lines, urinary catheters, tracheostomy cannulae, and ventilator hoses; enforcement of precautions for new joint prostheses; avoidance of trauma from motor restlessness; and surveillance to avert wandering into unsafe situations.

13. What other nursing interventions are indicated to manage delirium?
Beyond immediate safety measures, nursing staff can be instrumental in reducing confusion by setting a calendar and clock in the patient's field of vision, providing frequent verbal reorientation cues, surrounding the patient with familiar personal possessions, pictures, and objects from home, and enlisting the help of family and friends in providing comfort and reassurance. Adjustment of the level of sensory stimulation may also be helpful, increasing the amount of stimulation for patients who have sensory impairment or deprivation and reducing the level for those who are overwhelmed by external stimuli. Nursing staff can also employ sleep hygiene measures to manage the disruption of sleep-wake cycles that typically occurs in patients with delirium.

14. Describe the follow-up care that should be provided after delirium has resolved.
Delirium is a traumatic experience for most patients. Although some are amnestic for events that occur during the course of delirium, many have distressing memories of their confusional state. Even after their acute confusion has resolved, their recollections of illusions, hallucinations, and delusions may be confusing and upsetting, and they may harbor misunderstandings about events and treatment, sometimes attributing malicious intentions to caregivers and family members. For those patients who are not persistently confused due to underlying dementia, it is usually helpful to conduct a debriefing session. This gives the patient an opportunity to express residual concerns, fears, and anger, and it gives the health care provider a chance to provide a medical explanation for the confusional state and to counsel the patient and family. It is especially important to reassure patients about the resolution of their confusion and to discuss prognosis, emphasizing that they are not expected "to go crazy" or "lose their mind," though they may be at risk for recurrence of confusion if exposed to similar circumstances in the future. Therefore, patients and families should be advised to inform future health care providers about their history of confusion and any known causal or precipitating factors. This history can be extremely valuable for prevention.

BIBLIOGRAPHY

1. Breitbart W, Marotta R, Platt MM, et al: A double-blind trial of haloperidol, chlorpromazine, and lorazepam in the treatment of delirium in hospitalized AIDS patients. Am J Psychiatry 153:231–237, 1996.
2. Diagnostic and Statistical Manual of Mental Disorders, 4th ed. Washington, DC, American Psychiatric Association, 1994, pp 123–133.
3. Inouye SK, Charpantier PA: Precipitating factors for delirium in hospitalized elderly persons. JAMA 275: 852–857, 1996.
4. Levkoff SE, Evans D, Liptzin B: Delirium: The occurrence and persistence of symptoms among elderly hospitalized patients. Arch Intern Med 152:334–340, 1992.
5. Lipowski ZJ: Delirium in the elderly patient. N Engl J Med 320:578–582, 1989.
6. Liptzin B: Delirium. In Sadavoy J, Lazarus LW, Jarvik JF, Grossberg GT (eds): Comprehensive Review of Geriatric Psychiatry II, 2nd ed. Washington, DC, American Psychiatric Press, 1996, pp 479–495.
7. Practice guideline for the treatment of patients with delirium. Am J Psychiatry 156(Suppl):1–20, 1999.
8. Rabins PV: Psychosocial and management aspects of delirium. Int J Psychogeriatr 3:319–324, 1991.
9. Trzepacz PT, Wise MG: Neuropsychiatric aspects of delirium. In Yudofsky SC, Hales RE (eds): American Psychiatric Press Textbook of Neuropsychiatry, 3rd ed. Washington, DC, American Psychiatric Press, 1997.

5. FATIGUE

Stephen I. Chavin, M.D.

1. Patients often present to their primary care physicians with a complaint of tiredness or weakness. What symptoms do these terms describe?

Features Distinguishing between Fatigue and Weakness

FATIGUE	WEAKNESS
Feeling of extreme exhaustion not preceded by extraordinary physical activity	Usually accompanied by decreased muscle strength in single tasks
Difficulty concentrating on physical and mental tasks	Reduced endurance in repetitive muscle activity
	Often associated with ≥ 1 objective physical abnormalities of the neuromuscular system
Generalized inability to accomplish necessary daily activities	

Patients use a bewildering variety of terms to describe what appears to be the same subjective symptom complex. The terms include fatigue, exhaustion, tiredness, and weakness, in addition to malaise or lassitude. These terms are usually synonymous with **fatigue**, defined as the presence of one or more features listed in the above table.

Other patients use the term fatigue to describe what appears to be a **weakness**, or diminution of muscle strength and muscle function. In some instances, patients can accurately describe the nature of their complaint. In other cases, the physician must carefully probe both the patient and family members in order to elicit the history and formulate a differential diagnosis.

2. In the general population, how prevalent is fatigue?

A national survey completed more than 20 years ago showed that fatigue was the 7th most common complaint reported by patients. In a more recent study of 1159 consecutive adults attending two primary care clinics, 24% of patients reported fatigue as a major problem, although fatigue was not invariably the reason for the clinic visit. Of the 1159 patients surveyed, 31% were aged 65 years or older. In this group of elderly people, 34% of the women and 18% of the men reported fatigue as a major complaint. These prevalences were not significantly different from those in younger members of the cohort.

Other surveys of primary-care patients complaining of fatigue have indicated prevalences ranging from as low as 2–9% up to 17–47%. Overall, a reasonable estimate is that 1–11 million patient visits to physician offices per year are related to the symptom of fatigue.

3. Why do some patients with fatigue fail to report this symptom to the physician?

Some patients, because of personality or culture, may simply deny the presence of a symptom. Other patients remain unaware of the developing fatigue and unconsciously may reduce their levels of physical activity. Among these patients, there is no intention to deceive; they simply have modified their lifestyle to accommodate the fatigue. To identify such cases, the physician must have a suspicious mind and ask the patient detailed questions, e.g., about changes in amount and kinds of daytime physical and mental activities and alterations in sleeping habits.

4. Can fatigue and life events be associated?

Some life events, such as death, spousal illness, or concerns about personal finance, may lead to feelings of fatigue. Furthermore, the mere self-awareness of growing older may cause symptoms of fatigue. Finally, poor nutrition or extreme reduction in the amount of physical exercise also may lead to this symptom. The biochemical or physiologic mechanisms by which life events cause fatigue can only be speculated at this time. Clearly, a careful history plus the development of a mutually trusting relationship between patient and physician will facilitate identification and perhaps alleviation of the relevant factors.

5. Is depression often associated with fatigue?

Yes. Fatigue is included in the operational definitions for a number of psychiatric disorders, including major depression and dysthymia according to the *Diagnostic and Statistical Manual, 4th ed.* (DSM-IV). The symptom is also assessed in various depression rating scales used for elderly patients, such as the Beck, Yesavage, and Hamilton instruments. The Center for Epidemiologic Studies Depression Scale (CES-D) and the Profile of Mood States (POMS) are two especially useful tools because they separate fatigue-related questions from the total scale.

The inclusion of fatigue on these scales attests to the high prevalence of fatigue and related somatic symptoms in patients with psychiatric disorders, but it does not explain the etiologic relationships. Although considerable observational and experimental evidence links the hypothalamic–pituitary axis to both fatigue and depression, the physiologic mechanisms of the linkage remain obscure. The important point is that the physician must seek out evidence of psychiatric disease in a patient complaining of fatigue.

6. What kinds of medical diseases are associated with fatigue?

In a study of 300 cases of "weakness and fatigue" in an urban referral medical clinic, 20% (61 patients) were found to have physical causes for the fatigue. These causes included chronic infection, metabolic disease such as diabetes mellitus, neurologic disease, and heart disease. Among the 61 patients with identifiable physical causes, 46% had an obvious disease, 21% had equivocal diagnostic findings, and 33% had occult disease. The remaining 80% of the 300 patients, for whom no physical causes could be identified, were given diagnoses of "nervous exhaustion or fatigue, psychoneurosis, or depression" (no demographic information was provided about these patients).

Thus, a variety of diseases have been linked to fatigue. In some, such as cardiac failure or atrial fibrillation, inadequate perfusion of peripheral tissues is the likely cause. In sleep disorders, an impairment of the reticular activating system may reasonably be inferred. In the majority of medical conditions—such as hypo- and hyperthyroidism, diabetes mellitus, hepatitis, cancers, lymphoma, tuberculosis, electrolyte disturbance, chronic obstructive pulmonary disease, and acute infection—plausible mechanisms often are not obvious. In fact, a multiplicity of mechanisms may operate through a small number of common pathways and effectors, such as interleukin-6 and tumor necrosis factor.

7. Can medications cause fatigue?

Pharmacologic therapies are a common and often unpredictable cause of fatigue. The number of medications that have been linked to fatigue is legion, and few classes of drugs have escaped this notoriety. Nonetheless, accurate studies of incidence or prevalence are difficult to find in the literature.

In some cases, such as antihistamines, sedative tricyclic antidepressants, hypnotics, and psychotropic drugs, the cause–effect relationship between the drug's use and the development of fatigue is well-established, and plausible pharmacologic explanations are obvious. In the majority of cases, however, the causal connection may only be suspected, and this problem is compounded if the adverse effect is an idiosyncratic one. Even placebos have been associated with fatigue, indicating that the pharmacodynamics may involve a synergism between the drug and patient. The nearest one can come to proving that a medication has caused fatigue is to demonstrate a chronologic relationship between the start of therapy and the appearance of symptoms, as well as cessation of symptoms following discontinuation of the medication.

Agents That May Cause Fatigue

Alcohol	Dopamine and dopamine agonists (e.g.,
Anticholinergic agents	bromocriptine)
Anticonvulsants	H$_2$ receptor antagonists
Antiviral agents (e.g., amantidine)	Hypnotics
Beta-blockers, esp. lipophilic ones	Neuroleptic agents
Biologic response modifiers, e.g. interferons	Nonsteroidal anti-inflammatory agents
Caffeine	Retinoic acid derivatives
Calcium channel blockers	Tricyclic antidepressants
Chemotherapeutic agents, antimetabolites	Vasodilators
Chemotherapeutic agents, cytotoxic drugs	

8. Is anemia a common cause of fatigue in the elderly?

This is a widely held misconception. In fact, a low hemoglobin concentration is an *uncommon* cause of fatigue. As a general rule, symptoms from anemia seldom appear until the hemoglobin has fallen to levels considerably < 50% of normal. Also, with chronic anemias, their development may be slow enough to allow time for physiologic adaptions to ensure delivery of adequate O$_2$ and other nutrients to the peripheral tissues, thereby preventing symptoms.

When significant symptoms are noted in a patient with only moderate anemia, the physician should suspect some underlying pathology that either is interacting synergistically with anemia (e.g., congestive heart failure with poor cardiac output) or is itself causing both the symptoms and anemia (e.g., metastatic cancer). Anemia, however, may be directly responsible for the symptoms when it has developed acutely (e.g., severe autoimmune hemolytic anemia) with inadequate time for compensatory mechanisms to appear. A somewhat different situation occurs when the anemia has developed quickly as a result of blood loss; in this case, the signs and symptoms are those of hypovolemia, poor cardiac output, and inadequate perfusion of essential organs, such as brain and liver.

The definitive test for anemia as the cause of fatigue is a therapeutic trial transfusion of packed red blood cells adequate to raise the hemoglobin to a level of 7–8 gm/dl. A positive result is a significant reduction in the patient's symptoms sustained for the duration of the hemoglobin elevation (usually many days). If the beneficial effects are only transient (1–2 days), it is unlikely that a low hemoglobin concentration per se is causing the fatigue. Before choosing a therapeutic transfusion trial, the physician and patient should consider the risks and benefits of this approach, taking into account the severity of the symptoms, possibility of volume overload, and infectious complications.

9. Is it possible to distinguish between fatigue from physical causes and fatigue from psychological ones?

Fatigue, like pain, is subjective and possesses no objective or easily demonstrable attributes or correlates. Therefore, the two types of fatigue are indistinguishable unless a cause can be identified. In another sense, however, certain characteristics may point toward one or the other etiology.

PHYSICAL FATIGUE	PSYCHOLOGICAL FATIGUE
Worsens as day progresses	Varies unpredictably and rapidly in intensity
Diminished or eliminated after rest or sleep	Most severe on awakening
May be objectively demonstrated by muscle weakness, esp. after muscle use	May improve as day progresses
	No measurable muscle weakness or relation to muscle use

Finally, patients who appear to be fatigued but who deny or minimize the complaint are more likely to be suffering from a physical cause, whereas patients with psychological fatigue rarely deny the presence of fatigue and may even exaggerate it. An important caveat is that a patient may be suffering simultaneously from both psychological and physical causes of fatigue. For example, patients with lymphoma may suffer physical fatigue as well as depression.

10. Why should the primary care doctor pay serious attention to a common subjective complaint such as fatigue?

1. Patients with fatigue as a major complaint may have a persistent and striking degree of global dysfunction, comparable to that seen in patients with untreated hyperthyroidism or patients who have survived myocardial infarction. Thus, fatigue is not a trivial complaint but one with serious health implications.

2. The symptom may be a harbinger of a serious medical condition, e.g., chronic infection, overdose, or drug reaction, which may be diagnosed and treated at an early stage.

3. The attention paid to the patient's complaints may foster an improved patient–doctor relationship.

11. How should fatigue be evaluated in an ambulatory primary care setting?

When the patient presents initially with a complaint of fatigue, a minimal work-up should include a comprehensive history (physical and psychological) and physical exam. If these investigations are unrevealing, then it probably is reasonable to defer further extensive laboratory testing until the fatigue has persisted for 4–8 weeks.

12. How do laboratory tests help elicit the causes of chronic fatigue?

In a survey of 102 patients (mean age = 57) with fatigue, the following laboratory tests were done: hematocrit, erythrocyte sedimentation rate (ESR), serum creatinine concentration, serum potassium concentration, urinalysis, serum thyroxine and triiodothyronine concentration, serum thyroid stimulating hormone, chest x-ray, monospot test, and stool for occult blood. Only the ESR showed a significant difference in fatigued versus control subjects; 12% of the fatigued subjects compared with 4% of controls had abnormally elevated ESRs, although unequivocal causes for the elevation could not be found. Thus, in the absence of any cause readily identifiable from the initial history and physical examination, random laboratory investigations usually are not helpful in evaluating the causes of fatigue. In such cases, the best approach is periodic follow-up and clinical reassessments.

BIBLIOGRAPHY

1. Allan FN: The differential diagnosis of weakness and fatigue. N Engl J Med 231:414–418, 1944.
2. Engel GL: Nervousness and fatigue. In MacBryde CM, Blacklow RS (eds): Signs and Symptoms: Applied Pathologic Physiology and Clinical Interpretation, 5th ed. Philadelphia, J.B. Lippincott, 1970, pp 632–649.
3. Huyser BA, Parker JC, Thoreson R, et al: Predictors of subjective fatigue among individuals with rheumatoid arthritis. Arthritis Rheum 41:2230–2237, 1998.
4. Ingles JL, Eskes GA, Phillips SJ: Fatigue after stroke. Arch Phys Med Rehabil 80:173–178, 1999.
5. Kroenke K, Wood DR, Mangelsdorff AD, et al: Chronic fatigue in primary care: Prevalence, patient characteristics, and outcome. JAMA 260:929–934, 1988.
6. Lloyd AR: Chronic fatigue and chronic fatigue syndrome: Shifting boundaries and attributions. Am J Med 105(3A):7S–10S, 1998.
7. Matthews DA, Manu P, Lane TJ: Evaluation and management of patients with chronic fatigue. Am J Med Sci 302:269–277, 1991.
8. Mendoza TR, Wang XS, Cleeland CJ, et al: The rapid assessment of fatigue severity in cancer patients: Use of the Brief Fatigue Inventory. Cancer 85:1186–1196, 1999.
9. National Center for Health Statistics: The National Ambulatory Medical Care Survey: 1975 Summary, United States, January–December 1975. In Vital and Health Statistics series 13, no. 36 [DHHS publ no. (PHS)84-1717]. Hyattsville, MD, Public Health Service, 1978.

6. DIZZINESS AND VERTIGO

Lesley Carson, M.D., Dana L. Suskind-Liu, M.D., and Glenn W. Knox, M.D.

1. What is the clinical difference between dizziness and vertigo?

Dizziness is a common and often complicated complaint in geriatric patients. It is one of the most common reasons for physician visits in patients over 75 years of age and the third most common reason in patients over 65 years. Dizziness can be subtyped into vertigo, presyncopal lightheadedness, and dysequilibrium; it is often multifactorial and difficult to describe. It also may have psychogenic features. Vertigo, which refers to a sense of rotational movement and spinning, suggests vestibular pathology. Presyncopal lightheadedness describes an impending faint and is due to cerebral hypoperfusion. Dysequilibrium describes a feeling of imbalance and unsteadiness of body, not of head, which may result from pathology in the motor control system (visual, vestibulospinal, proprioceptive, somatosensory, cerebellar, motor) and vestibular system (inner ear, middle ear, brainstem, cerebellum).

2. Can dizziness be a normal part of aging?

Presbystasis is the term used to describe the dysequilibrium of aging. It is thought to result from an overall decline in vestibular, visual, proprioceptive, and neuromuscular function. Although functional decrease in vestibular activity in elderly people is slight, the overall decline in compensatory mechanisms (i.e., proprioception, vision, and neuromuscular) leaves them vulnerable to unstable conditions to which a younger person could easily adapt. Presbystasis is a diagnosis of exclusion. Nearly all causes of dizziness are pathologic. The elderly patient with symptoms of vertigo or dizziness often has a definable etiology. Patients diagnosed with presbystasis are prime candidates for vestibular rehabilitation, during which they learn methods of compensation.

3. What major etiologies should be considered in vertigo or dizziness in the elderly?

Vertigo—acute
    Vertebrobasilar event
    Toxic (drugs/illness)
    Infectious
    Trauma
    Tumor
    Seizure
    Transient ischemic attack
    Cerebrovascular accident
    Cardiac arrhythmia
Vertigo—recurrent
    Meniere's disease
    Migraine
    Hypothyroidism
    Multiple sclerosis
    Presbylabyrinth
    Syphilis
    Diabetes mellitus
        Small vessel
        Peripheral neuropathy

Vertigo—positional
    Benign paroxysmal positional vertigo
    Infection
    Trauma
    Cervical vertigo
    Central causes
Imbalance
    Medication toxicity
    Sensory impairment
    Cervical spine dizziness
    Presbystasis
Presyncope
    Orthostasis
    Hyperventilation
    Muscle weakness

Adapted from Mader SL: Dizziness and syncope. In Yoshikawa T (ed): Ambulatory Geriatric Care. St. Louis, Mosby, 1993, pp 305–315.

4. How do you differentiate among vertigo, lightheadedness, and dysequilibrium?

	COMMON EXAMPLES	TIME FRAME	CHARACTERISTIC FEATURES
Vertigo	Benign positional vertigo	Short and episodic, < 1 minute	Rapid head movements, precipitate, recurrent
	Vertebrobasilar insufficiency • Transient ischemic attack • Medullary dysfunction • Cerebellar infarcts	Longer and episodic, 20 min–2 hr or continuous	Associated neurologic symptoms, such as diplopia, hallucinations, and dysarthria, as well as nausea and vomiting
	Meniere's disease	Even longer episodes, 2 hr–2 days	Fluctuating hearing loss, tinnitus, pressure in ear
	Neurolabyrinthitis	Episodic for days	Associated with nausea, vomiting and acute onset with recent upper respiratory infection
Lightheadedness	Vasovagal episodes	Episodic	Induced by strong emotion; fall in heart rate and blood pressure
	Orthostatic hypotension	Continuous (may occur daily)	Precipitated by rapid change to standing position; medications, volume loss, autonomic dysfunction implicated
	Cardiac arrhythmia	Episodic or continuous	Syncope of sudden onset
	Valvular heart disease	Continuous or episodic	Murmur of aortic stenosis
Dysequilibrium	Multiple neurosensory deficits	Continuous	Worse with standing or walking; multiple deficits, including degenerative joint disease, medication, decreased vision
	Physical deconditioning	Continuous	Decreased activity, after recent fall, <1 wk bedrest
	Peripheral neuropathy	Continuous	Associated with acoustic neuroma, diabetes mellitus, renal failure Worse in dark
	Cerebellar disease	Continuous	Accompanied by intention tremor, incoordination, dysarthria

5. Which aspects of the physical exam need to be evaluated during the work-up for dizziness in the elderly?

Initial evaluation should include traditional orthostatics, full cardiovascular exam, and a complete neurotologic work-up. Blood pressure and pulse should be measured in the lying, sitting, and standing positions, because orthostatic hypotension is a common cause of dizziness in the elderly. Orthostatic hypotension is defined as a drop in systolic blood pressure of > 20 mmHg from lying to standing position. However, in the elderly orthostatic symptoms may occur without the 20-mmHg drop in systolic pressure even 10–30 minutes after the assumption of erect posture. Cardiovascular exams are performed to identify possible cardiac arrhythmias, significant valvular heart disease, and carotid bruits.

A complete neurotologic exam should be performed, beginning with an otologic exam and including a cranial nerve exam, evaluation of the external and middle ear, and a fistula test. The fistula test is performed by applying pressure to the ear and evaluating for vertigo and nystagmus. A positive result indicates the presence of a fistula of the labyrinth due to cholesteatoma or infection. Evaluation for nystagmus, an objective finding that accompanies vertigo, is also important. Spontaneously induced nystagmus may indicate central or peripheral vestibular dysfunction. Nystagmus is named according to the direction of the rapid component. Fixation inhibits peripheral spontaneous nystagmus with the slow phase toward the abnormal side and the fast phase toward the normal side. The Dix-Hallpike or Nylen-Barany maneuver evaluates positional nystagmus. Nystagmus with latency time of 3–10 seconds until onset, less than 1-minute duration, fatigability on repeat testing, and a rotatory nature with a vertical or horizontal component can be found in peripheral nervous system disorders. A Weber-Rinne test is performed to assess for sensorineural or conductive hearing loss. The Romberg test and tandem gait tests evaluate vestibular, proprioceptive, and cerebellar components.

6. Which basic and adjunctive tests should be ordered to evaluate the dizzy or vertiginous patient?

Routine lab tests include an electrocardiogram (EKG), blood sugar, and complete blood count. An EKG suggests the presence or absence of an arrhythmia. Anemia and hypoglycemia can be detected by a complete blood count and blood sugar.

Adjunctive tests may greatly facilitate a diagnostic work-up. They should be obtained, however, with a systematic rather than a "shotgun" approach. A complete audiogram should be obtained in all patients complaining of hearing loss and vertigo and in all patients with abnormal neurotologic exams. Electronystagmography (ENG), which evaluates the vestibular system by recording nystagmus, aids in differentiating central from peripheral vestibular dysfunction. It should be obtained in patients complaining of vertigo or patients with neurotologic findings such as nystagmus. Patients should avoid all vestibular suppressants for at least 48 hours before testing. Auditory brainstem-evoked responses should be obtained in patients with asymmetric sensorineural hearing loss to rule out acoustic neuroma. Magnetic resonance imaging (MRI) may be considered in selected patients. MRI examination of the temporal bone is often ordered in patients suspected of having acoustic neuromas or other cerebellopontine angle masses. Computed tomography (CT) of the temporal bones also may be obtained when cholesteatomas or other middle ear lesions are suspected.

Cervical spine radiographs should be obtained if cervical dizziness is suspected, whereas an echocardiogram, carotid and vertebral artery Doppler scans, tilt-table testing, and a 24-hour Holter monitor are obtained if presyncope is diagnosed.

7. What is vestibular rehabilitation? Who is a candidate?

Vestibular rehabilitation is a form of physical therapy designed specifically to help dizzy patients to cope in their environment through vestibular compensation. It is a multidisciplinary treatment program that uses vestibular provocation as well as conditioning and control exercises. It teaches the patient to use existing visual or proprioceptive cues. Although vestibular suppressants may be used as adjunctive therapy, preferably patients should avoid such medication during vestibular rehabilitation. Vestibular rehabilitation is used most often in patients with benign paroxysmal positional vertigo (BPPV) and dizziness secondary to presbystasis, vestibular surgery, or traumatic head injury. Although elderly patients make slower progress in vestibular rehabilitation than younger patients, they often derive significant benefit. Vestibular rehabilitation is inappropriate for patients in whom the cause of dizziness has not been identified. In addition, long-term benefits have not been found in patients with Meniere's disease.

8. What is Meniere's syndrome?

Meniere's syndrome is characterized by episodic vertigo, aural fullness, tinnitus, and fluctuating hearing loss. The pathophysiology is thought to be secondary to endolymphatic hydrops, possibly due to bacterial, viral, or syphilitic causes. The hearing loss is unilateral and involves the low-frequency range. The episodes of vertigo typically last minutes to hours, at times with nausea and vomiting. A sensation of unsteadiness may persist for days thereafter. Diagnosis is made on the basis of the typical clinical history and documentation of fluctuating hearing loss as well as episodic vertigo. Medical management includes acute management with antivertiginous medication, prophylactic salt restriction, and diuretics in an effort to reduce the hydrops. Surgical treatments, such as labyrinthectomies, vestibular nerve sections, and endolymphatic shunts, are not recommended in elderly patients, who tend to have more difficulty adapting after such procedures. Vestibular rehabilitation results in minimal improvement.

9. Define BPPV. How is it diagnosed?

BPPV is one of the most common causes of vertigo in elderly patients. It occurs usually after trauma or an episode of viral labyrinthitis. The pathophysiology is thought to be due to the release of otoconia (small calcium carbonate crystals in the saccule) into the posterior semicircular canal. With head movement the crystals are displaced, resulting in vertigo and nystagmus. Patients develop vertigo that occurs with positional changes and lasts less than 1 minute. BPPV is diagnosed by a suggestive history and a positive Hallpike maneuver on physical examination. Extensive diagnostic testing is not required. Although 90% of cases resolve spontaneously within a few months, exacerbations may last for years.

The Hallpike maneuver is used to evaluate for BPPV. Nystagmus and vertigo are assessed after the head is turned to the left and the patient is quickly lowered from a sitting to a supine position. The head is held in the supine position for 1 minute. The procedure is repeated with the head turned to the right. The test should be repeated several times on the side that is most symptomatic to check for fatigability. A positive Hallpike test classically provokes the patient's symptoms and elicits nystagmus on the affected side.

Treatment is directed toward active provocation of the vestibular system with the goal of vestibular habituation and resolution of symptoms. The Epley maneuver repositions free-floating endolymphatic particles in the posterior semicircular canal. The patient is placed in the provocative head-hanging position and remains there for several minutes. The patient is then rotated to the opposite side, with the head turned 45° downward. The patient should be aware that dizziness is exacerbated initially during the exercises but will subside with time. Theoretically this maneuver allows the floating particles to continue their course through the common crus into the utricle by rotating the posterior semicircular canal 180° in the plane of gravity. Meclizine may be useful in the short term for control of symptoms.

10. What is the role for vestibular suppressants such as lorazepam and meclizine in elderly vertiginous patients?

The use of vestibular suppressants is not contraindicated in the elderly. An antiemetic may also aid patients with severe nausea and vomiting. Elderly patients, however, may be extremely sensitive to vestibular suppressants. In addition, they may be taking other medications that interact with or affect the metabolism of such medications.

11. Which medications are possible causes of dysequilibrium?

Geriatric patients are often on polypharmacy that may either cause or exacerbate baseline dizziness or vertigo. It is extremely important to obtain a thorough medication list, including as-needed prescriptions.

CLASS OF DRUG	TYPE OF DIZZINESS	MECHANISM
Alcohol	Positional	Cerebellar dysfunction
Sedatives	Disorientation	Depression of central processing
Antihypertensives	Lightheadedness	Orthostatic hypotension
Anticonvulsants	Dysequilibrium	Cerebellar dysfunction
Aminoglycosides	Dysequilibrium, oscillopsia/vertigo	Damage to labyrinthine hair cells
Diuretics	Positional	Orthostatic hypotension

12. How does the time frame of the symptoms relate to the diagnostic etiology?

The time frame of the patient's symptoms may give an indication of the etiology. BPPV usually resolves within 30 seconds to a minute after the provoking positional change. In patients with vascular etiologies, such as transient ischemic attack, symptoms last for 20 minutes to several hours. Episodes of vertigo in Meniere's disease usually last from minutes to hours. The episodes of vertigo with neuronitis and labyrinthitis continue for days. The more continuous the symptoms, the more carefully one should consider psychological states, medications, or diseases that cause permanent structural damage, such as stroke and peripheral neuropathy.

13. Describe a general approach to the diagnosis of dizziness.

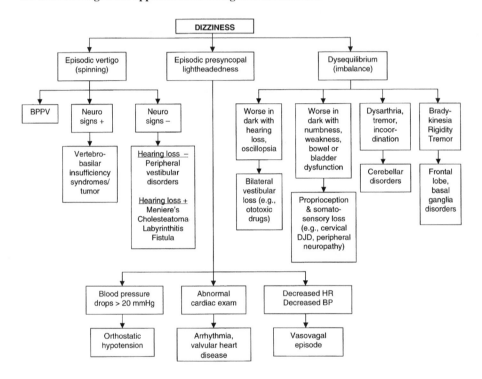

BIBLIOGRAPHY

1. Aronow WS: Dizziness and syncope. In Hazzard WR, Blass JP, Ettinger WH, et al (eds): Principles of Geriatric Medicine and Gerontology, 4th ed. New York, McGraw-Hill, 1999, pp 1519–1524.
2. Baloh RW: Dizziness in older people. J Am Geriatr Soc 40:713–721, 1992.
3. Baloh RW: Approach to the evaluation of of the dizzy patient. Otolaryngol Head Neck Surg 112:3–7, 1995.
4. Cohen H, Rubin AM, Gombash L: The team approach to treatment of the dizzy patient. Arch Phys Med Rehabil 73:703–708, 1992.
5. Cohen H: Vestibular rehabilitation reduces functional disability. Otolaryngol Head Neck Surg 107:638–643, 1992.
6. Gomez CR, et al: Isolated vertigo as a manifestation of vertebrobasilar ischemia. Am Acad Neurol 47:94–97, 1996.
7. Katsarkas A: Dizziness in aging: A retrospective study of 1194 Cases. Otolaryngol Head Neck Surg 110:296–301, 1994.
8. Lempert T, Gresty MA, Bronstein AM: Benign positional vertigo: Recognition and treatment. BMJ 311:489–491, 1995.

9. Mader SL: Dizziness and syncope. In Yoshikawa T (ed): Ambulatory Geriatric Care. St. Louis, Mosby, 1993, pp 305–315.
10. Sloan PD: Evaluation and management of dizziness in the older patient. Clin Geriatr Med 12:785–801, 1996.

7. INVOLUNTARY WEIGHT LOSS IN THE ELDERLY

Mary Ann Forciea, M.D.

1. What is significant weight loss in older patients?

A documented fall in weight of 4–5% in 1 year is the best standard to use in outpatients over age 65. In a prospective study of a population of community-dwelling men over age 65 who were eligible for care through the Veterans Administration (VA), Wallace et al. have demonstrated that a 1-year documented weight loss of > 4% was the best single predictor of death within 2 years. Other standards used in the literature have ranged from 7.5–10% over 6 months, but these higher limits have not been as carefully correlated with future mortality as has the 4–5% limit. In Wallace et al.'s 2-year follow-up, mortality rates were 28% in weight losers, as compared with 11% in controls.

2. Is weight loss in the elderly different from that in other medical patients?

Diseases identified as the cause of weight loss in older patients are the same as those identified in middle-aged adults: **unknown causes** (approx 25% in most studies), **depression**, and **cancer** being the three most common diagnoses. The widely held belief that weight loss in older patients is more often due to malignant causes has not been validated in studies to date. Morley and others suggest that social or functional disorders that limit access to food (poverty, immobility, and isolation) may be more prevalent in older patients who lose weight than in younger persons.

Thompson and Morris have suggested that involuntary weight loss may be less serious in elderly outpatients than in younger patients. They found a 2-year mortality of 9% in their study of 45 elderly primary care patients who had lost 7.5% of their baseline body weight in the 6 months prior to the study. Wallace et al., in a VA clinic-based study, found a 2-year mortality of 28%, closely approximating mortality levels reported in younger patients losing weight. Differences in disease burden in the two populations may well explain the difference in mortality seen.

3. What is the differential diagnosis of involuntary weight loss in the elderly?

Common causes of weight loss in elderly outpatients can be more easily remembered with the portentous mnemonic **DEAD** (which refers of course to the outcome of excessive weight loss): drugs, eating, access, and disease.

Drugs. Medications can produce anorexia, xerostomia (e.g., anticholinergics), and nausea, all of which curb appetite. Taste and smell can be altered by a variety of medicines. Drugs such as antibiotics often result in diarrhea and caloric loss. In addition, the physical fact of taking 4 or more tablets shortly before a meal (once-a-day meds being ingested with breakfast) may inhibit normal appetite. Refer to the table on the following page for examples of specific medications.

Eating. Elderly patients may lack the manual dexterity to cut food or use standard silverware due to stroke, arthritis, or confusion. The amount of time required to consume a meal may leave the food cold and unappealing. Patients may have adopted unusual diets either to promote health or by overly enthusiastic efforts to reduce salt or cholesterol. Sullivan et al., in a study of elderly patients admitted to a VA evaluation unit, found > 80% of patients to be affected by oral health problems that could interfere with normal mastication.

Access to food. Older patients can lose weight because they are too poor to buy enough nourishing food, too immobile to shop for food, or too confused to prepare appealing meals. They may be unaware of community assistance programs, such as "meals on wheels," or too proud to use such services. Liquid food supplements are not covered by federal (Medicare) or most state (Medicaid) assistance programs.

Disease. In the 75% of cases of weight loss where a cause is identified, a wide variety of illnesses may present (see question 5).

Medications that May Affect Appetite and Digestion

Decreased appetite
    Anorexia—amphetamines (Ritalin), selegiline, selective serotonin reuptake inhibitors (SSRIs)
    Xerostomia—anticholinergics, e.g., oxybutynin (Ditropan), flavoxate (Urispas), trihexyphenidyl
      (Artane), benztropine (Cogentin), pilocarpine
    Nausea—digoxin, quinidine

Altered taste and smell—antibiotics, steroid nasal sprays

Diarrhea—antibiotics, nonsteroidal anti-inflammatory drugs

---

4. List some oral problems seen in the elderly that may affect appetite and digestion.
    Absent teeth
    Missing teeth
    Poorly fitting dentures
    Dental caries with or without pain
    Gingival infection or inflammation
    Mucous membrane infection (candidiasis)
    Temporomandibular joint pain

5. Which diseases are usually associated with weight loss in the elderly?

Depression was the most frequent single cause found by Thompson and Morris in their elderly family practice patients. Elderly patients must still be screened for alcohol use and certainly may be active alcoholics.

Malignancies, especially lung and gastrointestinal (GI) tumors, are frequent causes of weight loss. Chronic leukemias and lymphoma also may be seen. Physiologic products of malignant cells, such as tumor necrosis factor, a cytokine, can interfere with the body's metabolism and caloric requirements.

Cardiopulmonary disorders, such as congestive heart failure or chronic obstructive pulmonary disease, can be associated with weight loss in late stages ("cardiac cachexia").

Renal failure and uremia may present with anorexia as one of the earliest symptoms.

Infection, especially with tuberculosis, is still seen in older patients, particularly those with compromised immune function. HIV should certainly be considered in patients with risk factors.

Endocrine disorders may manifest with weight loss as a presenting symptom. Hyperthyroidism is the most notorious endocrine cause of weight loss, and in the variant of hyperthyroidism known as "apathetic hyperthyroidism," weight loss may be the presenting symptom. Patients with diabetes mellitus may lose weight from osmotic diuresis with severe hyperglycemia. In the late stages of either type I or type II diabetes mellitus, patients may lose weight due to a combination of renal disease, abnormal protein metabolism, and depression, but weight loss rarely is the presenting symptom at this stage of the illness.

6. What information from the history is pertinent in evaluating weight loss?

Documentation of the weight loss is ideal: Marton et al. described an inaccuracy rate of nearly 50% in patients complaining of weight loss. Evidence of weight change from the medical records is preferred but often unavailable. Many states require weight reporting on the drivers' license; although this is a self-report, the number can give some indication of "usual" weight. Evidence from clothing, such as wear on belt holes or safety pins on waist bands, can also support recent weight loss. Photographs are often useful, as is history provided by family.

Dietary review is important but often difficult. Older patients may be unwilling to complete dietary logs, and their recall of meal composition is unreliable. Caregivers may be more helpful in supplying dietary information.

Social information addressing the issues in access to food will be helpful. Information on **alcohol** use and **smoking** history are always relevant. Past **surgical history** can be important, especially if it concerns the GI tract.

7. Which components of the physical exam are relevant?

Documentation of the **weight** is necessary, either to quantitate loss or to establish a new baseline. **Blood pressure** recordings should include orthostatic alterations, which might indicate dehydration as well as weight loss. **Temperature** should be recorded.

The **skin** should be examined for confirmation of weight loss and for jaundice, rash, or petechiae. Palpation of **lymph nodes** in the submandibular, supraclavicular, axillary, and inguinal regions is important, as is estimation of size of the **liver** and **spleen**.

Examination of the **eyes** may signal thyroid disease. Careful examination of the **oral cavity** is especially important. Sullivan et al. found that the number of general oral problems was the best predictor of involuntary weight loss in the year preceding inpatient geriatric assessment in a group of elderly veterans.

The **thyroid** gland should be examined for size and consistency; a bruit overlying an enlarged gland usually indicates increased blood flow as is seen in Graves' disease. **Chest** exam may disclose evidence of consolidation or obstruction. **Abdominal** examination should include assessment of organ size and consistency. **Pelvic** and **rectal** examinations are especially important in pursuing occult malignancy.

Neurologic assessment must include an evaluation of mental status, as well as muscle tone and strength as it pertains to mobility.

8. What constitutes a cost-effective work-up?

In Thompson and Morris' study of elderly outpatients, the initial history and physical examination revealed a source for the weight loss when an organic cause was evident. Although no case-control studies have been conducted in the elderly, most authors recommend laboratory testing to include complete blood count, erythrocyte sedimentation rate, urinalysis, multiphasic chemistry panel (blood sugar, creatinine, liver function tests, calcium, phosphorus, and electrolytes), thyroid stimulating hormone, chest x-ray, and HIV testing (if risk factors are present). The role of the prostate-specific antigen screening test in elderly men has not yet been defined but is being offered in many practices as part of periodic screening in older men.

Specialized laboratory studies are sometimes ordered to evaluate whether weight loss has led to actual malnutrition. Measurement of serum albumin is often an initial screen; levels of transferrin, retinol-binding protein, or prealbumin have been proposed as indicators of visceral protein stores. Cutaneous delayed hypersensitivity is reduced in malnutrition, as are the numbers of total lymphocytes.

9. How can I treat weight loss?

If no specific cause of weight loss is identified (as happens in approximately 25% of patients), watchful waiting is best. In Thompson and Morris' study, 27% of patients stabilized their weight during the 2-year study period.

In patients in whom an organic cause is identified, clearly treatment should be offered. Medication regimens should be altered, when possible, if side effects are responsible. Dental referral is indicated for patients with contributing oral problems.

Collaboration with a skilled social worker can not only help to address societal services, such as meal service or homemaker services, but also help to educate patients and families about caregiving skills. Formal consultation with a dietitian is of great value in educating families and patients about a nutritious diet and in addressing special problems such as modified diets (low-salt or diabetic diets), texture-specific diets (soft, puréed), and the use of liquid dietary supplements. (See also Chapter 17.)

BIBLIOGRAPHY

1. Gazewood JD, Mehr DR: Diagnosis and management of weight loss in the elderly. J Fam Pract 47:19–25, 1998.
2. Marton KI, Sox HC, Krupp JR: Involuntary weight loss: Diagnostic and prognostic significance. Ann Intern Med 95:568–574, 1981.
3. Morley JE, Mooradian AD, Silver AJ, et al: Nutrition in the elderly. Ann Intern Med 109:890–904, 1988.
4. Pamuk ER, Williamson DF, Madans J, et al: Weight loss and mortality in a national cohort of adults, 1971–1987. Am J Epidemiol 136:686–697, 1992.
5. Reife CM: Involuntary weight loss. Med Clin North Am 79:299–313, 1995.
6. Sullivan DH, Martin W, Flaxman N, Hagen JE: Oral health problems and involuntary weight loss in a population of frail elderly. J Am Geriatr Soc 41:725–731, 1995.
7. Thompson MP, Morris LK: Unexplained weight loss in the ambulatory elderly. J Am Geriatr Soc 39:497–500, 1991.
8. Wallace JI, Schwartz RS: Involuntary weight loss in elderly outpatients. Clin Geriatr Med 13:717, 1997.
9. Wise GR, Craig D: Evaluation of involuntary weight loss. Postgrad Med 95(4):145–151, 1994.

8. SEXUAL FUNCTIONING

Fran E. Kaiser, M.D.

1. How does the sexual response cycle change with aging?

Changes in Human Sexual Response with Aging

PHASE	MALE	FEMALE
Excitement	Reduced scrotal vasocongestion Decreased testicular elevation Delayed penile erection	Reduced breast and genital vasocongestion Diminished vaginal secretions Delayed arousal
Plateau	Prolonged Diminshed pre-ejaculatory secretions	Reduced elevation of uterus and labia majora
Orgasm	Short duration Reduction in prostatic and urethral contraction	Short duration Fewer and weaker uterine and vaginal contractions
Resolution	Rapid detumescence and testicular descent Prolonged refractory period	Rapid reversal to prearousal stage

As defined by Masters and Johnson, the stages of sexual response change with aging, although these changes do not preclude sexual activity. In 1992, the National Institutes of Health (NIH) defined erectile dysfunction as "the inability of the male to attain and maintain erection of the penis sufficient to permit satisfactory intercourse." Erectile dysfunction has replaced the emotionally charged term *impotence.*

2. Are loss of sexual function and erectile dysfunction normal consequences of the aging process?

No. While some older adults experience a decrease in sexual activity with age, many individuals remain sexually active. Erectile dysfunction, though common with age (occurring in 52% of all men aged 40–70 and > 95% of diabetic men > 70), indicates underlying organic disease. An estimated 30 million men in the United States have erectile dysfunction.

3. Is the most common cause of erectile dysfunction psychogenic?

No. Prior to the 1980s, it was thought that 90% of erectile dysfunction was due to psychogenic causes. Although underlying organic etiologies are more common than psychogenic problems, one cannot discount a psychological overlay to a chronic problem. Depression, performance anxiety (fear of failure), and "widower's syndrome" (a widower's entering a new relationship may evoke guilt about the deceased partner, as bereavement may not be completed) may occur.

We now know that the most common cause of erectile dysfunction is vascular. Over 50% of men have vascular dysfunction, which can relate to poor arterial inflow, excessive venous outflow, or a combination of these factors. Neurologic, hormonal, and medication effects can also play a role. Neurologic problems such as stroke, multiple sclerosis, spinal cord lesions/traumas, and peripheral and autonomic neuropathy may cause erectile dysfunction. Diabetes, hypo- and hyperthyroidism, hyperprolactinemia, and Cushing's syndrome are associated with erectile dysfunction. No one knows the frequency of these conditions—it depends on the setting. An endocrinologist will see more hormonal problems than an internist, and a psychiatrist may see more depression than another specialist. More information about the physiology of erection is now known. Altered nitric oxide, vasoactive intestinal peptide, and neuropeptide Y are implicated in erectile function.

Etiology of Impotence

Vascular	**Psychologic**	**Medications** *(cont.)*
Arteriosclerotic	Depression	Antidepressants
Venous leakage	"Madonna" syndrome	H$_2$ blockers
Arteriovenous malformations	Performance anxiety	**Systemic defects**
Local trauma	Widower's syndrome	Renal failure
Nervous system	Stress	Chronic obstructive pulmonary
Central	**Endocrine**	disease
Stroke	Diabetes mellitus	Cirrhosis
Multiple sclerosis	Hypogonadism	Leprosy
Temporal lobe epilepsy	Hyperprolactinemia	Myotonia dystrophica
Spinal cord	Hypothyroidism	**Nutritional disorders**
Trauma	Hyperthyroidism	Obesity
Tumor	Cushing's syndrome	Protein-calorie malnutrition
Peripheral	**Medications**	Zinc deficiency
Autonomic neuropathy	Antihypertensive agents	**Peyronie's disease**
Sensory neuropathy	Anticholinergics	**Prostatectomy**

4. What is the role of medication in causing erectile dysfunction?

Ten percent of commonly prescribed medications result in erectile dysfunction. In nearly 25% of men with erectile dysfunction, medications play a role. *All* antihypertensives, regardless of class, have been associated with impotence. The most common medications to cause potency problems are thiazide diuretics. These drugs drop penile pressures and lower testosterone and bioavailable testosterone levels.

5. How does hypogonadism cause erectile dysfunction?

Hypogonadism can be defined as a low testosterone level (generally < 300 ng/dl) and a low bioavailable testosterone level. Bioavailable testosterone is the fraction of testosterone not bound to sex hormone-binding globulin (SHBG) and is the "testosterone equivalent" of the relationship of the free thyroxine index to total thyroxine. That is, since testosterone is bound to SHBG, a measure of the total testosterone alone is not especially helpful in defining gonadal status. Low testosterone and low bioavailable testosterone levels are linked to low libido (sex drive) but not, per se, to erectile dysfunction. Young men who have been castrated may get erections. However, improvement in libido with testosterone treatment may be enough to overcome lack of sexual interest and erectile problems in some individuals.

6. What tests are helpful in diagnosing and determining the cause of erectile dysfunction?

All patients should be screened for sexual problems. A nonjudgmental question such as "Do you have any difficulty with your ability to have sex?" may be a good opener.

A careful sexual, medical, and medication history and a depression assessment using the Beck Depression Inventory or the Yesavage Geriatric Depression Scale are all beneficial. Penile tissue should be examined for fibrous plaques or bands that would occur with Peyronie's disease (plaques or bands causing penile bending). Small or soft testicles, gynecomastia, and increased hip girth suggest hypogonadism. Decreased penile sensitivity or abnormal cremasteric or bulbocavernosus reflexes suggest neuropathy. Penile Doppler testing can be helpful to diagnose abnormal vascular status, especially when an exercise component is added. This test measures pressure in the penis and compares it to pressure in the arm. A ratio < 0.65 (penis to brachial pressure) is diagnostic of vascular problems.

Testosterone, bioavailable testosterone, and luteinizing hormone should be measured. Thyroid function tests should be obtained. Nocturnal penile tumescence testing (sleep study of erectile function) is not especially helpful in those over age 50, as it is often impaired in older subjects despite an ability to get and maintain erections adequate for intercourse.

7. How can you treat erectile dysfunction?

When an etiology such as hypogonadism with decreased libido or depression is found, management is clear. In most cases, however, the etiology is multifactorial, and various alternatives are available. Noninvasive choices include sildenafil and vacuum tumescent devices. **Sildenafil** (Viagra), an oral type V phosphodiesterase inhibitor, results in penile vasodilation when stimulation occurs. It is contraindicated in patients taking nitrates and also may impair color vision. Care and caution should be used in patients with known or suspected cardiac disease, even if they do not take nitrates. **Vacuum tumescent devices** (the creation of negative pressure using a pump attached to a plastic tube placed over the penis) create an erection. A band or ring is then placed at the base of the penis, the vacuum is released, and the tube is removed. The erection lasts 15–30 minutes. **Penile injection therapy** (prostaglandin E1, alprostadil [Caverject]) is used when the man wishes to get an erection. **Surgery** or the implantation of bendable or inflatable rods into the penis is another method of treatment. Each method has benefits as well as problems, and often individual lifestyle and preference dictate therapeutic choice.

8. What is the effect of estrogen loss in women?

Estrogen deficiency is associated with a reduction in vaginal blood flow, decreased vaginal lubrication, and increased vaginal fragility with thinning of vaginal mucosa. These changes can result in dyspareunia (painful intercourse). To treat estrogen deficiency locally, Estrace cream (or its equivalent) is inserted into the vagina 2–4 gm once daily for 2 weeks and then as maintenance 1 gm 1–3 times a week. Estrogen and progesterone have minimal effects on libido, and levels do not predict desire, sexual function, or sexual response. Estrogen has a positive and beneficial effect on vaginal lubrication and tissue strength (stronger and less friable) and from that aspect can improve sexual function. Testosterone does seem to play a major role in libido in women.

9. Is hysterectomy associated with an alteration in sexual function?

Hysterectomy is the most commonly performed surgery in women, with one-third of women over age 60 having had this procedure. However, it tends not to be associated with a decline in sexual function. For women who feel that sex is primarily a procreative function, the loss of the uterus may impact on the psychological importance and influence sexual response. For women in whom uterine contractions play an important role in orgasm, hysterectomy may impair orgasmic sensation but generally does not result in anorgasmia.

10. Does medication use affect sexual function in women?

This is essentially unknown, because few studies of medication effect explore sexual function in women.

11. What reasons do older women give for changes in their sexual activity?

- Lack of a partner
- Partner erectile dysfunction
- Personal health problems
- Vaginal dryness

Masturbation is a common form of sexual expression, especially when one does not have a partner or the partner's health or abilities are impaired. Many older individuals find this an acceptable and enjoyable experience.

12. What about sexuality in a long-term care setting?

There is no age at which sexual activity and expression ends. It is important to recognize that a nursing home is still home. Staff need to provide opportunities for privacy for mutually desired sexual activities or for masturbation. The only true problem is coercive or aggressive behavior.

BIBLIOGRAPHY

1. Bretschneider JG, McCoy NL: Sexual interest and behavior in healthy 80- to 102-year-olds. Arch Sex Behav 17:109–129, 1988.
2. Diokno AC, Brown MB, Herzog AR: Sexual function in the elderly. Arch Intern Med 150:197–200, 1990.
3. Feldman HA, Goldstein I, Hatzchristou G, et al: Impotence and its medical and psychosocial correlates: Results of the Massachusetts Male Aging Study. J Urol 151:54–61, 1994.
4. Goldstein I, Lue TF, Padma Nathan H, et al: Oral sildenafil in the treatment of erectile dysfunction. N Engl J Med 338:1397–1404, 1998.
5. Kaiser FE, Viosca SP, Morley JE, et al: Impotence and aging: Clinical and hormonal factors. J Am Geriatr Soc 36:511–519, 1988.
6. Kaplan HS, Owett T: The female androgen deficiency syndrome. J Sex Marital Ther 19:13–24, 1993.
7. Krane RJ, Goldstein I, de Tejada IS: Impotence. N Engl J Med 321:1648–1659, 1989.
8. Morley JE, Kaiser FE: Impotence: The internist's approach to diagnosis and treatment. Adv Intern Med 38:151–168, 1993.
9. Rendell MS, Rajfer J, Wicker PA, et al: Sildenafil for treatment of erectile dysfunction in men with diabetes. JAMA 281:421–426, 1999.
10. Roughan PA, Kaiser FE, Morley JE: Sexuality and the older woman. Clin Geriatr Med 1:87–106, 1993.

9. CONSTIPATION

William F. Edwards, M.S.N., R.N., C.S., CRNP

1. What is constipation?
From a medical perspective, constipation is often defined as a frequency of < 3 bowel movements a week. From the individual's perspective, constipation can mean that stools are difficult to expel, too hard, or too small, or there may be a sensation of incomplete evacuation. Although it is important to teach the patient about normal bowel function, successful management requires that the clinician also respect the patient's concerns.

2. Is constipation a normal part of aging?
The frequency of bowel movements in healthy older populations is essentially the same as it is in the younger population. Despite this fact, the use of laxatives is more common in the elderly, even if they are not having infrequent stools.

3. List the causes of constipation.
For most elderly individuals, there are likely to be multiple contributing factors:

Dietary
- Inadequate caloric intake
- Poor fluid intake
- Low-fiber diet
- High-fat diet
- Refined foods
- Poor dentition
- Swallowing problems
- Tube feedings

Psychological
- Depression
- Confusion
- Emotional stress

Functional
- Inadequate toileting
- Poor bowel habits
- Weakness
- Immobility/lack of exercise

Colonic/anorectal disorders
- Ischemia
- Postsurgical obstruction
- Rectocele or rectal prolapse

Colonic/anorectal disorders *(cont.)*
- Tumors
- Volvulus or megacolon
- Barium or bezoars
- Fissures or hemorrhoids
- Fistula or abscess
- Radiation fibrosis
- Stricture
- Prostatic enlargement
- Diverticulosis

Neurogenic disorders
- Spinal cord lesions
- Parkinson's disease
- Cerebrovascular accidents
- Dementia

Endocrine/metabolic disorders
- Diabetes
- Hypothyroidism
- Hyperparathyroidism
- Hypokalemia
- Hypercalcemia

4. What medications can cause constipation?
Aluminum: antacids (Amphojel, ALternaGEL), sucralfate
Anticonvulsants: phenytoin, carbamazepine, phenobarbital
Antidepressants: amitriptyline, nortriptyline, venlafaxine
Antihistamines: diphenhydramine, chlorpheniramine
Antihypertensives: acebutolol, prazosin
Antilipemics: cholestyramine, colestipol
Antiparkinsonian drugs: bromocriptine, Sinemet, amantadine, benztropine, pramipexole
Antipsychotics: haloperidol, risperidone

Antispasmodics: oxybutynin, opiate or barbiturate compounds
Bismuth: Pepto-Bismol, Rectacort
Calcium: antacids (Tums), supplements (calcium carbonate)
Calcium channel blockers: verapamil, nifedipine
Diuretics: hydrochlorothiazide, furosemide, indapamide
Ganglionic blockers: trimethaphan
Iron supplements
Laxative misuse
Nonsteroidal anti-inflammatories: naproxen, sulindac, ketoprofen
Opiates: codeine, morphine, oxycodone
Phenothiazines: thioridazine, chlorpromazine, perphenazine
Sedatives: diazepam, flurazepam, thiothixene

5. Do all individuals complaining of constipation require a complete evaluation?
Individuals with a precipitous change in bowel habits (including the caliber or characteristics of the stool) require a thorough evaluation. For those with a history of constipation > 2 years, the focus should be on management. In obtaining the history, you must find out how the patient defines constipation and whether the patient has had a change in bowel function or is dealing with a long-term problem. Many elderly were reared with the idea that daily movements were essential to good health and that failure to move the bowels led to the buildup of dangerous toxins.

6. What other aspects of the history are most important?
- In patients with recent onset of constipation, the history should focus on excluding underlying causes such as malignancy, intestinal obstruction, or irritable bowel syndrome.
- Exacerbation or complications of a known illness must be considered.
- A thorough evaluation of recent changes in diet, medications, emotional state, and level of activity is warranted.
- In evaluation of the diet, total caloric intake, fiber content, and fluid intake should receive special attention.
- The clinician needs to inquire about problems related to chewing and swallowing.
- It is essential to evaluate the patient's complaint of constipation as thoroughly as possible.
- The color, amount, consistency, frequency, size, and symptoms experienced during defecation are key components of the history.
- Brief screening tests for cognitive function and mood assist the clinician in detecting non-physiologic causes of constipation.

7. Is a complete physical examination necessary in evaluating the patient with constipation?
If the patient is not known to the clinician, a complete physical exam is needed to rule out systemic causes. For most patients, the focus is on examination of the mouth, abdomen, and anorectal area and assessment for dehydration. The **oral** examination focuses on adequacy of dentition and detection of any lesions or tumors. The **abdomen** is examined for bowel sounds and detection of pain or localized masses. The **anorectal area** is evaluated for sphincter muscle tone; presence of stool in the vault; lesions such as hemorrhoids, strictures, fistulas, or masses; and prostatic enlargement. A neurologic examination can identify common systemic causes of constipation.

8. How do you decide when to do additional diagnostic testing?
If the symptom of constipation began < 2 years ago or if the patient has pain or any evidence of rectal bleeding, colonoscopy or sigmoidoscopy and barium enema are mandatory. In addition to detecting cancer, endoscopy also can reveal the presence of diffuse dark pigmentation, melanosis coli, which is caused by chronic use of laxatives such as cascara, senna, and aloe.

If the patient has liquid stool leakage or symptoms of impaction with an empty rectal vault, abdominal x-rays can detect a high impaction or other signs of obstruction. Additional diagnostic testing, such as colonic transit time and motility studies, is needed only if the patient does not respond to treatment for constipation. Blood work should include a complete blood count (CBC), electrolytes, glucose, and thyroid studies.

9. Are any serious complications associated with constipation?

Fecal impaction is the major complication, and it can be life-threatening. Fecal impaction can cause cognitive problems, malaise, fatigue, urinary retention, bowel and urine incontinence, anal fissure, hemorrhoids, stercoral ulcer, and intestinal obstruction. Watery diarrhea can occur around impacted stool. A mass of stool in the rectum can impair sensation and lead to the need for larger volumes of stool to stimulate the urge to defecate. Constipated patients, especially those who have chronically abused laxatives, can develop **megacolon** and **volvulus**. Straining during defecation affects cerebral and coronary circulation and can cause **transient ischemic attacks** and **syncope**, especially in the frail elderly. Finally, chronic constipation is a risk factor for **colon** and **rectal carcinoma**.

10. Discuss approaches to treating constipation.

The treatment of constipation is individualized for each patient according to the identified causes. The clinician must balance the need to make changes slowly with the patient's desire to get results quickly (as evidenced by the $400-million/year laxative industry). Patient outcome goals might include the passage of a soft formed stool at least 3 times a week without straining and the avoidance of complications associated with constipation.

1. The first step in managing constipation is to stop or switch any medications that may be contributing, including laxatives.

2. It is best to start a bowel program with an empty colon, which may require the use of enemas or even manual disimpaction. Aside from avoiding soap suds, there is no consensus on the best type of fluid to use for enemas. In patients who may require a series of enemas, normal saline is probably best. The temperature should be about 105°F, and the amount should not exceed 500 ml. For occasional use, the popular sodium phosphate enema is usually safe, but the amount should not exceed 120 ml.

3. Healthy bowel function requires an adequate **fluid intake**. If there are no fluid restrictions because of renal or cardiac problems, 2 to 3 liters/day is an appropriate goal. This needs to be done gradually to improve compliance. Water is the ideal fluid—caffeinated beverages and some fruit juices can cause diuresis, which can exacerbate constipation.

4. **Dietary fiber** should also be increased. This is done gradually to avoid unpleasant bloating and gas pains and to give the patient's colon a chance to adapt. The amount of additional fiber required to improve bowel function varies greatly, from 6 to 30 gm.

5. Regular **exercise** is an important component of healthy bowel function. Ambulatory patients should be encouraged to walk for 20 minutes daily. Even those elderly individuals who are bed- or chair-bound can benefit from an exercise program that involves turning from side to side, twisting the trunk, or exercising the arms.

6. The clinician should instruct the patient in the importance of establishing a **routine** that promotes normal bowel function. This includes taking advantage of the gastrocolic reflex, which for most individuals is most pronounced after breakfast or supper. Many individuals find it helpful to have a warm drink with breakfast. It is important that the patient have a private opportunity for about 10 minutes each day to attempt to have a bowel movement. It is also important to emphasize the need to respond as soon as possible to any urge to defecate. Proper position also facilitates bowel function. Squatting is the best position, but this is often not possible for the elderly who require high toilet seats. The squatting position can be emulated in these cases by using a foot stool. The patient should be instructed to lean forward and use the hand to apply firm pressure on the lower abdomen.

7. Institutionalized patients require close monitoring. It is not adequate simply to mark whether or not the person's bowels moved. It is important to note the amount, color, and consistency of the stool. Each care plan should include information about the individual's usual bowel habits, including the time of day that is most conducive to normal evacuation.

Comparison of Laxatives, Suppositories, and Enemas

LAXATIVES	USUAL DAILY DOSE	ONSET OF ACTION	COMMENTS/CONSIDERATIONS
Bulk laxatives			
Psyllium (Metamucil)	1 tbls up to 3 times/day	12–72 hr	Good for long-term use in ambulatory individuals who maintain adequate fluid intake. Psyllium can lower cholesterol, and methylcellulose and calcium polycarbophil are less likely to cause gas pain.
Methylcellulose (Citrucel)	1 tbls up to 3 times/day	12–72 hr	
	2–4 tabs every day	12–72 hr	
Polycarbophil (FiberCon)			
Hyperosmolar laxatives			
Lactulose (Chronulac)	15–30 ml qd qid	24–48 hr	Effective in ambulatory and immobile patients. Safe for diabetics and patients with renal failure. Sorbitol costs 10% as much as lactulose with the same efficacy. Polyethylene glycol is used for bowel preparation before a GI procedure.
Sorbitol	15–30 ml qd qid	24–48 hr	
Polyethylene glycol (Golytely)	240–480 ml	0.5–1 hr	
Stimulant laxatives			
Senna (Senokot)	2 tabs every day to 4 tabs 2 times/day	8–12 hr	Castor oil, aloe, and phenolphthalein should be avoided. The latter can impair vitamin D and calcium absorption and has been associated with dermatitis, Stevens-Johnson syndrome, photosensitivity reactions, and cancer in laboratory animals. Senna is safe for long-term use in the elderly and is a good choice for slow-transit constipation that does not respond to sorbitol.
Bisacodyl (Dulcolax)	10–30 mg at bedtime	6–12 hr	
Cascara	1 tab or 5 ml at bedtime	8–12 hr	
Saline laxatives			
Magnesium hydroxide (milk of magnesia)	5–30 ml every day, 2 times/day	1–3 hr	Commonly prescribed in hospitals because they empty the bowel in a few hours. Can cause electrolyte imbalance; magnesium levels should be monitored if used regularly. Avoid magnesium- and aluminum-containing products in patients with renal insufficiency. May be useful in patients with colonic hypomotility if stimulant agents are no longer effective.
Magnesium citrate	200 ml every day	1–3 hr	
Emollient laxatives			
Mineral oil	15–45 ml	6–8 hr	Avoid mineral oil in the elderly because of the risk of aspiration, interference with absorption of fat-soluble vitamins, and risk of leakage through anal sphincter. Stool softeners are popular, but there is little evidence for their efficacy. They should be avoided in patients with a large amount of soft stool in their rectum. Adding 8 ounces of water to the diet probably is more effective.
Docusate salts (Colace)	100 mg 2 times/day	12–72 hr	

Table continued on following page.

Comparison of Laxatives, Suppositories, and Enemas (Continued)

LAXATIVES	USUAL DAILY DOSE	ONSET OF ACTION	COMMENTS/CONSIDERATIONS
Suppositories			
Bisacodyl suppositories	10 mg suppository	5–30 min	For occasional use when stool is present in rectum. May cause cramping
Glycerin suppositories	3–4 gram suppository	15–60 min	and local irritation.
Enemas			
Soap-suds	500 ml	2–15 min	Reserve for constipation that does not
Mineral oil	100–250 ml	2–15 min	respond to other approaches. Soap-
Phosphate (Fleet)	100–250 ml	2–15 min	suds enemas can cause damage to
Tap water	500 ml	2–15 min	rectal mucosa and should be avoided.
Normal saline	500 ml	2–15 min	Mineral oil may be helpful for acute disimpaction. Phosphate enemas are generally well-tolerated with occasional use but can cause hyperphosphatemia. Normal saline is probably the safest for the elderly.

11. What are the most effective ways of adding fiber to the diet?

The best way to add fiber is by making subtle changes in the diet. The changes should be made gradually to avoid gas pains and bloating, which can occur with fiber. Switching to **whole-grain breads** and to **cereals** high in fiber may be the only change some individuals need to make. Lessons in label reading are often necessary because prominently advertised "wheat" breads are often not made of whole wheat.

Many brans have become popular, but wheat bran is the most effective type for promoting bowel function. For individuals who prefer hot cereals, wheat bran may be mixed in with the cereal. Institutional food is often low in fiber, and residents of such facilities may benefit from a **fiber supplement**. Supplements made from 2 parts wheat bran (sometimes given in the form of 100% bran cereal, which is more palatable but less effective than crude bran), 2 parts applesauce, and 1 part prune juice have been effective. The starting dose is 30 ml daily, and it costs significantly less than laxatives.

The common advice "eat more fruits and vegetables" may not be sufficient to add enough insoluble fiber to the diet. A dietary consultation may be appropriate to help an individual make changes that take into consideration traditional eating habits, cost, dentition, and taste.

12. Are there any precautions associated with adding fiber to the diet?

1. Fiber should not be added to the diets of individuals with **megacolon**. In fact, such patients should be on a fiber-restricted diet and may need to be managed with enemas.

2. Some elderly individuals are at risk for development of **bezoars**. Bezoars are hard, dense masses of fibrous materials that can cause irritation in the stomach or obstruction in the intestines. Individuals with poor dentition, history of surgery for peptic ulcer disease, or stomach cancer are at greater risk for bezoars.

3. Fiber should be avoided in patients with **intestinal stricture**.

4. Increased fiber can pose a hazard for **bed-bound patients** by increasing bulk in a colon that is already distended.

These exceptions aside, most elderly individuals who make dietary changes gradually to increase fiber will have no problem. Individuals who use fiber supplements should be told not to expect overnight results. They also should not double-up on supplements because this can cause diarrhea or even obstruction. The latter is most likely to occur if the patient does not drink enough water.

13. What is the role of laxatives in the management of constipation?

For most patients, laxatives and enemas should not be a part of routine bowel management but should be used only occasionally to prevent the complications associated with constipation. Individuals who have used laxatives for years will require education about the harmful effects of laxatives and their role in causing constipation. However, patients with megacolon or with a medical condition that requires that they avoid straining may need to use laxatives or enemas.

14. What considerations influence choice of laxatives?

The choice of laxative is determined by:
• The cause of the problem
• Nature of the constipation (is the stool hard or soft, high in the colon or in the rectum?)
• Other medical conditions
• Other medications the patient may be taking
• Cost of treatment
• Patient preference

15. Describe the different types of laxatives and considerations in their usage.

1. **Psyllium-based supplements** offer the benefit of lowering cholesterol, whereas **methylcellulose** and **calcium polycarbophil** are less likely to cause gas pain.

2. **Hyperosmolar laxatives** are effective in both the amulabory elderly and those in nursing homes. Sorbitol is much less expensive than lactulose and just as effective. Polyethylene glycol (Golytely) is often used for bowel preparation before colonoscopy or barium enema. It has been used in nursing home residents to treat impaction and is more effective than lactulose.

3. **Stimulant laxatives** are popular because of their efficacy, but many have toxic long-term effects and can damage the colon and cause electrolyte imbalance. Senna is safe for the elderly and did not cause problems in individuals over age 80 who used it daily for 6 months. Senna is a good choice for patients with more resistant slow-transit constipation who do not respond to sorbitol.

4. **Saline laxatives** are the most commonly prescribed laxatives in hospitals because they empty the bowel within a few hours. These products can cause electrolyte imbalance and magnesium levels should be monitored if a magnesium-based product is used regularly. Products containing aluminum or magnesium should be used with caution in individuals with poor renal function. Saline laxatives are useful for patients with colonic hypomotility if stimulant agents are no longer effective.

5. **Emollient laxatives** include mineral oil and docusate salts. Mineral oil should be avoided in the elderly because of the risk of aspiration, interference with absorption of fat-soluble vitamins, and risk of leakage through the anal sphincter. Stool softeners are popular, but studies of patients receiving them have shown no change in stool weight or water content, no increase in frequency of bowel movements, and no change in colonic transit time. They are especially ineffective in patients who have a large amount of soft stool in the colon. Stool softeners are often recommended in bed-bound patients with hard dry stool, in patients who must avoid straining, and as an adjunct to bulk agents. For most individuals, adding 8 oz of water to their daily intake would probably be more effective.

6. **Bisacodyl** and **glycerin suppositories** are appropriate for occasional use when stool is present in the rectum and are usually effective within an hour. They may cause cramping and local irritation. **Enemas** should be reserved for constipation that does not respond to other approaches.

BIBLIOGRAPHY

1. Friedman LS, Isselbacher KJ: Diarrhea and constipation. In Fauci AS, Braunwald E, Isselbacher KJ, et al (eds): Harrison's Principles of Internal Medicine, 14th ed. New York, McGraw-Hill, 1998, p 236.
2. Harari D: Constipation in the elderly. In Hazzard WR, Blass JP, Ettinger WH, et al (eds): Principles of Geriatric Medicine and Gerontology, 4th ed. New York, McGraw-Hill, 1999, p 1491.
3. Read NW, Celik AF, Katsinelos P: Constipation and incontinence in the elderly. J Clin Gastroenterol 20:61, 1995.
4. Romero Y, Evans JM, Fleming KC, et al: Constipation and fecal incontinence in the elderly population. Mayo Clin Proc 71:81, 1996.

10. INSOMNIA

Nalaka Gooneratne, M.D.

1. What changes occur in the typical sleep patterns of adults as they age?
Sleep is divided into five stages. Each stage is characterized by unique electroencephalogram (EEG) findings. The sleep of older adults is characterized by a decrease in stage III/IV sleep (slow-wave sleep), possibly the most restful phase of sleep. However, this may be due in part to a technicality: due to age-related changes such as atrophy, elderly subjects may continue to have stage III/IV sleep yet do not meet the technical definitions of stage III/IV sleep. In addition, the elderly have more frequent nocturnal arousals (awakenings) and their sleep efficiency (total time asleep ÷ total time in bed) is decreased.

Sleep Stages and Their Characteristics

SLEEP STAGE	CHARACTERISTICS	LENGTH (MIN)	CHANGE WITH AGING
I	Decreased muscle tone, slow eye movements	30	Increased
II	EEG with spindles and K-complexes	200	Stable
III/IV	Delta waves present on EEG	30	Decreased
REM	Rapid eye movements, decreased muscle tone, low amplitude EEG	150	Shortened time to first REM episode

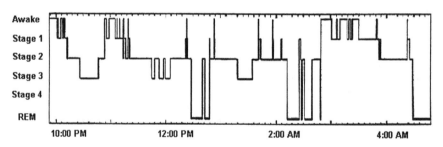

Graphic overview of a patient's sleep stages during the course of a sleep study.

Patients with Alzheimer's disease (even those with mild disease) have a generalized slowing of background EEG activity, a decrease in rapid eye movement (REM) sleep, a significant increase in nocturnal awakenings, reduction in slow-wave sleep, and altered stage I and II morphology. The decline in REM sleep often parallels the patient's intellectual decline. Patients with severe Alzheimer's disease may spend as much as 40% of their bedtime hours awake and up to 14% of their daytime hours asleep.

2. How is insomnia defined?
The term *insomnia* often is used loosely to describe the symptom of difficulty initiating or maintaining sleep. **Transient insomnia** refers to self-limiting cases that last < 1 month and usually do not require treatment. **Chronic insomnia** is defined as lasting > 1 month and is the focus of this chapter. The prevalence of the complaint of chronic insomnia in the elderly varies from study to study, with a range of 29.4% to 50%. There are many classification systems for insomnia, but most broadly distinguish between **primary insomnia** and **secondary insomnia** (insomnia due

to other causes). The *Diagnostic and Statistical Manual of Mental Disorders, 4th ed. (DSM-IV)* is primarily used in this discussion because it is straightforward and widely recognized. To satisfy the *DSM-IV* criteria for primary insomnia, a patient must have the following:

A. A predominant complaint of insomnia for ≥ 1 month
B. The sleep disturbance (or associated daytime fatigue) causes clinically significant distress
C. Insomnia does not occur during other sleep disorders (e.g., sleep apnea)
D. An absence of coexisting mental disorders (e.g., major depressive disorder)
E. The disturbance is not due to substance abuse or a general medical condition.

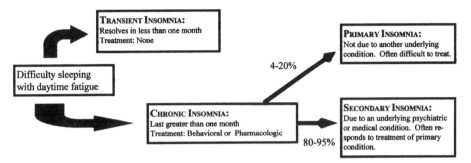

Types of insomnia and their relationship to one another.

Prevalences of primary insomnia may vary: in the elderly, it may constitute 4.1% of cases of insomnia (with a 1.2% population prevalence), but it may be as high as 20.2% of the total cases of insomnia. Secondary insomnia differs from primary insomnia in that criteria C, D, or E above may not be met. It accounts for the remaining 80–95% of insomnia cases. Women tend to have more complaints of insomnia than men.

A large discrepancy exists between the number of individuals who state they have difficulty sleeping and the clinical diagnosis of insomnia using the *DSM-IV* because of its more rigorous criteria in the classification paradigms. The elderly in particular are a diagnostic challenge and often report a lack of daytime repercussions of their insomnia complaint, thus failing to satisfy criterion B of the *DSM-IV* system; often they remain without a specific diagnosis to a greater degree than younger subjects. Fortunately, many of these patients will respond to the behavioral treatments outlined in question 8.

3. **What are the different types of secondary insomnia?**

Secondary insomnia may be due to psychiatric diseases or comorbid medical problems. The following is a list of their specific subtypes and incidences based on the *DSM-IV*:

- **Psychiatric diagnosis associated with an insomnia complaint.** In these cases, the patient has a primary psychiatric diagnosis, most commonly generalized anxiety disorder or major depressive disorder, and the insomnia is but one of many aspects of the disease. The insomnia often does not warrant specific attention and improves as the underlying problem is treated. Some studies suggest that more than one-half of all individuals who complain of insomnia fall into this category.

- **Insomnia due to an underlying mental disorder.** In certain situations the insomnia is the *main complaint* of a patient who actually suffers from a mood disorder; this insomnia is severe enough to warrant specific attention. Such patients often "focus on their sleep disturbance to the exclusion of the symptoms characteristic of the mental disorder, whose presence may become apparent only after specific and persistent questioning." Thus, this type of secondary insomnia is distinguished from psychiatric diagnosis associated with an insomnia complaint, in which case the insomnia is a minor (not the major) part of the symptom complex of another primary psychiatric diagnosis. Insomnia due to an underlying mental disorder affects 2.0% of people older than 65. It may account for up to 44% of cases of insomnia.

- **Sleep disorder due to a general medical condition, insomnia type.** In this case, the insomnia is severe enough to warrant attention and is due to a general medical condition such as arthritis, congestive heart failure, hyperthyroidism, or gastroesophageal reflux. Typically, sleep apnea, narcolepsy, and periodic leg movements are not included in this category. The specific prevalence is estimated to be 1.8% of the elderly.
- **Substance-induced sleep disorder, insomnia type.** (See table below.)

Substances That May Cause Insomnia

Alcohol	Diuretics (furosemide)	Caffeine (teas, soda, chocolate)
Beta-blockers	Levodopa/carbidopa	Withdrawal from sedatives
Bronchodilators (albuterol)	Methyldopa	Illegal drug use
Cimetidine	Nifedipine	
Corticosteroids	SSRIs	
Decongestants (pseudoephedrine)	Theophylline	

SSRIs = serotonin reuptake inhibitors.
Adapted from Ancoli-Israel S: Sleep problems in older adults. Putting myths to bed. Geriatrics 52:20, 1997.

- **Circadian phase disorders, such as delayed sleep phase type or jet lag type.** These disorders result from a mismatch between the subject's endogenous sleep-wake regulation system and fundamental demands. Currently, it rarely is diagnosed in the elderly; however, new research suggests that it may play a greater role than initially suspected.
- **Dyssomnia not otherwise specified.** This broad category includes:
  - **Sleep hygiene and sleep deprivation**. These refer to the environment in which sleep occurs. They may be impaired by elevated noise levels, frequent disruptions from family members, and uncomfortable sleeping conditions. Institutionalization often is accompanied by the development of insomnia.
  - **Periodic limb movements** (PLMs). PLMs are characterized by repetitive leg movements that occur every 20–40 seconds and cause an arousal that can lead to a perception of disrupted sleep; a patient must have > 40 per night to meet diagnostic criteria. PLMs may be associated with peripheral neuropathies, chronic renal failure, dementia, anemia, and tricyclic antidepressants and occur in up to 44% of elderly patients.

4. How is insomnia diagnosed?

The diagnosis of insomnia is primarily a clinical one and does not require lab testing for confirmation. As long as the patient's condition satisfies the criteria outlined in question 1, he or she meets the definition of primary insomnia. Note that patients who complain of insomnia have a tendency to over-report their problem; often a discrepancy is found between the objective sleep latency and sleep efficiency on objective sleep testing and the patient's subjective complaints.

5. When should a patient with insomnia have a formal sleep study (polysomnography)?

In a position paper on the role of nocturnal polysomnography in insomnia, the American Sleep Disorder Association (ASDA) recommends that a patient should have a polysomnogram when:

- The insomnia remains persistent despite behavioral or pharmacologic therapy.
- The insomnia may be due to precipitous arousals or violent behavior during sleep.
- The insomnia may be caused by circadian rhythm disorders.
- Other diagnoses (e.g., sleep apnea or PLMs) are highly suspected or the actual clinical diagnosis is unclear.

6. What are important aspects of the history and physical examination in an elderly patient with insomnia?

- **Clarify sleep habits.** In addition to standard questions, also ask about what he or she does before falling asleep (e.g., reading in bed or watching TV) and his or her coffee and/or nicotine consumption.
- **Check for any symptoms of sleep-disordered breathing**, such as snoring, witnessed apneas (although these patients usually do not complain of insomnia), or nocturnal leg movements.
- **Perform a review of psychiatric symptoms to screen for depression or anxiety.** Also determine if the patient has any prior experiences or expectations that may increase anxiety about sleep (e.g., "I always sleep poorly; I have grown to expect it").
- **Assess the severity of any comorbid medical problems** (e.g., dyspnea, pain, orthopnea, cough, nocturia).
- **Inquire about medications**, which may include prescription and over-the-counter drugs as well as alternative preparations (e.g., herbal).

The physical exam should screen for the severity of the patient's comorbid medical conditions (especially arthritis) and also evidence of hyperthyroidism, a rare but curable cause of insomnia.

7. Describe the etiology of insomnia in older adults.

Although insomnia is often due to underlying psychiatric or medical problems, there is a growing appreciation of the role of circadian rhythm abnormalities in promoting disrupted sleep in the elderly. The human body has an internal clock, which is located in the suprachiasmatic nucleus and relies on extrinsic stimuli such as light exposure and social cues to regulate the body's sleep-wake cycle. In elderly subjects, evidence shows that this clock is phase-advanced relative to younger subjects and may possibly have a weaker amplitude. The elderly may be inclined to go to bed sooner but wake up earlier, thus creating a sense of insomnia. The decrease in amplitude, as seen by a drop in melatonin levels up to one-tenth that of younger subjects, or ablation of their melatonin rhythm altogether may lead to a greater tendency to awaken from sleep. In patients with Alzheimer's disease, neuronal degeneration in the sleep-wake regulatory pathways may lead to impaired sleep as demonstrated by histologic studies of brainstem sections from patients with Alzheimer's disease.

Furthermore, many elderly are exposed to < 30 minutes of bright light per day, which may contribute to their altered circadian physiology. Long-term institutionalization also contributes to disturbed sleep because of the frequent nocturnal interruptions, noisy environment, increased nap time, limited bright light exposure, and the multiple psychosocial issues associated with institutionalization. Nocturnal light exposure in particular may serve to blunt melatonin rhythms that may contribute to fragmented sleep. The combination of weakened circadian rhythm and comorbid medical and psychiatric conditions possibly may interact to decrease the threshold of awakening in the elderly and thereby promote insomnia.

8. What is the treatment of insomnia in the elderly?

Successful treatment should begin with amelioration of the underlying condition in secondary insomnias, such as improved nocturnal pain control and treatment of underlying psychiatric disorders. If the insomnia persists, behavioral therapy should be initiated and then incorporated with pharmacologic therapy if the response to behavioral changes alone is suboptimal.

Behavioral Therapy

- **Sleep hygiene modification** involves educating the patient about the most effective sleep habits:
  - Avoid caffeinated products, alcohol, and tobacco after 6 PM.
  - Limit naps to 30 minutes or ideally stop daytime napping altogether.

  • Limit liquid intake near bedtime to reduce nocturia.
  • Strive to have a sleeping environment that is quiet and free from disruptions.
  • Establish a consistent bedtime.
  • Avoid watching TV or reading in bed.

In patients with Alzheimer's disease, limiting daytime napping can help improve nocturnal sleep.

  • **Sleep-restriction therapy** limits time spent in bed. It begins with asking the patient to estimate the amount of time he or she sleeps each night and then spend only 15 minutes more than that in bed for the first few nights. Fifteen minutes is then gradually added every few nights until a comfortable level of nocturnal sleep is reached. For example, if a patient states that he or she sleeps only 4 hours a night, instruct the patient to go to bed at 1:45 AM and awaken at 6:00 am. After the patient is able to sleep during this entire period (usually after a few days because of fatigue), instruct him to go to bed at 1:30 AM (15 minutes earlier than before), and so on.
  • **Stimulus control therapy** attempts to strengthen the association between the bed and sleeping. The patient is instructed to use the bed only for sleeping and to leave the bed if she is awake for more than 15–30 minutes, which helps remove any negative conditioning that might prompt a patient to paradoxically feel more awake when lying in bed.

Pharmacologic Therapy

The pharmacologic treatment of insomnia is complicated by the decreased rate of metabolism in the elderly, increased total body fat (increased volume of distribution for lipid soluble agents), the high rate of polypharmacy in the elderly, and their increased sensitivity to the central nervous system–depressant effect of some medications. In general, starting doses should be one-half that of the standard starting doses:

  • **Sedative/hypnotics** are recommended for short-term use only (< 3–4 weeks) and should not be prescribed if sleep apnea is suspected. For chronic insomniacs, sedative/hypnotics can be used intermittently (every 2–4 days) as needed, although little data verify this regimen. A short half-life is needed to minimize daytime sedation. If a patient complains of difficulty initiating sleep, then an agent with a very short half-life is appropriate (zolpidem tartrate [Ambien] with a 2.5 hr half-life, 2.5 mg starting dose); however, if the tendency is to wake up frequently or too early, an agent with a longer half-life may help (temazepam [Restoril] with a half-life of 10–17 hr, 7.5 mg starting dose).
  • **Tricyclic antidepressants** also can be used to treat insomnia because of the frequent association between depression and insomnia, and they have a role in patients in whom depression is a major component. Their use is limited by their anticholinergic effects; nortriptyline and desipramine are most useful for this reason.
  • **Over-the-counter medications** that are often used include analgesics such as Tylenol PM or sedating antihistamines. However, little data are available regarding efficacy of these agents.
  • **Melatonin** may help certain patients with insomnia who have abnormal melatonin rhythms. However, little data presently support its routine use. Also, melatonin is not FDA-regulated, and potencies and quality vary. Doses of 0.3–1 mg most closely mimic physiologic levels. Given concern about unregulated manufacturing and the equivocal efficacy data to date, routine use of melatonin is not recommended.
  • **Bright light therapy** has been shown to improve sleep quality in insomniacs in small studies and has a more well-established role in cases of seasonal affective disorder and early morning awakening insomnia. In Alzheimer's disease, some studies have shown a benefit, whereas others showed no improvement. Regimens include 2,000–10,000 lux for 2 hours usually administered in the early evening.
  • **Selective serotonin reuptake inhibitors (SSRIs)** primarily are used to treat depression, but interest is growing in the use of agents such as paroxetine (Paxil), 20 mg, for insomnia.

Research is ongoing in the field and complicated by the fact that some SSRIs may actually cause insomnia.

- **Periodic limb movements** can be treated with levidopa-carbidopa (100–600 mg of the L-dopa as needed), pergolide (Permax; start at 0.05 mg 2 hr before bedtime), or clonazepam (0.5 mg–3.0 mg).

9. What are the side effects of treatment with sedatives?

Sedative use notably increases in the elderly with insomnia: 37% of elderly insomniacs used sedatives regularly versus 10.3% of elderly noninsomniacs in one Australian study. The immediate side effects of sedatives are increased risk of daytime fatigue with an associated risk of falls and cognitive dysfunction. In addition, dependence occurs in 15–30% of long-term benzodiazepine users. Patients with respiratory disease may develop carbon dioxide retention and narcosis when using sedatives. When sedatives are withdrawn, patients are at risk of rebound insomnia (i.e., worsening of their insomnia), especially with short- and intermediate-acting benzodiazepines.

10. What are the sequelae of insomnia?

Insomnia has been associated with a significantly increased risk of developing major depression, alcoholism, and anxiety disorder. In addition, there is an associated increase in daytime fatigue and sleepiness which, along with the nocturnal disruptions, impairs quality of life. The caregiver stress associated with frequent nocturnal disruptions also is a factor that may contribute to the institutionalization of a demented relative.

BIBLIOGRAPHY

1. American Psychiatric Association: Diagnostic and Statistical Manual of Mental Disorders. 4th ed. Washington, DC, American Psychiatric Association, 1994.
2. Ancoli-Israel S: Sleep problems in older adults: Putting myths to bed. Geriatrics 52:20–30, 1997.
3. ASDA–Standards of Practice Committee of the American Sleep Disorders Association: Practice parameters for the use of polysomnography in the evaluation of insomnia. Sleep 18:55, 1995.
4. Buysse D, Reynolds CI, Kupfer D, et al: Clinical diagnosis in 216 insomnia patients using the International Classification of Sleep Disorders (ICSD), DSM-IV, and ICD-10 categories: A report from the APA/NIMH DSM-IV field trials. Sleep 17:630–637, 1994.
5. Feinsilver S, Hertz G: Sleep in the elderly patient. Clin Chest Med 14:405–411, 1993.
6. Henderson S, Jorm A, Scott L, et al: The morbidity of insomnia uncomplicated by psychiatric disorders. Gen Hosp Psychiatry 19:245–250, 1997.
7. Monane M: Insomnia in the elderly. J Clin Psychiatry 53:23–28, 1992.
8. Monk TH: Sleep disorders in the elderly. Ciracadian rhythm. Clin Geriatr Med 5:331–346, 1989.
9. Morin CM, Colecchi C, Stone J, et al: Behavioral and pharmacological therapies for late-life insomnia: A randomized, controlled trial [see comments]. JAMA 281:991–999, 1999.
10. Ohayon MM: Prevalence of DSM-IV diagnostic criteria of insomnia: Distinguishing insomnia related to mental disorders from sleep disorders. J Psychiatr Res 31:333–346, 1997.
11. van Someren E, Mirmiran M, Swaab D: Nonpharmacological treatment of sleep and wake disturbances in aging and Alzheimer's disease: Chronobiological perspectives. Behav Brain Res 57:235–253, 1993.
12. Vitiello M, Prinz P: Alzheimer's disease. Sleep and sleep/wake patterns. Clin Geriatr Med 5:289–299, 1989.
13. Wooten V: Sleep disorders in geriatric patients. Clin Geriatr Med 8:427–439, 1992.

11. SENSORY CHANGES

David Guha, M.D., and Eugenia L. Siegler, M.D.

1. What major changes does the eye undergo with aging?

Presbyopia, the loss of accommodative ability, is the best known of the age-associated ocular changes. This is due to hardening of the lens nucleus (nuclear sclerosis) and ciliary muscle atrophy. It begins at approximately age 40 and progresses; by the 60s, little, if any, ability to accommodate remains.

The eye undergoes other changes with age, as well. The retina receives less light as we age, because of increased light absorption by the lens, cornea, and vitreous. Pupils do not dilate as much when the environment darkens, which also reduces the amount of light that reaches the retina. Increasing opacity of the lens and other parts of the eye leads to reduction of contrast by scattering the light. At the retinal level, most elderly lose rods and, to a lesser extent, cones, as well as retinal ganglion cells. These changes can lead to some reduction in visual acuity, contrast sensitivity, dark-light adaptation, and functional peripheral vision, but the common ophthalmologic diseases have a far greater impact (see question 3).

2. What are the levels of visual impairment?

Legally blind: best corrected visual acuity in the better eye is ≤ 20/200 or the visual field is ≤ 20°.

Partially sighted: best corrected visual acuity in the better eye is ≤ 20/70 or the visual field is ≤ 20/50.

Functionally visually impaired: best corrected visual acuity in the better eye is ≤ 20/50.

3. What is the relationship between visual impairment and age?

In the Baltimore Eye Survey, the prevalence of visual loss (defined as < 20/40 in the better eye) was approximately 2% in whites and 8% in African-Americans in the 60–69-year age group; in those age 80 and older, the prevalence was 35% in whites and 40% in African-Americans. In a study conducted by the same group in nursing homes, the prevalence of poor vision was found to be almost 36% (of those participating in the study, 57% were white and 43% were African-American). Blindness, defined as visual acuity ≤ 20/200 in the better eye, appears to be far more prevalent in nursing homes than in the community. For example, the prevalences in those aged 70–79 (11.3% in whites and 18% in African-Americans) were 18.8- and 6.2-fold higher than in the corresponding community.

Significant numbers of community-dwelling and institutionalized elderly have refractive errors for which correction could improve vision. Improving vision (through refraction, cataract surgery, or other methods) leads to improved quality of life; the worse the initial vision, the greater the increase in quality of life with an improvement in vision. Individuals with visual impairments also may benefit from low-vision clinics, which can provide both counseling and adaptive devices.

4. Name the four most common ophthalmologic diseases in the elderly.

The Framingham eye study documented the prevalences of four diseases, and all increased with age (see table). These four are also the most common causes of blindness in community-dwelling elderly. In the nursing home, cataracts, corneal opacity, age-related macular degeneration, and open-angle glaucoma are the most common causes. Note that prevalence differs by race. Macular degeneration is the most common cause of visual impairment in caucasians, whereas glaucoma is the most common cause in African-Americans.

CONDITION	PREVALENCE IN THOSE AGED 75–85
Cataract (lens opacification)	46%
Age-related macular degeneration (resulting from deposition of drusen in the macular region)	28%
Open-angle glaucoma (retinal nerve damage due to sustained intraocular hypertension)	7.2%
Diabetic retinopathy (may be proliferative or nonproliferative)	7%

5. What are the potential adverse reactions of medications used to treat open-angle glaucoma?

Both oral and instilled glaucoma medications have significant side effects. Systemic side effects of the drops can be reduced by having the patient occlude the lacrimal puncta for 5 minutes while and after drops are instilled. It also is useful to check bottles to see if the preparation contains sulfites, which may cause allergic reactions.

Common Drugs for Glaucoma and Their Side Effects

CLASS	MECHANISM	PRODUCTS	SIDE EFFECTS
Beta-blockers	Decrease aqueous production	Timolol (Timoptic) Betaxolol (Betoptic) Levobunolol (Betagan)	Bronchospasm, bradycardia, hypotension, slowed conduction, worsened CHF, confusion
Miotics	Increase aqueous outflow		
Direct parasympathetic		Pilocarpine (Pilocar, Isoptocarpine, Ocucarpine) Carbachol (Isoptocarbachol)	GI, bronchospasm, bradycardia, confusion, poor night vision (worse with cholinesterase inhibitors)
Cholinesterase inhibitors		Demecarium (Humorsol) Echothiophate (Floropryl) Isoflurophate (Floropryl) Physostigmine (Isoptoeserine)	
Nonselective sympathetic agonists	Increase aqueous outflow	Dipivefrin (Propine) Epinephrine (Epifrin, Glaucon)	Dipivefrin is quite safe; epinephrine can be very cardiotoxic
Selective alpha$_2$ agonists	Decrease aqueous production; increase uveoscleral outflow	Brimonidine (Alphagan) Aproclonidine (Iopidine)	Drowsiness, hypotension (brimonidine); dry nose and mouth, follicular conjunctivitis (aproclonidine)
Carbonic anhydrase inhibitors	Decrease aqueous production	Oral Acetazolamide (Diamox) Methazolamide (Neptazane) Dichlorphenamide (Daranide) Topical Dorzolamide (Trusopt) Brinzolamide (Azopt)	GI, CNS, aplastic anemia, renal stones, acidosis, altered drug excretion. Topical preparations have fewer side effects
Prostaglandin analogues	Increase uveoscleral outflow	Latanoprost (Xalatan)	Muscle/joint pain, hyperemia, darkening of iris, changes in eyelashes

CHF = congestive heart failure; GI = gastrointestinal; CNS = central nervous system

6. How does the sense of taste change in the elderly?

Ageusia is the loss of the sense of taste. The sensation of a bad taste in the mouth is called **dysgeusia**. Weiffenbach and Bartoshuk describe a test to distinguish between peripheral (e.g., occurring in the mouth) and central dysgeusias. The patient should first try to rinse the taste away. If it does go away, even only briefly, the origin of the dysgeusia is probably oral. The clinician can then administer a local anesthetic to the mouth. If the dysgeusia gets stronger, the origin is probably in the central nervous system (CNS), and referral to a neurologist is indicated. These disorders can include temporal lobe tumors and damage to the chorda tympani.

Although thresholds for both detection of a substance and correct identification (recognition) increase with age beginning about age 60, these changes are of questionable clinical significance. Therefore, most people do not perceive a significant decline in taste with age. Many conditions, such as Bell's palsy, head trauma, chorda tympani damage from upper respiratory and ear infections, cancer, depression, hepatic and renal disease, zinc deficiency, hypothyroidism, malnutrition, and diabetes mellitus, can affect the sense of taste. Laryngectomy, local radiation therapy, and medications also can alter taste sensation.

7. Which drugs affect the sense of taste?

Of the hundreds of drugs that can change the sense of taste, the following are commonly used by the elderly:

Antibiotics
  Ampicillin
  Tetracyclines
  Metronidazole
Antihypertensives
  Angiotensin-converting enzyme (ACE) inhibitors
  Calcium channel blockers
  Ethacrynic acid

CNS active agents
  Carbamazepine
  Levodopa
  Lithium
  Phenytoin
Anti-gout medications
  Allopurinol
  Colchicine

8. How does the sense of smell change in the elderly?

Anosmia is the loss of the sense of smell. Those who complain of a persistent bad smell have a **parosmia**. The sense of smell (olfaction) declines far more dramatically with age than does the sense of taste. Some smell-like characteristics, such as pungency, are sensed by the trigeminal nerve and appear not to decline as much as true olfaction. The age-related decline in ability to recognize odors does have clinical significance; for example, elderly may have difficulty detecting that food is no longer edible or that natural gas is escaping from the stove.

Anosmia also has a major impact on quality of life. Much of the sensory stimulus that is perceived as taste is actually smell. A patient with anosmia can taste the sweetness of ice cream but, without visual cues of color, will not be able to determine the flavor. Such a chemosensory loss may have enormous impact on a patient's appetite or enjoyment of food. Unfortunately, little can be done to treat loss of smell and taste, except for discontinuation of medications that may be contributing to loss of smell. Counseling is another important option.

9. What diseases or conditions often seen in the elderly can affect the sense of smell?

Alzheimer's disease
Parkinson's disease
Head trauma
Renal and liver disease
Hypothyroidism
Diabetes mellitus

Rhinitis
Sinusitis
Asthma
Viral infections
Laryngectomy

10. What medications can affect the sense of smell?

Calcium channel blockers, antithyroid agents, opiates, and amphetamines.

11. What are the most common causes of hearing loss in the elderly?

Approximately 40% of elderly individuals have some form of chronic hearing impairment, defined as the inability to hear a pure tone softer than 40 dB at more than one frequency in one or both ears. The most common cause of bilateral hearing loss in the elderly is **presbycusis**, a sensorineural loss marked by difficulty hearing high-frequency tones and by impaired speech comprehension. Presbycusis may have both peripheral and central auditory processing components. Patients with presbycusis also may complain of **recruitment**, the perception that a sound has become dramatically louder despite only a modest increase in volume. Other causes of hearing loss in the elderly include cerumen plugs, otosclerosis, ototoxicity, Meniere's disease, and acoustic neuromas.

12. How can a primary care provider screen for hearing loss?

There are two basic kinds of screens.

1. **Measure the extent of hearing loss with a series of sounds or words:** One such tool is the Audioscope (Welch-Allyn, Inc., Skaneateles Falls, NY). The Audioscope resembles an otoscope and tests the patient's ability to hear pure tones. It emits a series of tones ranging from 500–4000 Hz into the ear. Standard pure-tone audiometers have been used for years but are less convenient to use. The Audioscope also enables visual inspection of the ear canal at the time of the test. The test can be deferred or canceled if excessive cerumen or pathology is found.

2. **Question the patient about the impact of hearing loss.** The Hearing Handicap Inventory for the Elderly–Screening Version (HHIE-S) consists of 10 questions that the patient answers either in response to a questioner or on a self-administered form. It measures the impact of hearing loss on social functioning. Scored on a 40-point scale, the test is considered positive for a severe handicap if the patient scores > 24 points. Another verbal handicap screen, the Self-Assessment of Communication (SAC), has also performed well in studies.

Despite their different approaches, these two types of screens have similar test characteristics. Sensitivities and specificities range from roughly 60–90% depending on the test cutoff points that are used. Unfortunately, compliance with advice at time of screening is poor, with only 15% of patients found to have a hearing impairment going on to buy a hearing aid. (See also Chapter 12.)

13. What kinds of devices can be used to improve hearing?

There are a wide variety of amplification devices. **Hearing aids** amplify and modify sound and deliver it directly to the canal. Since the early 1980s the most popular type has been worn in the ear. The version worn behind the ear is also popular and may be more easily manipulated by patients with visual impairments or arthritis. Hearing aids can be unilateral or bilateral and can be analog, digital, or hybrid. Despite the high prevalence of hearing loss, approximately 85% of hearing-impaired elderly lack hearing aids. The presence of an auditory processing disorder can reduce patient satisfaction and benefit from a hearing aid.

Assistive listening devices (ALDs) are used to connect the hearing-impaired individual directly to the source of the sound. They are usually found in special settings, such as theaters and places of worship. Another kind of ALD, a personal amplifier, can be purchased from electronics stores. Individuals speak directly into the amplifier, which transmits sound to the patient via earphones. These small devices are useful for those who cannot manipulate hearing aids or who need to communicate one-on-one in noisy areas.

A **cochlear implant**, which is a 22-channel electrode that is surgically implanted in the ear, is used only for sensorineural impairment. It may be helpful for severely hearing-impaired individuals.

14. What techniques can be used to communicate with those with hearing loss?

Speak clearly and slowly with a normal tone of voice. The hearing-impaired person may hear better if seated or standing against a wall. When the hearing-impaired person does not understand you, rephrase; don't repeat. Avoid competing noises by eliminating television, radio, and other background noises. Keep groups small so that the hearing-impaired individual can follow the conversation. Allow the hearing-impaired person to take advantage of visual cues: make sure your face can be easily seen, and use gestures when appropriate.

15. Do other sensory changes occur in the elderly?

Healthy elderly can show a number of subtle abnormalities on thorough physical examination. Kaye et al., in a cross-sectional study comparing healthy, community-dwelling elderly aged 64–75 years (young old) to those older than 84 years (oldest old), documented a high prevalence of many abnormalities in the oldest old, especially in gait, balance, and sensory function (vibration, proprioception, and stereognosis). They then used discriminant analysis to demonstrate that the oldest old performed more poorly than the young old in tests of olfaction, visual pursuit, one-leg standing with eyes closed, and heel-toe walking. Loss of vibratory sense also appeared to be important. These are "usual" aging changes. Elderly with comorbidities can be expected to have additional sensory changes.

BIBLIOGRAPHY

1. Alward WLM: Medical management of glaucoma. N Engl J Med 339:1298–1307, 1998.
2. Carter TL: Age-related vision changes: A primary care guide. Geriatrics 49:37–45, 1994.
3. Jerger J, Chmiel R, Wilson N, Luchi R: Hearing impairment in older adults: New concepts. J Am Geriatr Soc 43:928–935, 1995.
4. Kaye JA, Oken BS, Howieson DB, et al: Neurologic evaluation of the optimally healthy oldest old. Arch Neurol 51:1205–1211, 1994.
5. Kini MM, Leibowitz HM, Colton T, et al: Prevalence of senile cataract, diabetic retinopathy, senile macular degeneration, and open-angle glaucoma in the Framingham eye study. Am J Ophthalmol 85:28–34, 1978.
6. Lavizzo-Mourey RJ, Siegler EL: Hearing impairment in the elderly. J Gen Intern Med 7:191–197, 1992.
7. Schiffman S: Changes in taste and smell: Drug interactions and food preferences. Nutr Rev 52(II):S11–S14, 1994.
8. Schiffman S: Taste and smell losses in normal aging and disease. JAMA 278:1357–1362, 1997.
9. Tielsch JM, Javitt JC, Coleman A, et al: The prevalence of blindness and visual impairment among nursing home residents in Baltimore. N Engl J Med 332:1205–1209, 1995.
10. Tielsch JM, Sommer A, Witt K, et al: Blindness and visual impairment in an American urban population: The Baltimore Eye Survey. Arch Ophthalmol 108:286–290, 1990.
11. Weiffenbach JM, Bartoshuk LM: Taste and smell. Clin Geriatr Med 8:543–555, 1992.

12. PRINCIPLES OF SCREENING

Susan Day, M.D., M.P.H.

1. Why screen?

The fundamental principle behind screening is that the quality and duration of an individual's life can be improved by identifying early or asymptomatic disease, by modifying behavior to achieve a more healthy lifestyle, and by maximizing function when disease exists. Interventions for these purposes fall into three categories:

1. **Primary prevention** is targeted toward identifying and reversing risk factors that may lead to disease in the future. Examples of ways to reduce risk factors include improved nutrition, exercise, smoking cessation, and accident prevention. Interventions at this stage may involve counseling, immunizations, or chemoprophylaxis.

2. **Secondary prevention** efforts, including most screening programs, are aimed at preventing disease in the preclinical or asymptomatic phase. Hypertension and breast cancer screening are examples.

3. **Tertiary prevention** includes measures that prevent complications of existing disease. Cardiac and stroke rehabilitation programs fall into this category, as do the use of angiotensin-converting enzyme (ACE) inhibitors in patients with diabetes to prevent renal disease.

2. Why make separate recommendations for screening the elderly?

1. **The yield from screening/preventive interventions is greater in the elderly.** Because of the higher prevalence of disease in this population, more true-positive results will be obtained with a screening test. Of course, these tests may be less specific as well—a positive occult blood stool sample may be due to a spectrum of problems, ranging from benign to malignant.

2. **There is evidence of under-utilization of screening/preventive programs in the elderly.** Despite the benefit of screening in the elderly, evidence indicates that older individuals do not receive the recommended screening tests as often as they should. There are both provider and patient reasons for this underuse. Sociodemographic factors, such as race and education, socioeconomic status, and residence in a rural community, further affect access to screening services, making the indigent elderly an important target group for screening efforts.

3. **The measure of a successful program differs in the elderly.** In older patients, identifying reversible conditions that affect the quality of life may be more important than those that shorten life. In addition to morbidity and mortality, the ability to live independently and avoid nursing home placement, the number of acute care visits and hospitalizations required, and the psychological sense of well-being should be considered. All these factors have been shown to improve with an effective screening program.

4. **The level of intervention is different.** Primary prevention, with lifestyle modification, has the greatest impact on reducing disease for the population as a whole. In older patients, a broad approach to prevention is appropriate. Primary prevention is still crucial; the value of exercise in maintaining functional status, preventing osteoporosis, and reducing the risks of falls is a good example. However, secondary and tertiary prevention interventions become increasingly important. Efforts to maximize functional status in older patients with existing disease may have the greatest effect on the quality and duration of life.

3. What is the physician's role in screening?

The traditional role of a physician has been as healer, but as medical knowledge has grown, so has appreciation of the importance of preventing illness and maintaining health. Because patients are often unaware of the indications of screening, it usually is the physician who must take responsibility for teaching patients about healthy behaviors and ensuring that screening procedures are carried out in a timely fashion. Research supports the importance of physician counseling in areas such as smoking cessation and exercise, as well as in performing diagnostic screening procedures such as rectal and breast exams and Pap smears. Other health care personnel also play important roles: for example, nurse-initiated community-based screening for hypertension and breast cancer, counseling by nutritionists, and psychological screening by mental health providers.

4. What criteria are used to identify conditions suitable for screening?

Expert panels have reviewed the literature to formulate recommendations for timing and frequency of screening interventions. These panels have increasingly included the elderly as a group for whom distinct recommendations need to be derived. The following list includes elements generally agreed upon as being essential in the decision to screen.

1. **The condition must have a significant effect on the quality or quantity of a patient's life.** Screening should be targeted toward identifying conditions associated with significant morbidity, i.e. the "burden of suffering." Screening for hypertension and breast cancer helps reduce mortality and morbidity, and screening for glaucoma and hearing impairment in the older individual can improve the quality of life.

2. **The condition must be treatable.** Clinical interventions studied across a range of patient ages often demonstrate an age-related response to therapy. Evidence of effectiveness in older patients should be sought.

3. **The disease must have an asymptomatic period during which detection and treatment significantly reduce morbidity and/or mortality.** For any screening program to be effective, early detection of risk factors or disease must lead to an intervention that has a positive impact on outcome. Advancing detection of disease by 5 years only will be useful if the resulting treatment prevents or delays disease development by > 5 years.

4. **Tests for detection of disease must be affordable, safe, and have known test characteristics.** Both the cost of initial screening and the subsequent evaluation must be taken into account. The costs of evaluating a positive stool test for blood, an elevated serum prostate specific antigen, or an elevated serum CA-125 have been assessed and led to a general caution about using inexpensive but nonspecific tests that may lead to further expensive and risky diagnostic interventions.

5. **The incidence of the condition must be sufficient to justify the cost of screening.** No matter how dramatic the effect of early treatment in a specific condition, mass screening is not warranted if the disease is so rare that only a few individuals will benefit.

5. What are good test characteristics for a screening instrument?

1. **High sensitivity:** The ideal screening test should identify a high proportion of patients having the condition being sought. Since screening takes place at an early stage in the disease and because test sensitivity may vary according to the stage of disease, documentation of the sensitivity of the test in a given screening setting should be sought.

2. **High specificity:** The test should be normal in patients not having the condition being sought. In a low-prevalence situation, as often encountered in a screening setting, specificity is the key to reducing false-positive and false-negative results.

3. **High positive predictive value in the population being screened:** Some screening tests are designed to be used in low-prevalence situations, meaning that there will be many more people without the disease than with the disease. However, all patients who are told that their test is positive will need to receive further testing and/or treatment. The cost of follow-up of false-positive test results must be considered, in terms of both actual dollars and the psychological cost to the patient. The possibility of a false-positive result is reduced when the prevalence of disease increases.

4. **High negative predictive value:** A patient having a negative screening test should feel reassured that he or she does not have the condition of concern and not worry that the test could be in error. Thus, a normal result should be a reliable indicator that no disease exists. The cost of a false-negative test includes the loss of the benefit of screening (including, perhaps, a tendency to delay the reporting of symptoms) and the psychological costs of false reassurance.

6. How should general screening recommendations be applied to individual patients?

For people of all ages, screening programs must be adapted for the individual, taking into account the presence of risk factors and comorbid conditions. Public policy analyses, however, understate the risks and benefits to the individual patient, particularly the older patient. Functional status, presence of existing diseases, and attitudes toward screening can all appropriately influence the screening and preventive care interventions recommended for a given patient. It would not be reasonable to screen a 90-year-old woman with severe congestive heart failure for preclinical cervical cancer because her survival is already limited by her cardiac disease. However, screening for decreased visual acuity might result in an intervention that would improve that patient's eyesight and allow her to enjoy more sedentary activities such as reading. Similarly, an active 75-year-old woman should continue to be screened for cancer; her life expectancy is at least 10 years.

Patient preferences for treatment also must be considered. Recommendations for mass screening assume that an individual would pursue treatment, if indicated. Individuals may have very strong preferences about what treatments they would consider acceptable, and these preferences should be respected. A patient's ability to undergo treatment must also be taken into consideration. If the optimum cancer treatment is too toxic for a given individual, screening is not appropriate unless a less toxic alternative is available.

7. Why don't physicians comply with screening recommendations?

Physicians give several reasons when asked why they do not carry out the preventive services recommended in their patients:

1. **They are unaware of the recommendations.** The need for physician education has been a long-standing problem. In addition, because recommendations change frequently, physicians must be motivated to keep up to date on the frequency and indications for screening.

2. **They do not have the time.** Particularly in the elderly, patients often may have multiple active problems that must be addressed during each interval visit. Procedures such as pelvic or rectal exams, which involve disrobing and sometimes special examination rooms, require additional time. Counseling is also time-consuming, especially if patients and their families wish to discuss and review the recommendations or if the patient has any sensory or cognitive impairments.

3. **They forget.** Despite the best intentions, providers may not remember to include preventive measures into a routine health check, or if they do remember, they forget which measures are due for a given patient.

4. **They disagree with the recommendations.** Physicians sometimes disagree with formal recommendations if these differ from what they were taught or their current practice protocol. For example, a physician may be following the recommendations of the American Cancer Society, which are significantly more interventionist than those of the U.S. Preventive Services Task Force. Discrepancies among programs endorsed by expert panels and individual providers need to be resolved by careful review of the basis for the recommendations.

8. Why don't patients participate in screening programs?

In general, elderly patients are more likely than their younger colleagues to pursue healthy behaviors, such as regular blood pressure checks, dietary modifications, and accident prevention. They also appear to have a greater belief in the importance of lifestyle modification (diet, exercise, smoking) in reducing the risk of future morbidity, as well as heightened awareness of available interventions. Reasons leading to lower compliance include:

1. **Misunderstanding about normal aging:** The elderly may accept new symptoms as part of normal aging and consider the development of disease as inevitable.

2. **Cost of screening:** There has been progress in insurance coverage for some preventive health measures, such as flu shots, pneumococcal vaccines, bone mineral density measurements, and mammograms, which are now covered through Medicare. In addition, the increased participation of the elderly in managed-care systems that emphasize preventive measures has helped to reduce the cost of prevention to the individual. However, the costs (and availability) of transportation and subsequent testing must still be considered.

3. **Fear:** Patients may be reluctant to enter a program that may detect an illness. They may be apprehensive about the actual tests involved. Many patients dread mammograms and sigmoidoscopy because of lack of dignity and discomfort involved or because of negative experiences reported by others.

4. **Lack of a primary care provider:** Many elderly have been cared for by physicians older than themselves. When these physicians retire from practice, healthy community-dwelling patients may not have contact with a primary care provider who can ensure that they receive routine preventive care.

5. **Misperceptions/lack of information about screening:** Many elderly remain unaware of the value of screening tests or hold cultural values or beliefs that lead them to be fatalistic about a disease after it has been detected. On the other hand, many older people paradoxically believe themselves to be *less* susceptible to cancer.

9. What do you do when a patient refuses a screening procedure?

If a patient refuses a recommended screening test, the physician's responsibility is first to be sure that the patient understands the reason screening is being suggested and next to explore the patient's reasons. If the refusal is based on misinformation or logistic concerns, these should be addressed. Population-based estimates of disease should be translated into terms relevant to the individual; for example, what is the patient's risk of developing the condition, with and without screening? What are the chances of a false-positive or false-negative test? Does the patient understand the consequences of not participating? If an informed, competent patient refuses a screening test, the physician should respect that decision. The physician's recommendation and reasons for the patient's refusal should be documented on the patient's chart.

10. How can you improve the preventive care your elderly patients receive?

1. Work as a team to screen for preventable disease. Take advantage of community-based programs whenever possible.

2. Educate yourself and your patients about which conditions are worth screening for and what statistical rationales and emotional forces are involved. Explore your patients' health beliefs.

3. Integrate screening into routine visits when possible, but do not hesitate to schedule a separate visit if more time is needed.

4. Develop a reminder system and flow sheet that is part of each individual's record.

5. Find out what barriers exist for the individual (health beliefs, language, transportation, cost, need for a companion) and work to fix them.

11. What are the preventive interventions recommended for the general population aged 65 and older?

According to the 1995 recommendations of the U.S. Preventive Services Task Force, *asymptomatic* individuals 65 years and older should receive the following screening and counseling interventions as part of routine care. The frequency of services is left to clinical discretion, except where indicated, and should be adapted according to individual risk factors and comorbidity. Chapter 13 contains specific recommendations for cancer screening.

Screening
    Blood pressure
    Height and weight

Fecal occult blood test (annually) and sigmoidoscopy every 3–5 years

Mammography + clinical breast exam (every 1–2 years)

Papanicolaou test (all women who are or have been sexually active and who have a cervix. Consider discontinuation of testing after age 65 if previous regular screening provided consistently normal results.)

Vision screening

Assess for hearing impairment

Assess for problem drinking

Counseling

Substance abuse

    Tobacco cessation

    Avoid alcohol/drug use while driving, swimming, boating

Diet and exercise

    Limit fat and cholesterol

    Maintain caloric balance

    Emphasize grains, fruits, and vegetables

    Adequate calcium intake (women)

    Regular physical activity

Injury prevention

    Lap/shoulder belts

    Motorcycle and bicycle helmets

    Fall prevention

    Safe storage/removal of firearms

    Smoke detector

    Set hot water heater to < 120–130°F

    CPR training for household members

Dental health

    Regular visits to dental care provider

    Floss, brush with fluoride toothpaste daily

Sexual behavior (STD prevention)

    Avoid high-risk sexual behavior

    Use condoms

Immunizations

    Pneumococcal vaccine

    Influenza (annually)

    Tetanus-diphtheria (Td) boosters (every 10 years)

Chemoprophylaxis

    Discuss hormone prophylaxis (peri- and postmenopausal women)

BIBLIOGRAPHY

1. Asch DA, Hershey JC: Why some health policies don't make sense at the bedside. Ann Intern Med 122:846–850, 1995.
2. Fox SA, Roetzheim RG, Kingston RS: Barriers to cancer prevention in the older person. Clin Geriatr Med 13:79–95, 1997.
3. Hendriksen C, Lung E, Stromgard E: Consequences of assessment and intervention among elderly people: A three year randomized controlled trial. BMJ 289:1522–1524, 1984.
4. Leventhal EA, Prohaska TR: Age, symptom interpretation and health behavior. J Am Geriatr Soc 34:185–191, 1986.
5. Marton CP, Espino DU: Health screening in older women. Am Fam Physician 59:1835–1842, 1999.
6. McAlister FA, Taylor L, Teo KK, et al: The treatment and prevention of coronary heart disease in Canada: Do older patients receive efficacious therapies? The Clinical Quality Improvement Network (CQIN) Investigators. J Am Geriatr Soc 47:811–818, 1999.
7. Prohaska TR, Leventhal EA, Leventhal H, Keller ML: Health practice and illness cognition in young, middle aged, and elderly adults. J Gerontol 40:569–578, 1985.

8. Rubenstein LZ, Josephson KR, Nichol-Seamons M, Robbins AS: Comprehensive health screening of well elderly adults: An analysis of a community program. J Gerontol 41:342–352, 1986.
9. Sackett, DL, Haynes RB, Tugwell P: A Basic Science for Clinical Medicine. Boston, Little, Brown, 1985.
10. Soloman LJ, Mickey RM, Rairikas CJ, et al: Three-year prospective adherence ot three breast cancer screening modalities. Prev Med 27:781–786, 1998.
11. Sox HC: Preventive health services in adults. N Engl J Med 330:1589–1595, 1994.
12. U.S. Preventive Services Task Force: Guide to Clinical Preventive Services: An Assessment of the Effectiveness of 169 Interventions. Baltimore, Williams & Wilkins, 1995.

13. CANCER SCREENING

Angela DeMichele, M.D., Richard H. Greenberg, M.D., and David J. Vaughn, M.D.

1. Why screen for cancer in the elderly?

Cancer in persons older than 65 years accounts for the majority of cancer incidence (58%) and a disproportionate amount of cancer deaths (67%) in the United States. By the year 2030, the elderly's share of all cancer incidence will increase from the current 58% to 70%. The incidence of cancer per 100,000 population is 10 times greater for the elderly versus those < 65 years of age (2085.3 vs. 193.9). Thus, screening the elderly for cancer makes sense: screening tests are widely available, early detection improves the length and quality of survival in this population, and effective treatments are available for those malignancies detectable by screening. (See also Chapter 12, Principles of Screening.)

2. What diseases are appropriate for screening?

For a screening test to be useful, there must be a test or procedure that detects the disease in an early stage, and there must be evidence that earlier diagnosis results in an improved outcome. Breast, cervical, skin, prostate, and colorectal cancers are appropriate for screening in the elderly because the incidence rises with increasing age.

3. Why do the elderly get more cancer?

Many theories exist.

1. Aging generally leads to a **decline in immune function.** Involution of the thymus leads to T-cell deficiency, and interleukin-2 levels also decline with age. The overall decline in cell-mediated immunity is believed to impair immunologic surveillance against the appearance of spontaneous malignancies and to increase the susceptibility to environmental and infectious (e.g., viral) insults and carcinogenesis over time.

2. The appearance of cancer in response to **environmental exposures** may require long periods of time that favor an increased incidence in the elderly. Many known carcinogens require prolonged or cumulative exposures or lengthy time delays between the initial exposure and the appearance of the neoplasm. Strong evidence now exists to support the "multiple hit" hypothesis of carcinogenesis, in which a series of cumulative genetic mutations and alterations are necessary to transform normal tissues into malignancies.

3. The elderly also experience a wide range of **physiologic changes** that include alterations in hormone and enzyme levels that may influence normal cell growth and maturation; abnormalities of DNA transcription, proofreading, and repair; and alterations in the metabolic clearance of toxins. The telomere/telomerase hypothesis of aging and cancer is an example. Progressive telomere loss is a normal component of cellular senescence. This process, in conjunction with alterations in telomerase activity, may contribute to the transformation of normal cells into a malignant phenotype.

4. How does ageism affect cancer care?

Ageism is prejudice or discrimination against a particular age group, especially the elderly. Such attitudes, whether overt or subtle, often lead to an **ultraconservative** or **nihilistic** approach to the management of cancer in the elderly. Education of the public and health care providers and the implementation of properly designed studies can help to overcome some of the misconceptions that undermine the detection and care of cancer in the elderly.

5. Does age increase the extent of cancer at diagnosis?

In general, the stage of cancer at presentation is not significantly different according to age, with the exception of ovarian cancer in which older women are more likely to have more

advanced disease. However, when considering the yearly incidence of malignancy in the United States, the elderly account for a disproportionate number of cases:
- In men:
  84% of 200,000 annual cases of prostate cancer
  63% of 100,000 cases of male lung cancer
  70% of 75,000 cases of male colorectal cancer
  69% of the combined 66,000 cases of gastric, pancreatic, and urinary bladder cancers
    in men
- In women:
  50% of 182,000 annual cases of breast cancer
  76% of 74,000 cases of female colorectal cancer
  61% of 72,000 cases of female lung cancer
  65% of the combined 60,200 cases of gastric, pancreatic, ovarian, and urinary bladder
    cancers in women

Cancer in the elderly should not be considered less aggressive, less metastatic, or less of a public health problem than malignancies in younger patients.

6. With their frequent visits to doctors' offices, aren't the elderly adequately screened for cancer?

Despite having more physician visits and a progressively greater incidence of cancer than younger people, the elderly generally have a poorer participation in screening procedures. For example, more than half of women older than 65 years did not have a mammogram in the preceding year, and nearly 40% have *never* had a mammogram. Similarly, such women are less likely to have had a Pap smear in the preceding year than their younger counterparts (41% vs. 67%).

7. What are the current recommendations for cancer screening?

True consensus has not yet been reached for all tumor types, but general guidelines are as follows:

Breast	Breast self-exam monthly from age 20
	Physician breast exam annually from age 40
	Mammogram annually starting at age 40 (patients with a significant risk of carrying a breast cancer gene such as *brca*-1 or *brca*-2 or those with a known genetic alteration should begin screening earlier and should have mammography performed every 6 months) (see question 7)
Colorectal	Annual physician digital rectal exam from age 40
	Annual fecal occult blood testing and flexible sigmoidoscopy every 3–5 years from age 50
Uterine cervix	Annual Pap smear and pelvic examination starting at age 18–25 or at start of sexual activity in some populations
	Interval may be decreased to every 3 years after 3 negative yearly examinations
	Cessation of screening at any age is controversial; incidence continues to rise with age (see question 10)
Prostate	Annual digital rectal exam and serum prostate-specific antigen level determination starting at age 50 are recommended by some groups, but others debate the utility of this screening strategy in low-risk populations
	Some higher risk groups, such as men with family histories of prostate cancer or African-American men (2-fold higher incidence and mortality compared with whites) may warrant yearly screening starting at age 40
Lung	Routine chest x-rays or sputum cytology in asymptomatic populations are not currently recommended
	Smoking prevention/cessation should be encouraged

Skin	Complete skin examination for populations at risk (family history, increased sun exposure, presence of precursor lesions)
	Interval of screening: every 3 years for general population, over age 20; more frequently in people at increased risk; yearly exams are recommended in people over age 65
	Public education regarding minimizing sun exposure and skin self-examination
Ovary	No current recommendations for screening asymptomatic women other than examination of adnexa during a pelvic exam done for other reasons
	Ovarian palpation, pelvic ultrasound, and serum CA-125 levels have not been proved to be effective screening tools
Oral	Physician gloved examination of the oral cavity routinely (preferably yearly) for high-risk populations only (tobacco/alcohol use, presence of precursor lesions)
	Encourage regular dental examinations and cessation of risk exposures
Gastric	Upper GI barium fluoroscopy not generally applicable as a screening tool in the United States. (This study has proved useful in endemic areas, such as Japan.)
Urinary bladder, pancreatic	No recommendation

8. Is there justification to continue breast cancer screening past age 69?

Prospective trials have not yet answered this question. However, the incidence of breast cancer continues to rise past age 70 and remains high past age 85. Sensitivity and specificity of mammography and physician examination of the breast improve as the breast ages and glandular tissue is replaced by fat. Cost-effectiveness analysis supports physician breast examination annually and mammography every 2 years after age 65 and continuing indefinitely. Such surveillance would terminate only in those who are very ill and deemed to have a minimal life-expectancy.

9. How should colorectal cancer screening be applied to the elderly population?

Colorectal cancer incidence continues to rise steadily with age, particularly past age 65, with continued increases past age 85. Although the limitations of current screening techniques apply to the elderly population, the increased cancer incidence in this subgroup may make these screening methods somewhat more cost-effective. Current screening recommendations do not specify a particular age cut-off but generally favor application to patient populations considered at risk (due to positive family history, presence of prior colorectal cancer, or presence of adenomatous polyp of > 1 cm size or villous/tubulovillous histology). Future screening methods may utilize measures of colonic mucosal proliferation or the presence of genetic markers to stratify risk of future bowel neoplasia.

10. Is there justification to continue cervical cancer screening past age 64?

Between 1973 and 1991 the incidence of cervical cancer has risen among women born in the mid 1930s and later, particularly those of Caucasian and Hispanic ethnicity. In addition, almost 43% of deaths from cervical cancer occur in women older than 65 years. Cervical cancer in the elderly appears to progress more rapidly to invasive disease. In addition, many elderly women have *never* had a Pap smear. Surveillance for cancer of the uterine cervix should continue to the point of minimal life-expectancy, rather than an arbitrary age cut-off.

11. Does age influence the interpretation of the serum PSA level?

Prostate-specific antigen (PSA) concentrations correlate directly with age. The normal serum PSA concentration of a 60-year-old man increases approximately 0.04 ng/ml/yr. This rise is attributed to a typical increase in prostate volume of 0.5 ml/yr. Based on these trends, age-specific normal reference ranges for the serum PSA (based on the 95th percentile) for most modern assays are:

Age 40–49   0–2.5 ng/ml
50–59   0–3.5 ng/ml
60–69   0–4.5 ng/ml
70–79   0–6.5 ng/ml

Use of age-specific reference ranges makes the serum PSA level a more sensitive tumor marker in men < 60 years of age and a more specific tumor marker for men > 60 years of age.

12. How are serum PSA determinations and digital rectal exam (DRE) used in prostate cancer screening?

SERUM PSA LEVEL	DRE	DIAGNOSTIC ACTION
≤ Age-specific range	Negative	Continue annual serum PSA and DRE
> Age-specific range	Negative	Transrectal ultrasound Biopsy visible lesions Sextant biopsies of remaining prostate with two cores, including transition zone tissue
Any value	Positive	Transrectal ultrasound Biopsy palpable and visible lesions Sextant biopsies of remaining prostate

Recent data from the National Cancer Institute Surveillance Epidemiology and End Results (SEER) database indicate that since the late 1980s there has been a decrease in age and stage of disease at diagnosis with the advent of PSA screening. Others suggest that this approach may not be cost-effective in patients over age 75 or patients with serious comorbidities.

13. What socioeconomic barriers must be overcome to enhance cancer screening in the elderly?

This area has attracted increased research interest, particularly in light of the demographic shifts that predict increased elderly populations at risk for cancer in future years. The decline in physical mobility and financial resources associated with aging may be a significant barrier for access to or participation in screening efforts. Four factors have been identified as being important to the success of screening efforts in such a population:

1. **Education and recruitment:** Subpopulations at risk are identified and educational programs are introduced into local communities in a succinct and culturally sensitive fashion. Television is a particularly effective medium for reaching the elderly, especially the economically disadvantaged. Importantly, the format of the presentation may need modifications to be understood and remembered by a population who often has increased sensory or cognitive deficits. Recruitment to participate should be active and communicated through trusted community figures such as medical professionals, primary caregivers, community leaders, and friend/family "word of mouth." A common reason given for the failure of elderly individuals to participate in screening efforts is the lack of recommendations by their physicians. Specialists frequently visited by the elderly (e.g., ophthalmologists, rheumatologists) should share responsibility with primary care physicians to help educate and direct the elderly in proper cancer screening procedures.

2. **Accessible screening:** To be successful, the method of screening selected must be affordable and geographically accessible. The cost of testing and follow-up evaluation must not create a financial burden that would interfere with compliance. A recent study demonstrated that patients 65 years and older with supplemental fee-for-service private insurance in addition to Medicare were more likely to receive appropriate screening tests for cancer than those with Medicaid or Medicare alone. Patients should be informed of the screening benefits available to

them through their insurance or Medicare programs. Education regarding cancer prevention behaviors should be integrated into such an outreach program. Mobile vans are particularly useful to reach the elderly who often have difficulty traveling to remote screening sites due to physical and sensory handicaps. The screening sites must also be easily accessible to this population.

3. **Efficient diagnosis and treatment:** Geographic and chronologic integration of the interpretation of test results, provision of diagnostic studies, and initiation of definitive management are important components of a successful screening program for the elderly. Patient compliance is enhanced by decreasing time delays and providing management in a convenient manner that enhances bonding with a consistent health care team.

4. **Multidisciplinary treatment team:** Coordination of diagnosis, treatment, education, psychosocial support, and follow-up are important to a successful screening and treatment program for cancer in the elderly.

14. What misconceptions do the elderly have about screening?

Studies have identified a range of misconceptions that could deter an elderly person from participating in screening efforts. For example, many elderly persons believe that it is always "too late" when cancer is found and that cancer onset and curability are random processes or determined entirely by individual physiology and habits. They often do not perceive a potential benefit to be gained by early detection or recognize the distinction between treating cancer at early versus late or terminal stages. Some persons avoid cancer screening centers because they believe cancer is contagious, or they have concerns about privacy or embarrassment. Additionally, some persons believe that if they are pain-free, they cannot have cancer, and others dismiss symptoms such as pain, anorexia, weight loss, and fatigue as being caused by progressive age or comorbid conditions. Few older adults realize that they are actually at increased risk of developing a wide range of malignancies.

Clearly, the elderly must be convinced that they are appropriate candidates for screening and that they can safely benefit from participation. Educational programs to address these issues should be sensitive to the older patients' concerns about appearing or becoming vulnerable, losing empowerment to control their lives, and becoming a burden to their families.

BIBLIOGRAPHY

1. Costanza M: Issues in breast cancer screening in older women. Cancer 74:2009–2015, 1994.
2. Erghler WB, Congo DL: Aging and cancer: Issues of basic and clinical science. J Natl Cancer Inst 89:1489–1497, 1997.
3. Farkas A, Schneider D, Perrotti M, et al: National trends in the epidemiology of prostate cancer, 1973–1994: Evidence for the effectiveness of prostate specific antigen screening. Urology 52:444–448, 1998.
4. Littrup PJ, Kane RA, Mettlin CJ, et al: Cost-effective prostate cancer detection—reduction of low-yield biopsies. Cancer 74:3146–3158, 1994.
5. Oddone EZ, Feussner JR, Cohen HJ: Can screening older patients for cancer save lives? Clin Geriatr Med 8:51–67, 1992.
6. Potosky AL, Buren N, Graubad BI, Parsons PE: The association between health care coverage and the use of cancer screening tests. Results from the 1982 National Health Interview Survey. Med Care 36:257–270, 1998.
7. Rubenstein L: Strategies to overcome barriers to early detection of cancer among older adults. Cancer 74:2190–2193, 1994.
8. U.S. Preventive Services Task Force: Guide to Clinical Preventive Services: An Assessment of 169 Interventions: Report of the U.S. Preventive Services Task Force. Baltimore, William & Wilkins, 1989.
9. Vizcaino AP, Moreno V, Bosch FX, et al: International trends in the incidence of cervical cancer. I: Adenocarcinoma and adenosquamous cell carcinomas. Int J Cancer 75:536–545, 1998.

14. IMMUNIZATIONS

Sandeep Wadhwa, M.D., M.B.A., and Risa Lavizzo-Mourey, M.D., M.B.A.

1. Which immunizations are recommended routinely for persons over 65 years of age?

Influenza vaccine should be given annually during the fall to all persons over age 65. Because even healthy elderly persons have a reduced antibody response to the vaccine as compared with younger adults, it is recommended that the vaccine be given late in the fall—between Halloween and Thanksgiving. This timing allows a maximal antibody titer during the winter months of January and February, when the probability of influenza infection is greatest.

Pneumococcal vaccination should be given once at age 65 (with the 23-valent preparation). Data suggest that antibody levels begin to wane after 5–10 years. Revaccination is recommended at 5 years for those with the highest risk for fatal pneumococcal infection (those who are chronically immunosuppressed for any reason, including asplenic patients). The data are inadequate, however, to recommend revaccination for all elderly persons.

Tetanus and diphtheria should be given every 10 years during adulthood. It is important to obtain a Td vaccination history and give a booster in the elderly because reported cases of these illnesses occur predominantly in persons over 60 years. In addition, the vaccine is highly effective. Serologic surveys reveal that more than one-half of persons over 60 do not have protective antibody levels for tetanus or diphtheria.

2. Why is it especially important to immunize older people against influenza and pneumococcus?

1. Influenza and pneumococcal illness account for an enormous burden of preventable illness. Older persons are particularly **susceptible** to infections of the lower respiratory tract. Pneumonia and influenza are the fifth leading cause of death among the elderly. Even when respiratory infections do not cause death, they are associated with significant morbidity, including deconditioning, prolonged recovery times, and cardiac abnormalities such as arrhythmia. Elderly persons with cardiac disease, dementia, or chronic pulmonary diseases are particularly vulnerable. Furthermore, simple respiratory infections trigger decompensation of underlying chronic illnesses, such as congestive heart failure and diabetes, leading to excessive hospitalizations and death. Overall, 80–90% of the deaths caused by influenza occur in older persons. The incidence of pneumococcal pneumonia in persons over 65 is 50 cases/100,000 population compared with an overall incidence of 15–19 cases/100,000 persons/year in persons under 65.

2. The elderly are commonly in situations associated with **greater risk of exposure**. Examples include group settings such as nursing homes, retirement communities, assisted-living facilities, adult day care, and senior centers. Elders living in households with young or school-aged children are likely to be exposed to a variety of respiratory pathogens.

3. The vaccines for pneumococcal infection and influenza are **efficacious**. Based on case-control and epidemiologic studies, the efficacy of the pneumococcal vaccine is reported to be between 70 and 75% effective in preventing life-threatening pneumococcal diseases in the elderly. Similarly, the efficacy of influenza vaccine in preventing death in the elderly is about 85%. A recent meta-analysis confirms the cost-effectiveness of influenza vaccination in older persons. Finally, both vaccines are safe with relatively low risk of serious adverse reactions.

3. List the contraindications to influenza and pneumococcal immunizations.

- Severe allergic reaction to the pneumococcal vaccine in the past. This occurs in < 1% of the population.

- Anaphylactic reactions to eggs (hives, wheezing, or angioedema). The influenza vaccine virus is raised in egg media.
- History of Guillain-Barré syndrome or other neurologic syndromes after previous influenza vaccination.

4. **About which adverse reactions should one warn patients?**
   - **Soreness** at the injection site for up to 2 days occurs in less than one-third of patients.
   - **Mild, immediate hypersensitivity reaction** rarely may occur and is usually attributable to egg white allergy.
   - **Altered hepatic clearance** of certain medications (warfarin, theophylline, and phenytoin) may occur. This rarely is significant.
   - Recent placebo-controlled trials suggest that influenza vaccine is **not** associated with higher rates of systemic symptoms (fever, malaise, myalgia, headache) when compared to placebo injections.
   - Many older patients may remember the 1976 outbreak of **Guillain-Barré syndrome** (GBS) following the swine-flu vaccinations; although remote, the risk of GBS after flu vaccination should be addressed. In studies of the 1992–93 and 1993–94 flu seasons, investigators determined the relative risk of GBS to be 1.7, which is statistically significant; the attributable risk, however, is exceedingly small with an estimated one additional case of GBS per 1 million persons vaccinated. The demonstrated benefits of influenza vaccination dramatically outweigh the risks of vaccine-associated GBS.

5. **Are there any other vaccine-related issues about which one should counsel patients?**
   One cannot stress too strongly that these vaccines protect against *specific causes* of respiratory illness, not *all* viral infections or pneumonia. A common reason patients give for not seeking an annual flu shot is that "they got a flu shot one year and then got the flu anyway." The most likely explanation for such an occurrence is that the patient had already been exposed to the influenza virus at the time of immunization or that the patient was afflicted with a viral illness other than the flu. Similarly, the pneumococcal vaccine is antigen-specific: It does not protect against pneumonia caused by organisms other than pneumococcus.

6. **What are the most common misconceptions about contraindications to immunization in the elderly?**
   Contrary to common wisdom, immunization can be given in the following situations:
   - The patient has had a previous reaction to a vaccination consisting of mild to moderate local tenderness and swelling or fever < 40°C.
   - The patient experienced a mild acute illness following immunization.
   - The patient is currently receiving antimicrobial therapy or is recovering from an acute illness.
   - The patient has been recently exposed to an infectious disease.
   - The patient has an atopic history including allergies to some antibiotics.
   - The patient has a family history of allergies.
   - The patient is scheduled to receive both the influenza and the pneumococcal vaccines on the same day. (Different sites should be chosen.)

7. **Why is it necessary to immunize for influenza annually?**
   Three strains of influenza are currently circulating worldwide (two type A and one type B). The surfaces of these viruses are constantly changing. Influenza A viruses are categorized by subtypes based on two proteins: hemaglutinin and neuraminidase. Type A viruses undergo two kinds of genetic changes. One is antigenic drift whereby mutations gradually occur over time resulting in ineffectiveness of prior vaccines. The other change is known as antigenic shift, which is characterized by the sudden emergence of a new subtype. Changes in type B viruses occur by antigenic drift only. Typically the influenza vaccine includes the two subtypes of influenza A and the one type of type B strain that are predicted to be prevalent in that season. In addition to annual

changes in the makeup of the viruses, another reason why immunizations are recommended annually is that antibody levels decline over the year and generally are not sufficient for protection for more than one season.

8. **What underlying diseases put elderly patients at risk for death due to influenza or pneumonia?**
   • Chronic respiratory disease
   • Renal failure—especially those on dialysis
   • Hemoglobinopathies
   • Congestive heart failure

9. **What is the recommendation concerning influenza prophylaxis of long-term care residents and workers?**
   All residents and workers should be immunized annually. Eighty percent must be immunized to achieve "herd" immunity. Once herd immunity is achieved, unvaccinated individuals are at lower risk because the probability of infection within the whole group has been reduced. This includes residents of retirement communities, assisted-living facilities, and participants in senior daycare.

   Health care providers are a significant source of infection. Therefore, they must be immunized as well to achieve herd immunity. Because many health care providers are young women of child-bearing age, it is important to know that pregnancy and breast-feeding are not contraindications to immunization.

   When an exposure occurs before the 2 weeks required to achieve adequate antibodies titers (> 1:40), **antiviral prophylaxis** should be administered using amantadine or rimantadine. This prophylaxis can be discontinued:
   • After 2 weeks if the patient has been immunized.
   • When the flu season is over, if the patient has not been immunized. If the exposure occurs early in the season, simultaneous immunization is advised to limit the course of prophylaxis.
   • If exposure is known to be to influenza type B. Although amantadine or rimantadine are 70–90% effective in preventing influenza A, they are ineffective against type B.

   The maximum dose of amantadine is 100 mg/day, less if the patient has renal insufficiency. Rimantadine is usually dosed at 100 mg/day. Significant **neurologic symptoms** occur with both drugs, even at the recommended doses. As many as 30% of nursing home residents receiving prophylaxis have been reported to have psychosis, ataxia (with falls), seizures, or hallucinations. These are not benign medications in the frail, long-term care resident. However, an outbreak of influenza A is life-threatening to many residents.

10. **What are effective strategies for increasing immunization rates?**
    Data from 1995 suggest that, at best, 58% of elders got annual influenza vaccines, and only 40% received pneumococcal vaccines. Several strategies have been shown to improve immunization rates:
    1. A policy of immunizing against pneumococcal infection in all elders on discharge from the hospital, with clear documentation on the chart cover.
    2. Mailing pneumococcal vaccine reminder cards to everyone at age 65.
    3. Mailing flu shot reminder cards to all ambulatory elders annually in the fall.
    4. Having walk-in hours for influenza immunizations.
    5. Involving all staff (housestaff, office staff, nurses, and physicians) in a fall campaign to immunize elders against the flu.

11. **Do elderly travelers require any special immunizations?**
    No, not special ones. But older travelers should receive the World Health Organization–recommended immunizations or chemoprophylaxis for the area they plan to visit.

BIBLIOGRAPHY

1. Alagappan K, Rennie W, Kwiatkowski T, et al: Seroprevalence of tetanus antibodies among adults older than 65 years. Ann Emerg Med 28:18–21, 1996.
2. Arden NH, Cox NJ, Schonberger LB: Prevention and control of influenza: Recommendations of the Advisory Committee on Immunization Practices. MMWR 47(RR-6), 1998.
3. Lasky T, Terracciano GJ, Magder L, et al: The Guillain-Barré syndrome and the 1992–1993 and 1993–1994 influenza vaccines. N Engl J Med 339:1797–1801, 1998.
4. Margolis K, Nichol KL, Poland GA, et al: Frequency of adverse reactions to influenza vaccine in the elderly: A randomized, placebo-controlled trial. JAMA 307:988–990, 1990.
5. Nuroti P, Butler JC, Breiman RF: Prevention of pneumococcal disease: Recommendations of the Advisory Committee on Immunization Practices. MMWR 46(RR-8), 1997.

15. REDUCING CARDIOVASCULAR RISK

Bruce T. Liang, M.D., Daniel J. Rader, M.D., and Cheng-An Mao, M.D., M.P.H.

1. Why has the mortality rate for coronary artery disease (CAD) declined?

CAD remains the major cause of mortality and morbidity in the United States and the Western world. Nearly 5.4 million individuals are diagnosed as having CAD, and close to half a million deaths per year are attributable to coronary atherosclerosis. Estimates place the treatment of this disease at nearly $8 billion annually.

Fortunately, a variety of factors have contributed to the decline in the death rate from CAD over the past 25 years, as treatment programs designed to prevent modifiable risk factors have been developed. There has been a decrease in **serum cholesterol** levels in general and an improvement in the detection and treatment of **hypertension** over the past two decades. The proportion of patients, irrespective of gender or race, whose hypertension has been treated and controlled has increased, especially among African-Americans and women. **Cigarette smoking** in middle-aged men has declined, and there has been a remarkable increase in the general level of **physical activity**. There has been some change in **diet**, with a decrease in the consumption of saturated fats, certain red meats, eggs, butter, and cream as well as an increase in the use of vegetable fats and low fat milk.

Other factors contributing to the decline in CAD deaths include the early use of **thrombolytic therapy** in the treatment of acute myocardial infarction (MI) or the use of various adjunctive therapies such as **aspirin** and **heparin**. The availability of coronary care units as well as improved medical and surgical therapy for patients with acute coronary syndrome have also improved survival rates.

2. Define the various coronary risk factors.

Risk factors for CAD refer to conditions that predispose individuals to the morbidity and mortality of coronary atherosclerosis. The primary modifiable risk factors for CAD are:
- Hypercholesterolemia
- Hypertension
- Tobacco smoking
- Diabetes mellitus
- Low levels of high-density lipoprotein (HDL) cholesterol

Other potential risk factors whose importance is still being established include:
- Serum triglyceride levels
- Personality type
- Level of physical activity (see Chapter 16)
- Obesity and body habitus

3. How do lipid-lowering interventions affect blood flow and myocardial ischemia?

Often, patients without CAD have abnormal endothelial vasodilator function associated with elevated serum cholesterol levels, which may predispose them to myocardial ischemia. Studies demonstrate that cholesterol-lowering can improve endothelium-mediated vasodilator function, and this in turn may have important implications for reduced tendency toward myocardial ischemia. In addition to regression of coronary atherosclerosis, such results may explain the beneficial effect of cholesterol-lowering therapy.

4. How are lipids metabolized?

Lipids are circulated in the human body in complexes called lipoproteins, which can be separated by density during centrifugation. The degree of density is inversely related to lipid contents. The most important forms are:

Chylomicrons
Contain triglyceride and cholesterol obtained from dietary fat

Very-low density lipoprotein (VLDL)
  Contains triglyceride and cholesterol synthesized in the liver
Low-density lipoprotein (LDL)
  Generated from VLDL by the action of lipases
  Contains most of the plasma cholesterol
  Contributes to cholesterol plaque formation
  Significant risk factor for coronary artery disease (CAD)
High-density lipoprotein (HDL)
  Inversely correlated with CAD, which may be because HDL removes cholesterol from
    peripheral tissues

5. **What are the effects of aging on lipids?**
  In both men and women, total cholesterol (TC) levels increase from adolescence and
achieve the plateau in middle-age, then decline slightly after age 70 years. The levels are lower
in women than in men until menopause. In addition to TC, LDL-C levels are slightly lower in
older persons than in younger persons. HDL-C levels increase slightly in older people and are
higher in women than in men. A recent study in older persons reported that central fat deposition, glucose intolerance, obesity (in women), and use of ß-blockers (in men) are associated
with decreased HDL-C and increased TC. Higher LDL-C is also seen in obese patients and in
those with central fat deposition.

Lipoprotein Lipids in Older Persons, By Age

	MALE		FEMALE	
	> 70 YRS	50–69 YRS	> 70 YRS	50–69 YRS
TC	207	214	228	231
Triglyceride	130	141	132	125
HDL-C	51	48	60	59
LDL-C	143	146	149	152
TC/HDL-C	4.06	4.46	3.8	3.91

Cholesterol values given in mg/dl.

6. **In addition to age, what other elements influence plasma lipid levels in older patients?**
  Heredity
    Genetic abnormalities causing lower HDL-C or higher LDL-C increase the risk
      of atherosclerosis.
    Some families whose members usually live long lives show high HDL-C levels.
  Lifestyle
    Weight reduction can lower LDL-C and may raise HDL-C.
    Exercise increases HDL-C.
    HDL-C levels rise when a tobacco user quits smoking.
    Alcohol use raises triglycerides and HDL-C.
  Disease
    Cholesterol and LDL-C levels are elevated in hypothyroidism.
    Poorly controlled diabetes can increase triglyceride and cholesterol levels.
    Syndrome X is a condition associated with hyperglycemia, hypertension,
      hypertriglyceridemia, and low HDL-C.
    Nephrotic syndrome raises plasma lipid levels.
    Liver disease affects plasma lipid levels.
    Acute illness, such as infection or myocardial infarctions, can increase lipid levels.

7. **When should cholesterol levels be measured? How?**
  Clinical trials have demonstrated that lowering LDL-C and raising HDL-C can stop progression and even cause regression of coronary atherosclerotic lesions in middle-aged persons. It is

recommended that serum cholesterol levels be measured at least once every 5 years in all adults 20 years of age and above.

Because cholesterol levels can be influenced by acute illness, measurement should not be performed in acutely ill patients. High cholesterol should not be diagnosed from a single test indicating an elevated level of cholesterol; instead, repeated tests should be conducted after the initial reading to corroborate the results. A lipoprotein analysis is indicated when:

- HDL-C is < 35 mg/dl or TC > 240 mg/dl
- TC between 200 and 239 mg/dl, HDL-C < 35 mg/dl, or ≥ 2 risk factors.

The risk factors for increased levels are age (male > 45, female > 55), family history of premature CAD, current cigarette smoking, hypertension, low HDL-C (< 35 mg/dl), and diabetes mellitus.

8. How are cholesterol levels measured?

A lipoprotein analysis contains TC, triglyceride, HDL-C, and calculated LDL-C. The blood sample should be collected after a 12-hour fast as triglyceride (TG) levels are very sensitive to fat intake. LDL-C is calculated by using the following formula:

$$LDL\text{-}C = TC - (HDL\text{-}C) - (TG/5)$$

9. What cholesterol levels should be considered as treatment goals in the elderly?

Currently, there are not enough data to define the goal of cholesterol-lowering treatment in the elderly, especially when using drug therapy. More research is needed before definite recommendations can be given.

10. Summarize the types of hypolipidemic agents.

Major Drugs Used for Treatment of Hyperlipidemia

DRUG	MAJOR INDICATIONS	STARTING DOSE	MAXIMAL DOSE	MECHANISM	COMMON SIDE EFFECTS
Bile acid sequestrants Cholestyramine Colestipol	Elevated LDL	 4 mg/day 5 gm/day	 32 gm/day 40 gm/day	Increased bile acid excretion and increased LDL receptors in liver	Bloating Constipation Elevated TG
Nicotinic acid Immediate-release Controlled-release Niaspan	Elevated LDL, VLDL, low HDL	100 mg tid after meals 375 mg qhs	1 gm tid after meals 2000 mg qhs	Decreased VLDL synthesis	Cutaneous flushing GI upset Elevated glucose, uric acid, LFTs
HMG CoA reductase inhibitors Lovastatin Pravastatin Simvastatin Fluvastatin Atorvastatin Cerivastatin	Elevated LDL	 20 mg/day 20 mg qhs 10 mg qhs 20 mg qhs 10 mg qhs 0.2 mg qhs	 80 mg/day 40 mg qhs 80 mg qhs 80 mg qhs 80 mg qhs 0.4 mg qhs	Reduced cholesterol synthesis Upregulated hepatic LDL receptors Reduced VLDL production	Myalgias Arthralgias GI upset Elevated transaminases Sleep disturbances
Fibric acid derivatives Gemfibrozil Fenofibrate	Elevated TG, remnants	 600 mg bid 200 mg qd	 600 mg bid 200 mg qd	Increased lipoprotein lipase Decreased VLDL synthesis	Myositis GI upset Gallstones Elevated LFTs
Fish oils	Severely elevated TG	3 gm/day	12 gm/day	Decreased TG synthesis Enhanced TG catabolism	Diarrhea GI upset Fishy odor to breath

LDL = low-density lipoprotein, VLDL = very low density lipoprotein, HDL = high-density lipoprotein, TG = triglycerides, GI = gastrointestinal, LFTs = liver function tests.

11. What pharmacologic measures can be taken to prevent a second MI?

A number of specific pharmacologic interventions can reduce mortality *after* the onset of acute MI, including angiotensin-converting enzyme (ACE) inhibitors and beta blockers.

The CONSENSUS II study, conducted over 1 year at 103 Scandinavian centers enrolling 6,090 patients, demonstrated that patients receiving the ACE inhibitor **enalapril** within 24 hours of a confirmed MI failed to show improved survival during the next 6 months. However, there was a small but significant beneficial effect of enalapril on the progression of congestive heart failure. In the SAVE (Survival and Ventricular Enlargement) trial in the United States and Canada, 2231 patients with an ejection fraction ≤ 40% following an acute MI were randomized in a double-blind fashion to receive placebo or **captopril** and then were followed for an average of 42 months. Captopril-treated patients had a 19% reduction in risk of all-cause mortality and a 21% reduction in the risk of fatal and nonfatal major cardiovascular events. There was also a 25% reduction in risk for recurrent MI.

Beta blockers also may confer a survival benefit. Large clinical trials have shown that **atenolol**, **propranolol** and **metoprolol** improve survival in a wide spectrum of post-MI patients and reduce the incidence of sudden death and reinfarction. Results with **oxprenolol**, a beta blocker with intrinsic sympathomimetic activity, are far less encouraging; at least one trial shows a slight increase in mortality. Patients without contraindications to the beta blockers (e.g., asthma, moderate or severe congestive heart failure, arrhythmias) should receive prophylactic treatment with one after acute MI. Data are conflicting over the benefit of continuing this therapy beyond 2 years; but if beta blockers are well tolerated and if there is no reason to discontinue therapy, then they should be continued in most patients. For patients with an extremely good prognosis—e.g., those who have a first acute MI with good left ventricular function, negative stress testing, and no significant ventricular ectopy—beta blockers need not be given.

12. Does tobacco use predispose to CAD?

The use of tobacco products is a major risk factor in patients prone to the development of CAD (see Chapter 19). A number of mechanisms may be responsible:

- Decreased level of HDL
- Higher level of LDL
- Acute effect on blood pressure
- Higher fibrinogen level
- Increased platelet aggregability
- Prolongation in bleeding time
- Increased plasma norepinephrine levels

13. Describe the approach to elderly patients with hypertension. What lifestyle modifications can help lower blood pressure?

Hypertension is a major modifiable risk factor for the development of coronary atherosclerosis. The risk for developing coronary disease and heart failure is greater for elderly than for younger patients. Thus, effective antihypertensive therapy achieves greater reductions in cardiovascular diseases in elderly than in younger patients. In view of decreased bioreceptor sensitivity in the elderly, drugs causing postural hypotension should be avoided. Isolated systolic hypotension in the elderly is a serious risk factor for strokes. Diuretics, beta blockers, or calcium channel antagonists are usually effective. In elderly patients with coexisting hypertension and obesity, both effective antihypertensive therapy and weight reduction are important.

Although the precise correlation between high sodium intake and hypertension is not definitively established, clinical evidence suggests that a 100-mmol/day decrease in sodium intake leads to an average decline of 6 mmHg in blood pressure. An average American consumes 10–15 gm of salt per day, an amount that far exceeds the body's needs. In addition, both decreased consumption of saturated fat and increased intake of potassium contribute to a lowering of blood pressure. Another modification that helps lower blood pressure is avoidance of tobacco. When multiple lifestyle changes are made, an additive antihypertensive effect may be seen.

14. What evaluations are needed before an elderly person begins an exercise program? What is an appropriate level of exercise?

In general, long-term physical activity plays an important role in maintaining ideal body weight and muscle mass and perhaps in maintaining normal blood pressure and lowering lipid levels. However, people who have been sedentary and wish to start regular exercise must be cautious, because their sudden switch from a sedentary lifestyle to regular physical exercise may induce ventricular arrhythmias or acute MI. This concern is especially important in the elderly, because an age-related decline in physical activity may mean that symptoms of myocardial ischemia are not evident. Such patients should undergo a thorough physical exam and exercise stress test before undertaking a program of vigorous physical activity. However, many elderly patients may not be able to reach 85% of predicted maximal heart rate during an exercise stress test. In this case, a thallium perfusion scan following dipyridamole administration may provide equivalent information on the presence or severity of coronary disease.

The optimal level of exercise required to protect against CAD has not been established. Exercise expenditures of about 2000 kcal/wk, or the equivalent of running 20 miles/wk, correlate with protection from the development of CAD. If, after undergoing a thorough history, physical exam, and treadmill testing, the patient has no evidence or history of ischemic heart disease, then the exercise program probably does not need close monitoring. Another way to look at a desired level of exercise is that three sessions per week, each lasting 20–30 minutes, is necessary to bring about a significant improvement in aerobic capacity. Five sessions can produce the maximal result, which is usually achieved after weeks of training. In both men and women, there may be considerable additional reductions in risk factors for CAD if the level of physical activity exceeds the recommended guidelines.[11] The same general strategy should be applicable to the elderly, except that the intensity of exercise at each level of progression should be less; it should be individualized also on the basis of the results of screening procedures for coronary disease and the patient's general physical condition.

15. What is the relationship between obesity and CAD?

A National Institutes of Health consensus conference on obesity concluded that obesity is associated with poorer health and decreased longevity. Although the precise role of obesity as an independent risk factor for CAD is unclear, analysis of the Framingham data reveals its contribution to the overall risk for CAD. Blood cholesterol, blood pressure, glucose, and uric acid levels all increase with a greater body mass index. Obesity has a strong positive correlation with blood pressure, triglyceride, and insulin levels and is inversely related to the concentration of HDL cholesterol. All of these abnormalities are associated with an increased risk for coronary atherosclerosis. Weight reduction in obese individuals, in addition to helping the control of blood pressure, can also increase the threshold of angina pectoris.

16. Explain the relationship between family history and the risk for CAD.

There is a clear tendency for familial aggregation of CAD, likely due to aggregation of risk factors among family members. In an evaluation of siblings of patients with documented premature atherosclerosis, it was demonstrated that 48% of brothers and 41% of sisters were hypertensive and that 45% of brothers and 22% of sisters had a lipid abnormality. In addition to the risk of developing premature atherosclerosis from a positive family history, familial aggregation of risk factors implies a predisposition for development of CAD ultimately manifesting late in life. Fortunately, such risk factors in first-degree relatives of affected family members are mostly modifiable and lend themselves to preventive strategies aimed at reducing risk early on.

17. How should diabetic patients be treated to reduce their risk for CAD?

In diabetic patients, mortality associated with coronary atherosclerosis is increased. In the first National Health and Nutrition Examination Survey, age-adjusted death rates for diabetics were twice those seen in nondiabetics. Three-quarters of the increase in mortality among diabetic men was due to CAD. Type 2 diabetic patients with hyperinsulinemia are predisposed to coronary atherosclerosis. Insulin is a growth factor that enhances synthesis and uptake of lipids by smooth muscle cells. Epidemiologic studies have demonstrated that elevated fasting insulin levels predict the development of coronary atherosclerosis, even in nondiabetic patients, independent of all other CAD risk factors. Other studies demonstrate that hyperinsulinemia and insulin resistance, such as occur in type 2 diabetics, result in an increased frequency of CAD.

Hypertension and obesity also tend to be associated with diabetes and glucose intolerance. In fact, the frequency of hypertension is about twice that in patients with altered glucose tolerance.

Control of hypertension is particularly important in diabetic patients, as it leads to a decrease in microvascular complications. Because formation of glycosylated LDL has been implicated in the development of macrovascular disease, control of blood glucose may also help to reduce macrovascular or atherosclerotic complications in diabetics. Weight reduction can improve glucose-associated lipid abnormalities in type 2 diabetics. However, medications that decrease glucose tolerance, such as diuretics, should be avoided.

BIBLIOGRAPHY

1. Anderson TJ, Meredith IT, Yeung AC, et al: The effect of cholesterol-lowering and antioxidant therapy on endothelium-dependent coronary vasomotion. N Engl J Med 332:488–493, 1995.
2. Caspersen CJ, Bloemberg BPM, Saris WHM, et al: The prevalence of selected physical activities and their relation with coronary heart disease risk factors in elderly men: The Zutphen study, 1985. Am J Epidemiol 133:1078–1092, 1991.
3. Corti MC, Guralnik JM , Salive ME, et al: HDL cholesterol predicts coronary heart disease mortality in older persons. JAMA 274:539–544, 1995.
4. Jha P, Flather M, Lonn E, et al: The antioxidant vitamins and cardiovascular disease: A critical review of epidemiologic and clinical trial data. Ann Intern Med 123:860–872, 1995.
5. Levine GN, Keaney JF Jr, Vita JA: Cholesterol reduction in cardiovascular disease. N Engl J Med 332:512–521, 1995.
6. Lonn EM, Yusuf S, Jha P, et al: Emerging role of antiotensin-converting enzyme inhibitors in cardiac and vascular protection. Circulation 90:2056–2069, 1994.
7. Reaven GM, Lithell H, Landsberg L: Hypertension and associated metabolic abnormalities—The role of insulin resistance and the sympathoadrenal system. N Engl J Med 334:374–381, 1996.
8. Stein GH, Hamilton BP, Hamilton JH, et al: One year experience of elderly hypertensive patients with isradipine therapy. J Hum Hypertens 8:911–916, 1994.
9. Treasure CB, Klein JL, Weintraub WS, et al: Beneficial effects of cholesterol-lowering therapy on the coronary endothelium in patients with coronary artery disease. N Engl J Med 332:481–487, 1995.

16. EXERCISE IN THE ELDERLY: CAN IT IMPROVE FUNCTION?

Grace A. Cordts, M.D., M.S., M.P.H.

All parts of the body which have function, if used in moderation and exercised in labors to which each is accustomed, become thereby well developed and age slowly, but if unused and left idle, they become liable to disease, defective in growth and age quickly.

—Hippocrates

1. Can exercise improve functional status in the elderly?

Data from the Canadian Health Survey showed that an inevitable functional decline creates functional dependency starting 8–10 years before death. Most elderly people are totally dependent the year before death. The social and economic consequences of this dependency are staggering if one thinks of the projected increase in numbers of persons 65 years or older.

There is evidence that much of what was once viewed as aging is actually secondary to disuse. There are striking similarities between structural and functional declines associated with aging and the effects of enforced inactivity.

At age 65, women have an average of 19 more years of life, and men have an average of 15 more years. There is interest in looking at exercise as a potential way to minimize future functional decline or at least to compress the period of dependency into the last year of life—the concept of **compression of morbidity**. The potential benefit of improving quality of life is combined with the potential societal and economic benefits of decreasing institutionalization of our aging society.

Physical fitness is a determinant of functional status; intuitively, exercise should improve functional status. A preponderance of data supports this hypothesis. Exercise has been shown to improve multiple physiologic functions and has been used in the treatment of various diseases. Exercise improves cardiorespiratory capacity, muscle strength, endurance, flexibility, body composition (increases lean body mass and decreases fat), range of motion (ROM), sleep, and cognitive function. It has been shown to decrease patients' sensitivity to dyspnea and to improve lipid profiles. Exercise has been used to treat patients with cardiovascular disease, chronic obstructive pulmonary disease, diabetes mellitus, depression, osteoporosis, arthritis, Parkinson's disease, and falls, all with some degree of success.

Epidemiologic and observational studies show that people who exercise regularly require less support and institutionalization at any given age than nonexercisers. Abundant evidence indicates improvement in physical fitness when healthy older individuals take part in controlled, vigorous exercise.

The benefits of exercise in frail, elderly nursing home residents are not clear. Studies show that interventions are successful in increasing muscle strength, walking endurance, and grip strength. However, these improvements do not always translate into benefits in functional status and quality of life. The programs are time- and cost-intensive. Further investigation is needed to identify beneficial and cost-effective interventions in elderly nursing home residents.

2. What are the goals of an exercise program for the elderly patient?

Ward describes six objectives for an exercise program for the elderly:
1. Increased energy to cope with normal daily tasks
2. Improved capacity for unusual or unexpected demands
3. Quicker recovery from illness or stress
4. Improved balance
5. Greater opportunity to meet new people
6. More fun

3. When is it too late to start exercising?

It is not clear when it is too late to start exercising or if it is ever too late to start. Certainly the epidemiologic data suggest that people 70 years or older who report low levels of exercise have an increased risk of death. People who maintain activity in their lives do better. In a randomized trial, Posner took healthy older sedentary adults and showed that exercise reduced new cardiovascular events in the next 2 years. A study of nursing home residents found that people even in their 90s can improve functional capacity, grip strength, chair-to-stand time, and self-ratings of depression. There certainly are anecdotal reports of people starting to exercise in their 80s and doing well into their 90s and 100s. Even bedridden individuals can be given ROM exercises to prevent contractures or bed mobility exercises that facilitate the tasks of caregivers.

4. Who should be assessed for cardiovascular risk before initiating exercise?

How detailed an exam and how much testing are needed before starting an exercise program are controversial. Some believe that all people should have a complete physical exam and cardiopulmonary stress test before initiating exercise, whereas others believe that exercise is a normal part of life and that no screening is required for asymptomatic healthy individuals. The American Heart Association recommends an exercise stress test for sedentary men over 45 years of age, sedentary women over 50, and anyone with hypertension or heart disease. The Royal College of Physicians and British Cardiology Society recommend minimal use of special evaluations and believe that a medical exam is not necessary before starting an exercise program as long as the work-out begins at a low level and progresses slowly.

The degree of work-up depends on the patient and the intensity of the program to be undertaken. Asymptomatic patients who are beginning a low level of activity that gradually builds intensity probably do not need special evaluation. Patients with active cardiopulmonary symptoms or a history of angina, myocardial infarction, or palpitations should undergo a thorough history and physical exam, focusing on cardiac and pulmonary symptoms. These patients and asymptomatic older persons who are planning to take up a competitive sport or to become involved in a vigorous exercise program should have a stress test. If the stress test is positive, further evaluation is necessary before exercise is undertaken.

5. Are any medical conditions a contraindication to exercise?

Patients with aortic stenosis, severe congestive heart failure, hypertrophic cardiomyopathy, or uncontrolled hypertension should be cautioned against exercise because of the adverse consequences or may need special continuous supervision during exercise (as in a cardiac rehabilitation program).

6. How do exercise programs for the elderly differ from general exercise programs?

Physical fitness is the goal of exercise programs for younger individuals. Although physical fitness is an important aspect of all exercise programs, focusing on performance of activities of daily living and quality of life are more important for the elderly.

7. What does an exercise prescription include?

The content of an exercise prescription depends on whether its purpose is to increase physical fitness or improve, maintain, or regain functional status. Historically, an exercise prescription for physical fitness included the type, intensity, and frequency of exercise. Exactly what should be included to alter functional status is unknown, largely because it is not known what level of physical fitness is necessary to maintain functional status.

Most agree that improvement in physical fitness requires at least 20 minutes of aerobic exercise 3 times per week. For optimal benefit, the heart rate should be maintained at 60–80% of its maximum for the person's age for 20 minutes. A quick calculation for maximal heart rate is 220 minus age. For a prescription that focuses on the health benefits of exercise rather than physical fitness, the Centers for Disease Control and Prevention and the American College of Sports Medicine recommend regular participation in activities of moderate intensity for 30 minutes a day.

8. What should be included in an exercise program for the elderly?

The ideal program should include a warm-up period, an aerobic period, and a cool-down period. Flexibility exercises and strengthening exercises round out the program. The warm-up and cool-down periods should be extended, because steady state levels of blood pressure, heart rate, and ventilation are reached more slowly. The warm-up and cool-down periods should be about 20 minutes in duration.

9. What kind of exercise is best?

Walking is probably the cheapest and easiest form of exercise. Incorporating recreational activities into exercise helps to maintain compliance and participation. Water activities such as swimming, water aerobics, or water walking can be beneficial for patients with musculoskeletal problems. Water activities, however, do not have the beneficial effects of gravity for increasing bone density.

The type of exercise must take into account the patient and his or her potential problems as well as maximize safety, compliance, and enjoyment. Frail elders may have poor vision, unsteady gait, or musculoskeletal problems that limit the type of activity in which they can participate. In general, activities should be enjoyable and affordable, involve low impact with less force on joints, and use skills the patient already has. One study of exercise and mobility showed that any physical activity, including gardening, was beneficial as long as it was done 3 or more times per week.

Muscle-strengthening exercises should involve low resistance to prevent orthopedic injuries. They should be done with caution to avoid straining against a closed glottis to prevent cardiovascular complications. The patient should be instructed to exhale while performing the active phase of exercise and to inhale while relaxing. This strategy prevents straining against a closed glottis.

Isometric exercises should be avoided because they increase blood pressure and cardiac workload, creating the potential for adverse cardiac events.

10. What are the recommended intensity, frequency, and duration of exercise for elderly people?

The recommendations for achieving physical fitness in healthy younger people are well known. For cardiovascular fitness, the American Heart Association recommends activity 3 days per week for 20 minutes at 50% of $\dot{V}O_2$ max. The American College of Sports Medicine recommends activity 3–5 days per week at 60–90% of maximal heart rate or 50–85% of $\dot{V}O_2$ max. For the elderly who want to improve physical fitness, the intensity of exercise should be reduced and the duration and frequency increased to prevent injury. The same level of physical fitness can be achieved; it will simply take longer. Some evidence indicates that the intensity can be 40–50% of $\dot{V}O_2$ max and still have an effect. Future studies must address the issue of how intense a work-out is necessary.

From a practical standpoint, a good rule of thumb to monitor intensity is to tell patients that if they cannot talk during exercise, they are doing too much. The exercise program should leave the person feeling pleasantly aware of their muscles the next day. The amount of exercise should be increased gradually each week.

11. Do the elderly sustain more injuries and adverse effects from exercise?

No direct evidence addresses this question. If an exercise program is undertaken prudently, risk of injury or adverse complication should be minimized. The risk of injury seems to be related to high-intensity training and high-impact activities. Reviews of cardiovascular complications in cardiac rehabilitation programs show relatively low rates of adverse events: 1 in 112,000 patient hours for cardiac arrest; 1 in 294,000 patient hours for myocardial infarction; and 1 in 784,000 patient hours for death. The following recommendations may help to prevent injury:
- Emphasize warm-up period.
- Strengthen weakened joints, especially rotator cuff and wrists, if golf or tennis is to be undertaken.
- Emphasize low-impact activities, such as walking, bicycling, rowing, and cross-country skiing.

- In hot weather, exercise in air conditioning; in cold weather, exercise indoors.
- Ensure adequate hydration.
- Avoid exercising on hard surfaces.
- Use adequate footwear.
- For exercising in pools, make sure that adequate hand rails and nonslip decks are available.
- If balance is poor, avoid exercises such as cycling or skiing, which require balance skills.
- If symptoms occur, stop the activity immediately and contact a physician; go to the emergency department if symptoms do not resolve when exercise is stopped.
- Take antianginal medication before exercise.

12. How do you motivate and help patients comply with an exercise regimen?

Motivating patients and encouraging participation in exercise are major challenges. Emphasizing the benefits in terms of maintaining and increasing functional status is probably most successful. Specific examples include being able to get down on the floor to play with grandchildren, possibly preventing institutionalization, and recovering from illness quickly. Despite the lack of controlled studies, the following characteristics probably make an exercise program more appealing:

- Formal structure
- Demonstration of objective improvement (e.g., by keeping logs)
- Slow increase in exercise so that patient does not overdo it or become frustrated
- Easy ways to monitor intensity of work
- Grouping people according to ability and disability
- Use of enjoyable activities
- Supervision by older rather than young instructors

13. What community resources are available?

Because of a greater interest and emphasis on physical activity, more exercise programs aimed at older persons are being offered by various organizations. Local colleges and universities, community centers, YM or YWCAs, and rehabilitation hospitals with community outreach programs are good resources. The National Association for Human Development, American Physical Therapy Association, American Association of Retired Persons, and American College of Sports Medicine are valuable sources of information.

14. Is there a role for exercise in elderly hospitalized patients? What is the role of rehabilitation hospital or outpatient programs for the elderly?

Often immobilization and bedrest are prescribed for hospitalized elders; both can cause an acute deterioration in function, which at times may be impossible to reverse. Elderly patients should be mobilized as soon as possible. ROM exercises should be initiated immediately to promote activity and to prevent contractures. Physical therapy and occupational therapy should be initiated as soon as medically possible to help prevent functional decline. Bedrest should not be prescribed unless it is essential for recovery from illness. Elderly patients who have had any acute or semiacute deterioration in function may benefit from a rehabilitation program as an inpatient or outpatient.

15. Does Medicare reimburse for rehabilitation?

Medicare reimburses for rehabilitation if the benefit from the program is functionally significant. For example, programs that teach patients how to toilet themselves or to fix a meal—skills that allow them to remain at home—and programs that teach family members how to transfer a bedridden patient so that the patient can be maintained at home are covered. The patient has to show improvement. Medicare reimburses for inpatient and outpatient services. Programs include in-home services, rehabilitation hospitals, skilled nursing facilities, and outpatient services. The type of program depends on patients' needs and their abilities to participate in activities. For inpatient programs to be reimbursed, the patient must need medical supervision and 24-hour nursing care as well as be able to participate in 3 hours of physical therapy, occupational therapy, or speech therapy 5 days per week. This intensity of activity may be too taxing for some patients.

The Balanced Budget Act changed how skilled nursing facilities (SNFs) are reimbursed by Medicare. Many elderly patients debilitated from hospitalization went to SNFs for rehabilitation because they could not tolerate the intensity of an inpatient rehabilitation hospital. The new payment system, called the Medicare Prospective Payment System, includes an annual financial limitation for rehabilitation services. This reimbursement system will have an effect on patients moving from hospitals to SNFs. Exactly how is difficult to predict because the system was just implemented. It is anticipated that modifications will occur as ramifications of this system become clear.

16. What is the role of the primary care physician or geriatrician in promoting exercise?

Geriatricians and primary care physicians should take an active role in encouraging people to maintain physical activity or to begin an exercise program at any age. They can point out the benefits of exercise, know what community resources are available, help motivate patients, and know who needs further testing before initiating an exercise program. The physician should ask about physical activity at every office visit, including any symptoms associated with exercise, and encourage continued participation.

BIBLIOGRAPHY

1. Buchner DM, Beresford SA, Larson EB, et al: Effects of physical activity on health status in older adults. II: Intervention studies. Annu Rev Public Health 13:469–488, 1992.
2. Casperson CJ, Kriska AM, Dearwater SR: Physical activity epidemiology as applied to elderly populations. Baillieres Clin Rheumatol 8:2–27, 1994.
3. DiPietro L: The epidemiology of physical activity and physical function in older people. Med Sci Sports Exerc 28:596–600, 1996.
4. Elward K, Larson EB: Benefits of exercise for older adults. Clin Geriatr Med 8:35–51, 1992.
5. MacRae PG, Asplund BS, Schnelle JF, et al: A walking program for nursing home residents: Effects on walk endurance, physical activity, mobility, and quality of life. J Am Geriatr Soc 44:175–180, 1996.
6. Pate RR, Pratt M, Blair SN, et al: Physical activity and public health. A recommendation from the Centers for Disease Control and Prevention and the American College of Sports Medicine. JAMA 273:402–407, 1995.
7. Pollock ML, Graves JE, Sewart DL, Lowenthal DT: Exercise training and prescription for the elderly. South Med J 87:588–595, 1994.
8. Shephard RJ: The scientific basis of exercise prescribing for the very old. J Am Geriatr Soc 38:62–70, 1990.
9. Wagner EH, La Croix AZ, Buckner DM, Larson EB: Effects of physical activity on health status in older adults. I: Observational studies. Annu Rev Public Health 13:451–468, 1992.

17. NUTRITION

Marie Bernard, M.D.

1. Name the most common nutritional problem among elderly individuals.

In studies of elderly individuals in hospitals and nursing homes, **protein-calorie malnutrition** is found in 30–50% of the population. Borderline protein-calorie malnutrition is common in elderly outpatients. Multiple epidemiologic studies have demonstrated that elderly individuals commonly consume less than two-thirds of the recommended daily allowance (RDA) for multiple nutrients. This, combined with the effects of accumulated illnesses, medications, and social circumstances, depletes body caloric reserves for the stress of acute illness or surgery. Thus, with hospitalization, elderly individuals often have developed protein-calorie malnutrition and its associated morbidity and mortality. Elderly outpatients are much less likely to have overt malnutrition, unless they are recuperating from an acute illness.

2. Why do many elderly have reduced calorie intakes?

A number of factors contribute to elderly individuals' becoming protein-calorie malnourished:

1. As one ages, the senses of smell and taste diminish, thus rendering foods less palatable.

2. Accumulated illnesses and medications may suppress the appetite or impair the absorption of nutrients.

3. Many elderly individuals suffer from functional problems, making it difficult to get proper access to food or to prepare food properly.

4. Many elderly individuals suffer from social factors, such as decreased income, social isolation, and depression, that impair their ability to obtain food or their desire to consume it.

All of these factors combine to lead to suboptimal intake among elderly individuals, often leading to protein-calorie malnutrition upon their presentation to a hospital or long-term care institution.

Risk Factors for Poor Nutritional Status

Inappropriate food intake	Dependency/disability	Chronic medication use
Poverty	Acute/chronic diseases	Advanced age
Social isolation	or conditions	

Modified from The Nutrition Sceening Initiative, a project of the American Academy of Family Physicians, The American Dietetic Association and the National Council on the Aging, Inc., and funded in part by a grant from Ross Laboratories, a division of Abbott Laboratories.

3. How does malnutrition affect outcome of care in the elderly?

In protein-calorie malnourished patients, the length of stay in the hospital, cost of hospital care, and mortality are all 30–100% greater than in normally nourished individuals. Malnourished elderly outpatients also have poorer health and greater morbidity than normally nourished individuals. Morbidity associated with protein-calorie malnutrition includes increased infections, longer recovery time for wound healing, and less recovery of function.

4. When should you evaluate the nutritional status of elderly individuals? How?

Nutritional assessment can be difficult in elderly patients because aging and disease cause decreases in lean body mass that can mimic those seen with malnutrition. Although weight loss is seen with aging, recent unintentional weight loss—especially if it is > 5–10% of one's usual weight or > 10 lbs in 6 months—is significant.

An expert panel of nutritionists and gerontologists has developed a consensus regarding the nutritional assessment of elderly individuals. Their Nutrition Screening Initiative provides the first generally agreed-on standards for determining the nutritional status of elderly individuals. They also recommend proper interventions once risk factors for malnutrition are identified.

5. When should nutritional intervention be initiated for elderly individuals?

Most experts would not advise allowing a thin, frail, elderly person to go for 10 days with suboptimal intake. There are no firm guidelines, but the more underweight the patient and the greater the metabolic stress (particularly if the albumin level is < 3.5 gm/dl), the earlier nutritional intervention should be considered. Early identification of patients with intake significantly below 1000 kcal/day is therefore necessary.

A registered dietitian often is helpful in guiding the assessment of the nutritional needs of hospitalized or institutionalized elderly individuals and in assessing how closely spontaneous intake approximates those needs. This task is more difficult in ambulatory elderly. However, the guidelines of the Nutrition Screening Initiative for the Level 1 screen may help in identifying elderly individuals at risk for borderline intake.

Medicare does not pay for a home nutritional assessment. However, such assessments can be performed easily by a number of individuals.

- Checklists of risk factors can be administered by lay persons or home health aides. These should be considered for every elderly individual.
- Level I screens can be performed by nurses, social workers, and other health professionals in regular contact with elders. This screen should be performed if an elder is found to be at risk of nutritional deficiency, based on responses to the checklist.
- The Level II screen is intended for physicians to evaluate elderly individuals who appear nutritionally deficient based on the checklist and Level I screen.

(See figures on pages 84–87.)

6. What is unique about providing dietary supplements to elderly individuals?

Supplementation of the diet with enteral formulas is the first intervention to be provided (after problems with depression, social isolation, and/or difficulties with access to food have been addressed). Unfortunately, no medications have been identified that are clearly beneficial in stimulating appetite in the elderly. Food supplements have limited benefit in many elderly, due to the development of early satiety and/or taste fatigue. In addition, many elderly substitute enteral formulas intended for diet supplementation for their usual intake, thus deriving no net benefit from the intervention. In cases when spontaneous and supplemented intake cannot bring calorie and protein intake to goal levels, nutritional support via a nasoenteric or enteric tube is indicated.

7. How are the enteral nutrition formulas classified?

A plethora of formulas is available for nutritional support of the elderly. Each formula claims special properties that purportedly benefit diverse populations. However, based on review of the literature, there are few indications in the elderly for specialized formulas.

Formulas can be classified according to **protein form** as polymeric (blenderized), elemental, or free amino acids. Polymeric formulas are preferable to elemental formulas for simple diet supplementation, because they are more palatable. Polymeric formulas appear to be better tolerated in most elderly than elemental or amino acid formulas, which are more costly and unnecessary in most instances. The source of the protein does not appear to affect tolerance of feedings, with the exception of milk-based formulas. (The elderly have a higher prevalence of lactase deficiency than younger individuals, making milk-based formulas poorly tolerated by many.) Formulas that are high in osmolality and/or fiber do not appear to influence the occurrence of diarrhea. A study with a very small number of patients suggests that elemental formulas are beneficial for diarrhea in hypoalbuminemic patients because of their easier absorption. (See table, top of next page.)

8. How is an appropriate formula selected?

In general, the elderly require 0.8–1.0 gm protein and 25 kcal/kg body weight. Patients recuperating from hip fracture or major surgery may have higher protein needs, up to 1.0 gm/kg body weight. Thus, you should select a formula that provides an appropriate quantity of calories and protein over the course of 24 hours in an isosmolar form or more concentrated form if there are concerns regarding fluid retention. Formulas that have a mixture of carbohydrate, long-chain

Enteral Formula Comparison Chart

	BLENDERIZED		ELEMENTAL	FIBER-CONTAINING		LACTOSE-FREE
Product	Compleat Regular	Vitaneed	Travasorb	Enrich	Ensure Plus	Isocal
Cal/ml	1.07	1.0	1.0	1.1	1.5	1.06
mOsm/kg water	450	300	560	480	690	270
Calories to meet 100% RDA for vitamins and mineratls	1600	1500	2000	1530	2130	2000
Flavors	Natural food	Natural food	Unflavored	Varied	Varied	Unflavored
Cal/protein per 8-oz can	250/9	250/8	250/11	250/9	360/13	250/8

triglycerides, and intact protein (i.e., formulas that mimic real food) are usually well-tolerated. Although the elderly have a high prevalence of disorders of the GI tract that can affect fat absorption, data suggest that many elderly individuals can tolerate enteral formulas with as much as 67% of calories provided.as fat.

In intensive care unit patients, a low non-protein calorie to nitrogen ratio (e.g., 97:1) may be beneficial in promoting nitrogen retention. In metabolically stable patients, there also may be a role for providing more nitrogen-dense formulas to compensate for the fact that patients often do not receive the full amount of enteral nutrition prescribed (e.g., due to technical difficulties, cessation of feedings for diagnostic testing).

9. Is nutritional intervention effective in elderly individuals?

Few studies actually have demonstrated the efficacy of nutritional intervention in this or any age group. One study evaluated a group of 122 "thin" and "very thin" elderly women with hip fractures. In the randomized, controlled trial, 1000 cal and 28 gm of protein were provided by overnight tube feeding, in addition to a regular diet throughout the day. This intervention led to more rapid ambulation than in control patients. Another study demonstrated similar benefit of simple oral supplementation in 59 elderly hip fracture patients. In a prospective, controlled trial, the daily addition of 250 cal and 20 gm of protein to the usual diet resulted in fewer hospital complications, increased mobility, and fewer nursing home placements at 6-month follow-up than in the controls.

Several studies of long-term feedings in chronically ill elderly in nursing homes have failed to show the benefits demonstrated in shorter studies of elderly who have undergone surgical procedures. However, many of the long-term evaluation studies are retrospective, without clear documentation of the degree to which nutritional needs were matched with the nutrition support provided.

In sum, nutritional deficits would appear to be reversible in many cases. Adverse outcomes associated with malnutrition in the elderly are well-documented. Thus, the potential benefits of nutritional intervention appear worthy of the effort.

Benefits and Risks of Enteral Nutritional Support

BENEFITS	RISKS
Nutritional repletion	Aspiration pneumonia
Hydration	Diarrhea
Decreased morbidity	Tube displacement
Decreased mortality	Clogged tube
Fewer complications than parenteral therapy	Electrolyte disturbance
Lower cost than parenteral therapy	Infection of feeding formula

Level 1 Screen

Body Weight

Measure height to the nearest inch and weight to the nearest pound. Record the values below and mark them on the Body Mass Index (BMI) scale to the right. Then use a straight edge (ruler) to connect the two points and circle the spot where this straight line crosses the center line (body mass index). Record the number below.

Healthy older adults should have a BMI between 24 and 27.

Height (in):_____
Weight (lbs):_____
Body Mass Index:_____
(number from center column)

Check any boxes that are true for the individual:

☐ Has lost or gained 10 pounds (or more) in the past 6 months.

☐ Body mass index <24

☐ Body mass index >27

For the remaining sections, please ask the individual which of the statements (if any) is true for him or her and place a check by each that applies.

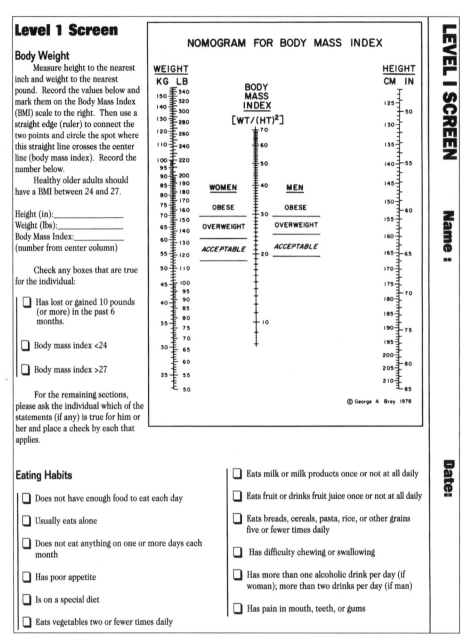

NOMOGRAM FOR BODY MASS INDEX

© George A Bray 1978

LEVEL I SCREEN   Name: Date:

Eating Habits

☐ Does not have enough food to eat each day

☐ Usually eats alone

☐ Does not eat anything on one or more days each month

☐ Has poor appetite

☐ Is on a special diet

☐ Eats vegetables two or fewer times daily

☐ Eats milk or milk products once or not at all daily

☐ Eats fruit or drinks fruit juice once or not at all daily

☐ Eats breads, cereals, pasta, rice, or other grains five or fewer times daily

☐ Has difficulty chewing or swallowing

☐ Has more than one alcoholic drink per day (if woman); more than two drinks per day (if man)

☐ Has pain in mouth, teeth, or gums

The level I and II screens. Reprinted with permission of the Nutrition Screening Initiative, a project of the American Academy of Family Physicians. The American Dietetic Association, and the National Council on the Aging, Inc., and funded in part by a grant from Ross Laboratories, a division of Abbott Laboratories.

(Figure continues on following pages.)

It should be noted that enteral therapy cannot be relied upon to meet the full hydration needs of a patient. If enteral feedings are the sole source of nutrition and hydration, 500–1000 cc of free-water supplementation also must be provided, depending on the patient's clinical condition

---

A physician should be contacted if the individual has gained or lost 10 pounds unexpectedly or without intending to during the past 6 months. A physician should also be notified if the individual's body mass index is above 27 or below 24.

Living Environment

☐ Lives on an income of less than $6000 per year (per individual in the household)

☐ Lives alone

☐ Is housebound

☐ Is concerned about home security

☐ Lives in a home with inadequate heating or cooling

☐ Does not have a stove and/or refrigerator

☐ Is unable or prefers not to spend money on food (<$25-30 per person spent on food each week)

Functional Status

Usually or always needs assistance with (check each that apply):

☐ Bathing

☐ Dressing

☐ Grooming

☐ Toileting

☐ Eating

☐ Walking or moving about

☐ Traveling (outside the home)

☐ Preparing food

☐ Shopping for food or other necessities

If you have checked one or more statements on this screen, the individual you have interviewed may be at risk for poor nutritional status. Please refer this individual to the appropriate health care or social service professional in your area. For example, a dietitian should be contacted for problems with selecting, preparing, or eating a healthy diet, or a dentist if the individual experiences pain or difficulty when chewing or swallowing. Those individuals whose income, lifestyle, or functional status may endanger their nutritional and overall health should be referred to available community services: home-delivered meals, congregate meal programs, transportation services, counseling services (alcohol abuse, depression, bereavement, etc.), home health care agencies, day care programs, etc.

Please repeat this screen at least once each year--sooner if the individual has a major change in his or her health, income, immediate family (e.g., spouse dies), or functional status.

---

and the tonicity of the formula. Additionally, although enteral feedings have fewer complications and lower cost than parenteral feedings, there are risks associated with enteral nutritional therapy, including aspiration pneumonia and diarrhea. Tube displacement and clogging can become significant clinical issues for patients with gastrostomies and jejunostomies. Unmonitored patients on enteral feedings can develop a vast array of electrolyte disturbances, generally relating to insufficient free water accompanying the feedings. Patients receiving enteral feedings that are mixed from powders are at risk for receiving infected feedings if good aseptic technique is not maintained or if feedings are allowed to hang for more than 24 hours. This is potentially problematic for frail older individuals with impaired immune responses.

10. What type of enteral feeding tube is preferable for short-term use in elderly patients?

Patients anticipated to require enteral nutrition support for a short time should have a **small-bore, pliable, nasoenteric tube** placed. These are often weighted to facilitate placement and identification by x-ray. Before feedings are initiated, the tube tip must be confirmed to be in the stomach, either by aspiration of gastric contents or by x-ray. Inadvertent placement of the feeding tube into the tracheobronchial tree may not induce coughing in the elderly. Nasoenteric tube malposition may occur in up to 1.3% of the population receiving tube feedings, and as many as 35% of tube-fed patients may have clogged tubes. Such clogging may be resolved with water or

Level II Screen

Complete the following screen by interviewing the patient directly and/or by referring to the patient chart. If you do not routinely perform all of the described tests or ask all of the listed questions, please consider including them but do not be concerned if the entire screen is not completed. Please try to conduct a minimal screen on as many older patients as possible, and please try to collect serial measurements, which are extremely valuable in monitoring nutritional status. Please refer to the manual for additional information.

Anthropometrics

Measure height to the nearest inch and weight to the nearest pound. Record the values below and mark them on the Body Mass Index (BMI) scale to the right. Then use a straight edge (paper, ruler) to connect the two points and circle the spot where this straight line crosses the center line (body mass index). Record the number below; healthy older adults should have a BMI between 24 and 27; check the appropriate box to flag an abnormally high or low value.

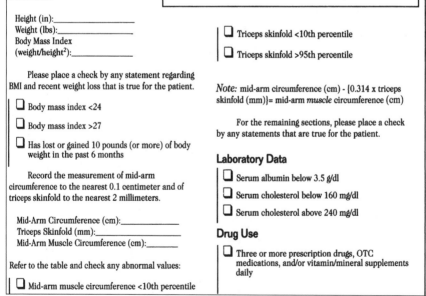

NOMOGRAM FOR BODY MASS INDEX

© George A Bray 1978

Height (in):_____
Weight (lbs):_____
Body Mass Index
(weight/height^2):_____

Please place a check by any statement regarding BMI and recent weight loss that is true for the patient.

☐ Body mass index <24

☐ Body mass index >27

☐ Has lost or gained 10 pounds (or more) of body weight in the past 6 months

Record the measurement of mid-arm circumference to the nearest 0.1 centimeter and of triceps skinfold to the nearest 2 millimeters.

Mid-Arm Circumference (cm):_____
Triceps Skinfold (mm):_____
Mid-Arm Muscle Circumference (cm):_____

Refer to the table and check any abnormal values:

☐ Mid-arm muscle circumference <10th percentile

☐ Triceps skinfold <10th percentile

☐ Triceps skinfold >95th percentile

Note: mid-arm circumference (cm) - {0.314 x triceps skinfold (mm)}= mid-arm *muscle* circumference (cm)

For the remaining sections, please place a check by any statements that are true for the patient.

Laboratory Data

☐ Serum albumin below 3.5 g/dl

☐ Serum cholesterol below 160 mg/dl

☐ Serum cholesterol above 240 mg/dl

Drug Use

☐ Three or more prescription drugs, OTC medications, and/or vitamin/mineral supplements daily

pancreatic enzyme. At least one case report has described an elderly individual post-stroke who became an obligate nasal breather, leading to an inability to tolerate nasoenteric feedings.

11. Which type of enteral feeding tube is preferrable for long-term use?

In an individual who may require feedings for a prolonged period, **percutaneous endoscopic gastrostomy** (PEG) is the preferred method of feeding. **Surgical gastrostomies** are reserved for

Clinical Features

Presence of (check each that apply):

☐ Problems with mouth, teeth, or gums

☐ Difficulty chewing

☐ Difficulty swallowing

☐ Angular stomatitis

☐ Glossitis

☐ History of bone pain

☐ History of bone fractures

☐ Skin changes (dry, loose, nonspecific lesions, edema)

Percentile	Men 55-65 y	Men 65-75 y	Women 55-65 y	Women 65-75 y
Arm circumference (cm)				
10th	27.3	26.3	25.7	25.2
50th	31.7	30.7	30.3	29.9
95th	36.9	35.5	38.5	37.3
Arm muscle circumference (cm)				
10th	24.5	23.5	19.6	19.5
50th	27.8	26.8	22.5	22.5
95th	32.0	30.6	28.0	27.9
Triceps skinfold (mm)				
10th	6	6	16	14
50th	11	11	25	24
95th	22	22	38	36

From: Frisancho AR. New norms of upper limb fat and muscle areas for assessment of nutritional status. Am J Clin Nutr 1981; 34:2540-2545. © 1981 American Society for Clinical Nutrition.

Eating Habits

☐ Does not have enough food to eat each day

☐ Usually eats alone

☐ Does not eat anything on one or more days each month

☐ Has poor appetite

☐ Is on a special diet

☐ Eats vegetables two or fewer times daily

☐ Eats milk or milk products once or not at all daily

☐ Eats fruit or drinks fruit juice once or not at all daily

☐ Eats breads, cereals, pasta, rice, or other grains five or fewer times daily

☐ Has more than one alcoholic drink per day (if woman); more than two drinks per day (if man)

Living Environment

☐ Lives on an income of less than $6000 per year (per individual in the household)

☐ Lives alone

☐ Is housebound

☐ Is concerned about home security

☐ Lives in a home with inadequate heating or cooling

☐ Does not have a stove and/or refrigerator

☐ Is unable or prefers not to spend money on food (<$25-30 per person spent on food each week)

Functional Status

Usually or always needs assistance with (check each that apply):

☐ Bathing

☐ Dressing

☐ Grooming

☐ Toileting

☐ Eating

☐ Walking or moving about

☐ Traveling (outside the home)

☐ Preparing food

☐ Shopping for food or other necessities

Mental/Cognitive Status

☐ Clinical evidence of impairment, e.g. Folstein<26

☐ Clinical evidence of depressive illness, e.g. Beck Depression Inventory>15, Geriatric Depression Scale>5

Patients in whom you have identified one or more major indicator (see pg 2) of poor nutritional status require immediate medical attention; if minor indicators are found, ensure that they are known to a health professional or to the patient's own physician. Patients who display risk factors (see pg 2) of poor nutritional status should be referred to the appropriate health care or social service professional (dietitian, nurse, dentist, case manager, etc.).

individuals at risk of complications with PEG placement (e.g., morbid obesity, esophageal obstruction, bleeding diathesis). Both procedures are associated with minimal complications. Morbidity and mortality associated with placement of these tubes may be due to the frail state of elders generally selected for this form of feeding. Occasionally, life-threatening complications of gastrostomies may arise, such as wound dehiscence, sepsis, or peritonitis.

Percutaneous endoscopic gastrojejunostomies and surgical jejunostomies have been recommended in the past to limit problems with aspiration pneumonia, but these procedures do not necessarily limit aspiration. They are associated with a number of complications, such as bleeding, infections, and wound dehiscence.

12. How should enteral feedings be provided to the elderly?

Continuous enteral feedings are most commonly provided for individuals receiving nasoenteral feedings and often for individuals receiving gastrostomy or jejunostomy feedings. Continous feedings are more easily administered through small-bore tubes than intermittent feedings. They also may decrease nausea, vomiting, and diarrhea. They have in the past been thought to be associated with a lower risk of aspiration pneumonia than intermittent feedings, but more recent data challenge this assumption. Data suggest that intermittent feedings allow for better protein synthesis than do continuous feedings. However, at present, no conclusive evidence shows that one form of feeding should be preferred over another.

Continuous feedings are generally administered starting at 25–50 ml/hr and progressively increased to 100–125 ml/hr, depending on the predicted caloric needs of the individual and the caloric density of the formula. Intermittent feedings are generally started at 200 ml four times daily and progressively increased to as much as 400–500 ml every 4–6 hours, depending on caloric needs. Formulas with a high tonicity are often diluted initially and then progressively increased to full strength and eventually full volume.

13. What is the most dangerous complication of tube feeding in elderly individuals?

Aspiration pneumonia is the one complication that can lead to mortality. In the literature, its incidence ranges from 3–33%. In the past, experts believed that this complication could be limited by continuous feedings (which limit the volume of fluid in the stomach at any one time) and by feedings below the pyloric junction. However, more recent studies suggest that continuous feedings may in fact increase the risk of aspiration pneumonia. Risk factors for pneumonia associated with tube feedings appear to be a history of pneumonia, esophagitis, and/or advanced age. The present literature suggests that gastrostomies and jejunostomies do not necessarily protect against the development of aspiration pneumonia.

All elderly patients, and especially those at high risk, should be monitored for clinical signs of aspiration, such as shortness of breath, rales, increased leukocyte count or shift, or simple confusion in a previously alert individual. If possible, avoid continuous tube feedings in individuals at risk for aspiration (i.e., with a prior history of aspiration or stroke).

14. What is the most common problem associated with tube feeding in elderly individuals?

Diarrhea. The development of diarrhea is particularly risky in the elderly, because it can predispose to skin irritation and the development of pressure ulcers. Risk factors for diarrhea in tube-fed patients include low serum albumin, antibiotic usage, hypertonicity of the formula, or low fiber content of the formula. However, several studies have disputed the role of low serum albumin level, tonicity of the formula, and fiber content of the formula. The major risk factor appears to be antibiotic usage.

15. Can frail elderly become infected as a result of contaminated tube feedings?

Studies have shown that manipulation of formulas (e.g., mixing of powdered formulas) leads to contamination. However, contamination does not appear to be related to the development of diarrhea or sepsis. One series found that pneumonia developed in 2 patients out of 24, with the organism found in respiratory secretions being the same organism found in the enteral formula. In this study, similar organisms were also found on the hands of nurses caring for these patients. Several other studies have had similar findings.

BIBLIOGRAPHY

1. Casper RC: Nutrition and its relationship to aging. Exp Gerontol 30:299–314, 1995.
2. Dwyer J: Nutrition Screening Initiative. Washington, DC, Nutritional Screening Initiative, 1991.

3. Evans WJ, Cyr-Campbell D: Nutrition, exercise, and healthy aging. J Am Diet Assoc 97:632–638, 1997.
4. Gariballa SE, Sinclair AJ: Nutrition, aging and ill health. Br J Nutr 80:7–23, 1998.
5. Howard L, Malone M: Clinical outcome of geriatric patients in the United States receiving home parenteral and enteral nutrition. Am J Clin Nutr 66:1364–1370, 1997.
6. Morley JE, Glick Z, Rubenstein LZ: Geriatric Nutrition: A Comprehensive Review, 2nd ed. Philadelphia, Lippincott Williams & Wilkins, 1995.
7. Safadi BY, Marks JM, Ponsky JL: Percutaneous endoscopic gastrostomy. Gastrointest Endosc Clin North Am 8:551–568, 1998.

18. ALCOHOL

David Oslin, M.D.

1. Is alcohol use safe in late life?

Generally, most people over age 65 do not have problems associated with alcohol consumption. No evidence suggests that the responsible use of alcohol in moderate amounts is deleterious to one's physical health. In fact, it may reduce cardiovascular mortality and overall mortality in all age groups. Furthermore, in older community-dwelling elders, moderate alcohol use is associated with fewer falls and greater mobility when compared with persons who do not drink. Less is known about any associations between moderate alcohol intake and the risk for mental illnesses, such as cognitive impairment or affective disorders. In patients with chronic illnesses such as diabetes, hypertension, or major depression, even moderate alcohol use should be avoided. Small amounts of alcohol can interfere with pharmacologic treatment or exacerbate illness.

2. Define heavy and moderate alcohol use.

Moderate alcohol use in older persons is an average of 1 drink/day. The typical pattern of drinking for most people is to consume 2 or 3 drinks on the weekend or when dining out. Others may have 1 glass of wine or a nightcap every evening. Although this amount of drinking is typically nonproblematic, patients should be educated about and monitored for the development of any problems indicative of alcohol abuse. **Heavy** alcohol use is > 1 drink/day.

3. What is alcohol abuse or dependence, and how prevalent is it in late life?

Alcohol abuse is defined by DSM-IV as a maladaptive pattern of drinking that leads to significant impairment in a person's life, including health, legal, or occupational problems or disruption in social or family functioning. **Alcohol dependence** represents a greater severity of impairment as manifested by three or more of the following:
- Tolerance
- Withdrawal symptoms
- Drinking more than intended
- Persistent desire or attempts to cut down
- A great deal of time spent in acquiring or recovering from alcohol
- Important social, occupational, or recreational activities ignored
- Continued use despite adverse problems related to alcohol

Epidemiologic studies have shown that "heavy" drinking is present in 3–9% of people over 65, with the current prevalence of alcohol abuse or dependence in the elderly being between 2–4%. There is about a 5:1 male-to-female ratio for alcohol abuse or dependence.

Alcohol use disorders are much more prevalent in clinics and hospitals. The prevalence of alcohol abuse and dependence among older primary care patients ranges from 4–13% with a lifetime prevalence of 33%. The prevalence for a current diagnosis of alcohol abuse or dependence among older inpatients on medical or surgical units ranges from 5–43%.

4. Did older patients with alcohol problems always begin drinking when they were younger?

No. Patients with an alcohol use disorder can be divided into two categories: those who have had problems most of their lives (early-onset group) and those who started having problems after age 50 (late-onset group). About one-third of older persons who are alcohol-dependent have the onset of their disease in late life. The incidence of alcohol abuse and dependence in late life has been estimated at 0.63 cases/100 person-years. The late-onset group may start problem drinking in relation to life stressors, such as affective disorders, retirement, loss of a spouse, or financial problems, but these are not the entire cause.

5. What are some risk factors that cause a person to start drinking in late life or relapse?

Change in social situation	Demographic factors
Death of spouse	Caucasian
Retirement	Male
Death of friends	Higher income
Increased leisure time	Higher education
Change in financial status	

A family history of alcohol dependence is less common in late-onset alcoholism than early-onset.

6. How can late-onset alcohol use disorders be prevented?

Prevention of excessive alcohol use is enhanced by a good **physician-patient relationship**. Routinely asking a patient about alcohol use, about significant stressors or losses, and about major changes in a patient's life such as retirement or loss of independence are keys to recognizing the onset of many problems, including problems with alcohol use. Recognition of these risk factors is paramount in preventing the escalating use of alcohol. This type of clinical relationship is becoming difficult as less time is spent with patients and as patients transfer care between many physicians.

The **community** can also play a role in preventing alcoholism. Programs at senior centers, churches, or community colleges can provide educational activities as well as social support networks for all elders. Health care providers should routinely inquire about a patient's leisure time management and hobbies and help to support community involvement. An intact social group of non–alcohol-abusing peers is an important aspect to preventing late-onset problem drinking.

7. Do changes in alcohol metabolism and degree of intoxication occur with aging?

The older person is more likely to have a higher blood alcohol level and suffer more acute intoxicating effects, such as trouble with balance, changes in fine motor skills, and cognitive dysfunction. This effect may be more pronounced in older women than in older men but has not been thoroughly studied. This effect represents a change in the volume of distribution of alcohol and not changes in hepatic metabolism. Also, changes in body mass and fat distribution occur with aging that will cause an increase in the blood alcohol level for a given amount of alcohol. Age-associated changes in the blood-brain barrier may make an older person more vulnerable to the intoxicating effects of alcohol. The increased intoxicating effect seen with older people is consistent with findings that the quantity of consumption but not the frequency decreases as people age. The older individual may reduce the amount consumed because less alcohol is necessary to produce a similar effect as when the person was 20 years younger.

8. What is the best way to identify patients with alcohol problems?

The **clinical interview** is the best tool for identifying persons with alcohol-related problems. Alcohol abuse and dependence have been shown to be underdiagnosed among the elderly in hospitals and primary care clinics. Several easily administered screening instruments have both good sensitivity and specificity. The **CAGE** interview is recommended as quick and sensitive. The patient is first asked if he has ever drunk any alcohol in his life. If the patient answers "yes," he is asked the following four questions:

1. Have you ever had the desire or attempted to **C**ut down on your drinking?
2. Have you ever become **A**nnoyed at someone because they told you that you had a drinking problem?
3. Have you ever felt **G**uilty about your drinking?
4. Have you ever drunk before noon or had an **E**ye-opener?

If the person answers yes to any of these questions, a detailed alcohol use history should be taken, with careful attention to how alcohol use has affected the patient's life. The use of clinic brochures and educating clinic staff about alcohol use problems are also effective ways of recognizing early problems. Prevention is the key to treating late-onset alcoholism.

9. List the medical problems associated with alcohol use.

Alcohol-related medical problems can be one of the best ways of identifying patients with alcohol use disorders, which have been associated with toxic effects on almost every organ system.

Hepatic dysfunction
Gastrointestinal disorders (varices, gastritis, pancreatitis, esophagitis)
Central and peripheral nervous system dysfunction
Anemia (macrocytic)
Myopathy
Cardiomyopathy
Aspiration pneumonia
Malnutrition (specifically thiamine deficiency)
Cancer (hepatic, GI, head and neck)

10. What is the best treatment for acute alcohol withdrawal?

Acute alcohol withdrawal, alcohol withdrawal seizures, and alcohol withdrawal delirium are preventable disorders. Careful history-taking to identify patients at risk is the key to prevention. In the event that alcohol is not available to a patient, such as after admission to the hospital or when required to stop drinking for tests, proper detoxification can prevent significant morbidity to the patient. Onset of acute confusion or other mental status changes after several days in the hospital also should alert the clinician to the possibility of alcohol withdrawal. The standard treatment for detoxification or for treating withdrawal symptoms is the use of **benzodiazepines** such as oxazepam. The dose of benzodiazepine should be titrated for each individual. The clinician should avoid overmedicating the patient and can use autonomic signs, such as heart rate and blood pressure, to guide the treatment.

11. Discuss the best treatment plan for a patient with an alcohol use disorder.

After you recognize that a patient has an alcohol problem, most patients are best treated in a structured **outpatient addiction program**. Also recognize that for some patients, the stigma associated with being in an addiction program makes them refuse to participate in a program. There also is evidence that the late-onset alcoholic is much less likely to seek treatment, although such individuals do respond to treatment. Some of these patients can be managed as outpatients in a primary care clinic. If a patient does not achieve abstinence or remission of the abuse or dependence, then convincing the patient of the merits of a treatment program becomes a key element in overall care. Although being firm about recommending treatment is important, it also is important for the physician to maintain a relationship with the patient so that he or she can continue to work with the patient on treating the illness.

Although alcohol use disorders are chronic illnesses and patients are prone to remissions and exacerbations, the long-term outcome for patients can be good. With close attention to drinking, family support, and management of leisure time, patients can change drinking habits. The literature suggests that older patients are as likely as younger patients to respond to treatment. The benefits of abstinence are not only improved quality of life and improved relationships, but also that many of the toxic physical effects of alcohol are reversible.

12. Which types of medications should be avoided in patients with alcohol use problems?

Many medications interact with alcohol causing an increase in side effects or toxic effects. Medications that are hepatically metabolized or are active in the CNS should be used with caution in patients who are actively drinking. In patients with an alcohol use disorder that is in remission, it is important to realize that medications such as benzodiazepines and opiates are also addicting and have the potential for abuse or causing a relapse. However, these medications may be used to treat an illness that warrants their use, such as acute pain or anxiety disorders, or for the short-term relief of insomnia. The key to using these medications is the careful monitoring of both the medications and alcohol use.

Medications with potential drug–alcohol interactions include:

H$_2$ blockers	β-blockers	Antihypertensives
Aspirin	NSAIDs	Nitroglycerin
Warfarin	Acetaminophen	Certain antibiotics
Benzodiazepines	Oral hypoglycemics	

13. Should naltrexone or disulfiram (Antabuse) be prescribed?

Medications that reduce a person's craving for alcohol or cause adverse effects after drinking have been demonstrated effective only in the context of an addiction program. They should not be used as the sole method of treatment.

14. How can the clinician respect patient confidentiality while involving the family in treatment?

The family may be one of the best allies in identifying and treating patients with addiction problems. Patients have the right to refuse any discussions with family, and consent from the patient should be obtained before discussing issues about substance use with family members. Care providers should educate patients, however, about eliciting the assistance of family members. As with any chronic condition, emotional support from family members and close friends is an important predictor of treatment response. Patients and physicians also should realize that family members are usually aware of a patient's alcohol use, and refusal to allow family members to help is often a way for a patient to obstruct treatment consciously or unconsciously.

BIBLIOGRAPHY

1. Frances A: Diagnostic and Statistical Manual of Mental Disorders, 4th ed. Washington, DC, American Psychiatric Press, 1994.
2. LaCroix AZ, Guralnik JM, Berkman LF, et al: Maintaining mobility in late life. Am J Epidemiol 137:858–869, 1993.
3. Lakhani N: Alcohol use amongst community-dwelling elderly people: A review of the literature. J Adv Nurs 25:1227–1232, 1997.
4. Liberto J, Oslin D, Ruskin P: Alcoholism in older persons: A review of the literature. Hosp Commun Psychiatry 43:975–984, 1992.
5. Nelson HD, Nevitt MC, Scott JC, et al: Smoking, alcohol, and neuromuscular and physical function of older women. JAMA 272:1825–1831, 1994.
6. O'Loughlin JL, Robitaille Y, Boivin J-F, Suissa S: Incidence of and risk factors for falls and injurious falls among the community-dwelling elderly. Am J Epidemiol 137:342–354, 1993.
7. Oslin DW, Liberto JG: Substance abuse in the elderly. In O'Brien C (ed): Psychiatry. Philadelphia, J.B. Lippincott, 1995.
8. Reid MC, Anderson PA: Geriatric substance disorders. Med Clin North Am 81:999–1016, 1997.
9. Swift RM: Drug therapy: Drug therapy for alcohol dependence. N Engl J Med 340:1482–1490, 1999.

19. TOBACCO USE AMONG THE ELDERLY

Charles Spencer, M.D., Ph.D.

1. What is the prevalence of tobacco use among older adults?

Tobacco use is the leading preventable cause of death in the United States. The total number of smokers in the U.S. in 1995 was 47 million. Of these, 13% were 65 years or older. Most elderly tobacco users began at age 15–25 years and thus have a smoking history greater than 50 pack years. To discourage tobacco use, patients must be convinced that cessation increases longevity and improves quality of life.

Percentage of Adults Who Were Current Cigarette Smokers:
United States National Health Interview Survey, 1994, 1995

AGE	MEN (%)		WOMEN (%)	
	1994	1995	1994	1995
18–24	29.8	27.8	27.8	21.8
25–44	32.3	30.5	27.8	26.8
45–64	28.3	27.1	22.8	24.0
≥ 65	13.2	14.3	11.1	11.5

2. How prevalent is the use of smokeless tobacco among the elderly?

Smokeless tobacco use in 1991 was higher among people 18–24 years of age or 75 years or older. For women the use was highest (2.3%) among those 75 years or older. Men 75 years or older accounted for the second highest age group (5.8%). Women favored snuff over chewing tobacco, whereas among men snuff and chewing tobacco were equally distributed. Rural regions of the South had the highest prevalence of use of smokeless tobacco.

3. What are the health costs and financial burdens associated with tobacco use?

Tobacco use directly and negatively affects both health and financial status. The financial burden for society of smoking has long been recognized. However, only recently has the social burden of second-hand smoking been addressed. Health care expenditures have been estimated to be in excess of $65 billion in 1985 for the cost of smoking. These costs include extra expenditures for medical insurance, absenteeism from work, and injuries from fires due to cigarette smoking.

In 1994 the most common causes of death among the elderly were similar to those attributable to smoking-related diseases: coronary heart disease, cancer, cerebral vascular accidents, and chronic obstructive lung disease. Tobacco use substantially increases the relative risk of vascular diseases, such as strokes, heart attacks, sudden death, and ischemic peripheral vascular disease. In 1991 tobacco usage was associated with 85% of the 143,000 deaths due to lung cancer. The relative risk for cancer of the oral cavity, pharynx, esophagus, stomach, and bladder is increased by tobacco use. Pulmonary illnesses, such as bronchitis, pneumonia, emphysema, and obstructive lung disease, are strongly related to tobacco usage.

The alkaline constituents of smokeless tobacco are more readily absorbed through the oral and esophageal mucosa, whereas the more acidic cigarette smoke favors absorption through the bronchial airways. The acid-base balance and the method of use may contribute to the higher occurrence of oral lesions with smokeless tobacco.

Passive smoking has been related to heart disease and lung cancer in nonsmokers. Passive smoking also affects the birth weight of infants. The effects of tobacco use by grandparents or other older adults living with young children, infants, or pregnant women may be inferred to be detrimental, but they have not been investigated.

Osteoporosis and cataracts, diseases with particular significance to the well-being of the elderly, are exacerbated by smoking.

Dental health and denture condition are significantly impaired by tobacco use in the elderly. Reluctance to leave elderly tobacco users alone because of the increased risk of fires and burns also contributes to the health and financial burden.

Estimated Smoking-attributable Mortality, Relative Risk Attributable to Smoking (Current) Compared with Nonsmokers, 1990

	RELATIVE RISK	
	CURRENT SMOKER, MALE	CURRENT SMOKER, FEMALE
Disease (> 35 yr)		
Cancer		
Lip, oral cavity and pharynx	27.5	5.6
Esophagus	7.6	10.3
Larynx	10.5	17.8
Trachea, lung and bronchus	22.4	11.9
Cardiovascular		
Hypertension	1.9	1.7
Ischemic heart		
35–64	2.8	3.0
> 65	1.6	1.6
Strokes		
35–64	3.7	4.8
> 65	1.9	3.0
Atherosclerosis	4.1	3.0
Respiratory		
Pneumonia, influenza	2.0	2.2
Bronchitis, emphysema	9.7	10.5
Chronic obstructive lung	9.7	10.5

4. Is cessation of tobacco use beneficial in older adults?

Tobacco cessation is beneficial for both the young and the elderly. The health risk of cigarette smoking can be eliminated only by quitting; switching to lower "tar" and nicotine cigarettes is not a safe alternative. Fewer tobacco users survive to be elderly compared with people who have never used tobacco. Life expectancy is approximately 18 years shorter for a 30-year-old smoker. Cessation of smoking at any age increases longevity and has the potential to increase quality of life. For example, 65-year-old, one-pack-a-day smokers who quit can expect to increase their life expectancy by 2–3 years.

5. What characteristics distinguish the older smoker from a younger smoker?

Most older smokers were heavier smokers, smoked brands with higher nicotine content, had social contacts who also were smokers, did not believe that quitting would improve health (47%), and were the least likely to report that they wanted to stop smoking completely.

6. What is the best cessation strategy for older adults?

Because older smokers are heavier users of tobacco and often have a long smoking history, a multipronged approach is recommended to assist cessation. The physical addiction, psychological dependence, and habitual tendencies from tobacco use need to be addressed.

Nicotine substitutes in the form of gum, patch, or nasal spray have been advocated. Both approaches require a motivated individual to avoid concurrent tobacco use. Consideration of asymptomatic ischemic heart and peripheral vascular diseases is essential before prescribing nicotine replacement therapy in the elderly. Serious adverse events, including stroke and myocardial infarction, have been reported with high dosages of nicotine substitutes in the elderly. Nervousness, irritability, sleep disturbance, and difficulty with concentration are common symptoms among the elderly and need to be interpreted cautiously by caregivers familiar with the patient.

A non-nicotine aid in tobacco cessation is available. Bupropion in an oral sustained-release form has been approved for use either alone or in combination with nicotine substitutes. Bupropion also is prescribed as an antidepressant. One should be familiar with the manufacturer's list of contraindications (seizures, concurrent use of MAO inhibitors, eating disorders, concurrent use of bupropion, and allergies to bupropion). Cautious use is advised in elderly tobacco users who have excessive alcohol or benzodiazepine intake and in those taking medications that lower the seizure threshold (e.g., theophylline and antipsychotic medications).

Older smokers are less likely (14.7%) to succeed when they attempt to stop. Successful adults are usually younger (49.4% are 25–44 years old), more educated (42.2% have > 13 years of education) and less likely to use assisted methods of cessation. However, if older smokers succeed in stopping tobacco usage, they are less likely to relapse (5.7%).

The importance of physician input in smoking cessation is underscored by evidence that 70% of successful and relapse patients in all age groups were urged to stop by a physician. Support services are recommended for both nicotine substitutes and bupropion therapy.

7. Do withdrawal symptoms differ among the elderly?

Care providers need to be aware of atypical withdrawal symptoms among the elderly. Increased day-time naps and complaints of dyspepsia and rheumatism may be the equivalent of more typical withdrawal symptoms, such as headaches, sleep problems, and nausea.

8. What are the short-term benefits of smoking cessation?

Short-term benefits among the elderly are illustrated by anecdotal reports of less staining of dentures, improvement in breath odor, and fewer holes in clothes. The association of increased weight with cessation of tobacco may be beneficial among frail, elderly smokers.

9. What are the most effective ways of prescribing nicotine substitutes?

An estimate of tobacco dependence should be obtained before prescribing nicotine substitutes and bupropion (Zyban). Unstable cardiovascular diseases are a contraindication to the use of substitutes. The medication should be used cautiously in patients with uncontrolled thyroid disease, uncontrolled hypertension, peptic ulcers, severe renal impairment, severe liver disease, and uncontrolled diabetes. The patch should be avoided in patients with active skin problems. Nicotine substitutes should be used only after tobacco use has stopped

Bupropion therapy may be initiated 7–14 days before the quit date. Nonchewable nicotine substitutes placed in the cheek should be used with adjuvant behavior modification therapy. Nicotine chewing gums should be chewed only when there is an urge to smoke or on a schedule; the gum is not to be chewed continuously. Nicotine gums and patches are available over the counter without a prescription. The patches are used daily, with tapering dosage every 4–8 weeks. Behavior support should continue after nicotine substitutes are stopped.

10. Do behavior modification techniques work in the elderly?

Behavior therapy in concert with nicotine substitutes has had mixed results. The consensus is that behavior therapy does not increase the cessation rate. Subset analysis on such groups as older smokers, heavier smokers, educated smokers, and single vs. married smokers needs to be studied.

11. Is the recommendation to quit smoking ever unwarranted?

The recommendation to quit smoking is never unwarranted. Smoking cessation benefits both the individual and society. However, one can respect the individual's choice, especially in the hospice patient who is terminally ill.

BIBLIOGRAPHY

1. Bartecchi CE, MacKenzie TD, Schrier RW: The human costs of tobacco use (Pt 1). N Engl J Med 330: 907–912, 1994.
2. Burns D: Cigarettes and cigarette smoking. Clin Chest Med 12:631–642, 1991.
3. Centers for Disease Control: Cigarette Smoking Among Adults–United States, 1995. MMWR 46:1217–1220, 1997.
4. Centers for Disease Control: Cigarette Smoking Among Adults–United States, 1996. MMWR 45:588–590, 1996.
5. Cox J: Smoking cessation in the elderly patient. Clin Chest Med 14:423–428, 1993.
6. Fiore MC (ed): Cigarette smoking. Med Clin North Am 76(2), 1982 [special issue].
7. Fiore MC, Bailey WC, Cohen SJ, et al: Smoking Cessation: Information for Specialist. Clinical Practice Guidelines. Quick Reference Guide for Smoking Cessation Specialist. No. 18. Washington, DC, U.S. Department of Health and Human Services, Agency for Health Care Policy and Research and Centers for Disease Control and Prevention, 1996, AHCPR Pub. No. 96–0694.
8. Fiore MC, Norotny TE, Pierce JP, et al: Methods used to quit smoking in the United States: Do cessation programs help? JAMA 263:2760–2765, 1990.
9. Giovino GA, Henningfield JE, Tomar SL, et al: Epidemiology of tobacco use and dependence. Epidemiol Rev 17:48–65, 1995.
10. Giovino GA, Schooley MW, Zhu BP, et al: Surveillance for selected tobacco use behaviors, United States, 1900–1994. MMWR 43(No SS–3):1–43, 1994.
11. Henningfield JE: Drug therapy: Nicotine medications for smoking cessation. N Engl J Med 333: 1196–1203, 1995.
12. Hughes JR, Goldstein MG, Hurt RD, Shiffman S: Recent advances in the pharmacotherapy of smoking. JAMA 281:72–76, 1999.
13. Jorenby DE, Smith SS, Fiore MC, et al: Varying nicotine patch dose and type of smoking cessation counseling. JAMA 274:1347–1352, 1995.
14. Nelson DE, Kirkendill RS, Lawton RL, et al: Surveillance for smoking-attributable mortality and years of potential life lost, by state—United States, 1990. MMWR 43(No SS-1):1–8, 1994.
15. Spangler JG, Salisbury PL: Smokeless tobacco: Epidemiology, health effects and cessation strategies. Am Fam Physician 52:1421–1430, 1995.
16. Thorndike AN, Rigotti NA, Stafford RS, Singer DE: National patterns in the treatment of smokers by physicians. JAMA 279:604–608, 1998.
17. U.S. Department of Health and Human Services: The Health Consequences of Smoking. Nicotine Addiction. A Report of the Surgeon General. Washington, DC, U.S. Department of Health and Human Services, 1988, DHHS Publication No. (CDC) 99–8496.

20. HYPERTENSION

Areena Swarup, M.D., and Mary Ann Forciea, M.D.

1. What levels of blood pressure are diagnostic of hypertension in the elderly?

Two varieties of hypertension are seen in older patients: (1) **essential hypertension** (also called systolic-diastolic hypertension), in which systolic blood pressure (BP) is ≥ 140 mmHg and diastolic BP is ≥ 90, and (2) **isolated systolic hypertension**, in which systolic BP is > 140 mmHg and diastolic BP is < 90 mmHg. **Secondary** hypertension is an elevation in BP caused by another disease process, such as pheochromocytoma or renal artery stenosis. Disorders of secondary hypertension are rare in office practice.

2. How common is hypertension in the elderly?

A large community survey of 906 people aged 71–96 years revealed the following prevalence of hypertension:

Normotensive	39.4%	Isolated systolic hypertension	13.2%
Borderline isolated		Diastolic hypertension	9.5%
systolic hypertension	28.6%	Hypertensive by mixed criteria	9.3%

The prevalence of hypertension varies with race and age. Essential hypertension is seen in patients over 65 years of age in approximately 15% of whites and 25% of blacks. Isolated systolic hypertension is seen in 10% of patients > 70 years old and 20% of patients > 80 years old.

3. Is the etiology of hypertension different in older patients?

Changes in peripheral vascular resistance are central to the development of both essential and isolated systolic hypertension in older patients. Resistance may increase due to occlusion of a blood vessel lumen (as with atherosclerotic change) and/or changes in vascular smooth muscle. Decreasing responses occur in β-adrenergic smooth muscle dilatation during normal aging, but α-adrenergic-mediated vasoconstriction is largely unchanged. This alteration in balance of adrenergic-mediated vessel wall tone leads to a heightened tendency to vasoconstriction and to increased peripheral vascular resistance. A second mechanism for elevated BP is an expanded extracellular volume, which may develop especially in black and elderly hypertensives. Both groups of patients exhibit low plasma renin levels and high sensitivity to dietary sodium.

4. Are the complications of hypertension different in older patients?

Cardiovascular disease is strongly linked to hypertension at all ages, including late life.
- The incidence of **left ventricular hypertrophy** (LVH) correlates highly with systolic BP in older patients. The presence of LVH continues to predict arrhythmias.
- Both essential and isolated systolic hypertension correlate with future vascular events. In a longitudinal study of community-living adults, 70% of **strokes** in elderly women and 42% of strokes in older men were directly attributed to hypertension.
- Another large study of community-dwelling men has shown continued risk of **end-stage renal disease** with hypertension throughout all age ranges.
- Prolonged hypertension is associated with a 21–37% increase in **congestive heart failure.**

5. Can the complications of hypertension in elderly patients be avoided with treatment?

Several large studies have documented that cardiovascular mortality and morbidity can be reduced with treatment of hypertension, even in late life. Compared with outcomes in patients of all ages treated with placebo, patients > 60 years old show the same percentage reduction in events as patients < 50 years old. Because the number of events is much larger in older patients, the reduction in absolute numbers of events in older patients is larger. Applegate summarized the effects of treatment as follows:

Essential hypertension
  Diastolic BP 90–105 mmHg: reduction of 5–8 events/1000 patient-years of treatment
  Diastolic BP 105–115 mmHg: reduction of 20–30 events/1000 patient-years of treatment
Isolated systolic hypertension
  31% reduction in cardiovascular events
  35% reduction in stroke
  Reduction of 50 events/1000 patient-years of treatment

6. Explain how blood pressure is measured in the elderly patient.

Measurement of BP in older patients must be performed with special care to avoid artifactual elevation. The standard of measurement is described using a sphygmomanometer connected to a column of mercury (Hg). Aneroid manometers can be used but must be calibrated against a mercury standard every 6 months. Measurement techniques are based on the detection of vibrations produced by the arterial wall under pressure (**Korotkoff sounds**).

The arm is the usual site of measurement. The cuff used must be positioned correctly and be large enough that the air bladder compresses an adequate area of the brachial artery. The distal margin of the cuff should be at least 3 cm proximal to the antecubital fossa, with the midline of the bladder (usually marked on the cuff) over the palpable artery. The cuff should extend to at least the midpoint of the biceps. Use of a cuff that is too small can result in readings that are 10–15 mmHg higher than the actual BP.

The cuff is inflated to a level of Hg that is 30 mm over that at which the brachial pulse disappears. The valve is opened, and the level of Hg is allowed to fall slowly. The bell of the stethoscope is placed lightly over the artery. The level of Hg at which the first sounds appear is the **systolic** BP (SBP). The sounds remain loud for a considerable time. The level at which the sounds disappear is the **diastolic** BP (DBP). In many patients, a "muffling" of the sound appears shortly before the sounds disappear completely. In such cases, the point of muffling also should also be recorded (e.g., 140/85/80).

The listener should continue observations to the point of 0 mmHg. In some patients, the sounds will reappear. The silent period is called an **auscultatory gap**. The point of permanent disappearance of sound is most reflective of the true diastolic BP. In rare conditions, such as thyrotoxicosis and aortic insufficiency, the sounds may continue to 0. In that event, the point of muffling is the most accurate assessment of the diastolic pressure.

Measurement with the patient in the seated position with the back supported is again the standard. On an initial visit, BP should be measured in both arms. Atherosclerotic obstruction to flow in an arm may result in a lower BP reading. In patients with such a differential, the higher reading is the more accurate reflection of systemic pressure. An initial visit should also include readings in seated and standing positions, because of the frequency of orthostatic hypotension in elderly patients.

In some situations the patient's arms may be inaccessible. Pressure can be taken in the thigh, using an especially large cuff. Ideally, the patient lies prone. The cuff is wrapped so that it extends a few centimeters proximal to the popliteal fossa. Pressure is measured over the popliteal artery.

Many patients purchase home BP monitors. These machines vary in quality. Patients should bring the machines with them to their next office visit so that the machines can be calibrated against a mercury sphygmomanometer and so that the reproducibility of the home machine can be checked. In addition, the technique used to measure BP can be checked for adequacy.

7. What is the significance of measuring pulse pressure in the elderly?

Pulse pressure (PP), measured as the difference between SBP and DBP, rises with age because of a progressive rise in SBP and fall in DBP with arterial stiffening and decreased elasticity. Recent studies have shown that an elevated PP is a better predictor for risk of myocardial infarction, cardiovascular mortality, and heart failure than SBP alone.

8. How do you measure orthostatic hypotension (OH)? What is the significance of measuring OH in an elderly hypertensive patient?

OH is defined as a drop of 20 mmHg or more in the SBP or a drop of 10 mmHg or more in the DBP 1–3 minutes after standing from a lying position. OH is seen in about 6–30% of the population, and its prevalence increases with age. It is caused by impaired baroreceptor sensitivity, reduced vessel compliance, and decreased stroke volume. OH should be looked for in all older people; if present, vasodilating and volume-depleting drugs should be avoided.

9. What is white coat hypertension?

BP should be measured with the patient relaxed and comfortable. "White coat hypertension" is a condition of transient hypertension created by the anxiety of the office encounter. Hypertension should not be diagnosed in the mild or moderate stages on a single office visit. Pressures should be repeated on 2 or 3 visits before consideration of treatment. Severe BP elevations (diastolic readings of >110) should be treated immediately.

10. What is pseudohypertension?

Pseudohypertension is a condition of falsely elevated BP readings caused by calcification of the arteries. The condition can be suspected if mild BP elevation is seen, if no end-organ damage of hypertension is found, and/or if patients rapidly develop symptoms of volume depletion or hypotension on medications. The diagnosis may be confirmed with **Osler's maneuver:** the cuff is inflated above the disappearance of sounds, and the brachial artery is palpated. If the artery is easily felt, the diagnosis is confirmed. If necessary, the diagnosis can be confirmed with measurement of intraarterial pressure, although this method is rarely used. Such patients should be maintained at modestly higher BP levels before treatment is considered.

11. Which parts of the history and physical exam are most important in hypertensive patients?

Hypertension discovered in the office is notoriously free of symptoms in older as well as younger patients. Inquiry should be made into prior diagnoses of "high blood pressure." The presence of other risk factors for cardiovascular disease, such as smoking, should be determined. A careful listing of prescription and over-the-counter medications should be made both to determine whether medications may be elevating BP and to guard against medication interactions. Baseline determinations of mood, sexual functioning, and sleep habits should be made, since changes in these symptoms are often considered side effects of antihypertensive medication. Social situations such as poverty that might limit compliance should be ascertained.

The physical examination confirms the diagnosis of hypertension. BP determinations are accomplished as described previously (see question 6). Examination of the eye grounds can document the presence of retinal disease. Stages are:

1—Ratio of diameter of arterioles to veins is < 2:3 or 3:4 ("arteriolar narrowing")
2—Focal spasm of arterioles
3—Hemorrhages and exudates
4—Papilledema

Evidence of left ventricular hypertrophy should be sought. The characteristics of the cardiac apex should be noted, both in size and force of impulse. Because patients with hypertension are at risk for abdominal aortic aneurysm, careful palpation and auscultation of the abdomen should always be done. The neurologic examination should look for signs associated with stroke.

Secondary hypertension should be suspected in patients who develop new or sudden-onset hypertension with a diastolic BP > 105 mmHg, who have persistent elevations of diastolic pressures > 100 mmHg despite treatment regimens, or who develop accelerated elevations in readings. Such patients should be referred for specialty evaluations.

12. Which laboratory tests are important in the initial evaluation of a hypertensive patient?

All new patients should have measurements of complete blood counts, serum sodium, potassium, bicarbonate, chloride, glucose, blood urea nitrogen, creatinine, uric acid, and calcium. Cholesterol screening should be performed (see also Chapter 12), as should an electrocardiogram (EKG) and urinalysis. The role of routine chest x-ray remains controversial. One strategy is to do a baseline film, with subsequent films obtained only if clinically indicated.

13. What are the goals of treatment?

Treatment goals for most older patients should be systolic pressures of 130–140 mmHg and diastolic pressures of approximately 80–85 mmHg. It is important to remember that overtreatment of hypertension can be dangerous: hypotension may result in falls.

14. How should hypertension be treated?

Options for the traditional treatment of hypertension include **weight reduction** for those patients above ideal body weight, **dietary sodium restriction**, **exercise**, and **medications**. These treatments are often prescribed in combination. Applegate has described a program of weight loss, exercise, and sodium restriction that resulted in reductions of systolic BP of 6 mmHg and diastolic BP of 5 mmHg in older patients with mild hypertension.

Weight loss and **dietary sodium restriction** programs can often be best taught in consultation with a registered dietitian (available through most hospitals). In the elderly, some patients become so concerned with diet that malnutrition may result; dietary patterns should be regularly reviewed at office visits.

Exercise programs are highly acceptable to most elderly patients. To affect BP, the exercise regimen should be performed for approximately 30 minutes three times weekly. Initiation of the program should be gradual, with careful warm-up and cool-down periods. The benefits of regular exercise can extend beyond effects of BP (see also Chapter 16).

Alternative therapies for hypertension such as meditation and acupuncture have generated interest in some patients, but no studies have been done that demonstrate their efficacy in older patients. Patients with moderate or severe hypertension should be encouraged to accept traditional therapy while pursuing nontraditional cures.

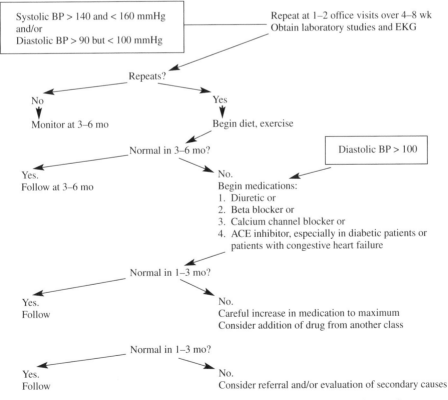

Protocol for management of hypertension in older patients without evidence of end-organ damage.

15. When is drug therapy used?

Drug therapy is initiated when elevated BPs are noted on multiple visits, when elevations of BP are moderate to severe, when nonpharmacologic methods (such as diet and exercise) have not brought BP levels into the desired range, or when evidence of end-organ damage is present, even in patients with high normal BP. Regimens should be kept as simple as possible.

Commonly Used Antihypertensive Medications

CLASS	DAILY DOSE	COST*
Diuretics		
Thiazides		
Hydrochlorothiazide (HCTZ)	12.5–50 mg	$ 1.04
Chlorthalidone	12.5–50 mg	$ 2.27
Loop diuretics		
Furosemide	20–320 mg	$ 1.73
Combinations		
HCTZ 25/triamterene	37.5, 1 tablet	$ 9.38
β-Adrenergic blockers		
Propranolol		
Regular	40–240 mg in 2 doses	$ 4.10
Extended release	80–240 mg in 1 dose	$23.18
Atenolol	25–50 mg in 1 or 2 doses	$20.26
ACE inhibitors		
Enalapril	2.5–40 mg in 1 or 2 doses	$19.09
Captopril	12.5–150 mg in 2 or 3 doses	$19.35
Lisinopril	20–40 mg once daily	$27.10
Angiotensin II receptor antagonist		
Losartan	50–100 mg	$32.20
Calcium channel blockers		
Diltiazem extended release	120–360 mg in 1 dose	$40.74
Verapamil extended release	120–480 mg in 1 or 2 doses	$36.62
Amlodipine	5 mg once daily	$37.70
Felodipine	5 mg once daily	$28.19

*Of lowest dose per 30 days, using wholesale price.
ACE = angiotensin-converting enzyme.

16. Do racial differences in response need to be considered in choosing initial therapy?

The Veterans Affairs Cooperative Study on Response to Antihypertensive Drugs showed that older black men responded best to a diuretic or calcium channel blocker, whereas older white men responded best to a beta blocker, calcium channel blocker, or angiotensin-converting enzyme (ACE) inhibitor. This difference in response may be explained by the low-renin profile in black patients compared with the medium-to-high renin profile in white patients.

17. Discuss the use of diuretics.

Diuretics were among the first classes of drugs shown to be effective in the treatment of hypertension, and they remain effective and in widespread use today. The efficacy of proximal-tubule diuretics, such as the thiazide group, in the reduction of BP in the elderly has been well documented. Thiazide diuretics can be ineffective in patients whose serum creatinine is > 1.5 mg/dl. Thiazide diuretics have been associated with hypokalemia, decreased glucose tolerance, hypercalcemia, impotence, and detrimental changes in serum lipids. These side effects may be transient or produce minimal change when compared to the drug's efficacy in lowering BP. Patients with serious or persistent alterations in lipids or glucose should be evaluated for change to another class of agents. Loop diuretics are used in patients with renal insufficiency, lipid abnormalities, or calcium elevations.

18. What are the drawbacks of β-blockers?

β-Adrenergic blockers are the next most widely used class of antihypertensive medications in general use. In the elderly and in African-American patients, in whom volume overload is a frequent contributor to hypertension, β-blockers may be less effective than they are in younger patients. Patients with congestive heart failure may be candidates for newer, selective beta blockers. Depression and orthostatic hypotension are frequent complications and can limit the usefulness of this group in older patients. However, in patients with coronary artery disease, beta blockers are the only antianginal drugs shown to improve cardiac mortality rates.

19. What are the compelling indications for using ACE inhibitors as a first-line drug in the elderly?

Diabetic nephropathy and hypertensive renal diseases are the two leading causes of end-stage renal disease. Patients with diabetes and hypertension now live longer because of improved treatments; thus, the number of elderly patients receiving dialysis is increasing. Numerous studies have shown that tighter BP control, with the goal of lowering blood pressure below 130/85, has slowed the progression of renal disease due to diabetes or hypertension. ACE inhibitors and possibly nondihydropyridine calcium antagonists may have additional benefit, independent of their blood pressure–lowering effects, in halting progression of renal disease. ACE inhibitors also have been shown to decrease mortality in patients with congestive heart failure and myocardial infarction, both of which are more prevalent in the elderly population.

20. Are any precautions necessary when using the ACE inhibitors?

ACE inhibitors are effective and generally safe if used carefully. In diabetic patients, this class of agent has been shown to preserve renal function. Side effects include nonproductive cough in approximately 10% of elderly patients, hyperkalemia in patients with impaired renal function, and actual deterioration in renal function in those patients with impaired renal blood flow. Patients with high renin levels (as in volume depletion or congestive heart failure) may also develop abrupt and severe hypotension in response to ACE inhibition. Clearly, this class of antihypertensive must be initiated with caution in older patients. A new group of drugs called angiotensin-2 receptor blockers may be considered in patients who are intolerant of ACE inhibitors because of cough.

21. Discuss the use of calcium channel blockers.

Calcium channel blockers have been widely used in the treatment of coronary artery disease. They cause vasodilatation and decreases in peripheral vascular resistance, which have made them attractive in the treatment of hypertension. Certain members of the class (e.g., nifedipine and isradipine) are associated with increases in heart rate. Verapamil and diltiazem are not associated with tachycardia but may slow conduction in the heart. Recent studies have demonstrated an increased rate of death in patients using the short-acting preparation of nifedipine. Data about the death rate in patients using the sustained-release forms of nifedipine are not yet available. The newer group of calcium channel blockers is being used with increasing frequency as monotherapy because of their low-risk profile.

22. When can antihypertensive medications be safely withdrawn?

Many experts now believe that careful withdrawal of antihypertensive medications can be attempted if:

1. The original level of BP was in the mild to moderate range.
2. The patient's BP has been in good control for a sustained period (at least 12 months).

Monitored withdrawal of medication may be most successful in those patients who have been successful in weight loss, dietary modification, and exercise.

BIBLIOGRAPHY

1. Allman RM: Basic evaluation of older persons with hypertension. Clin Geriatr Med 5:717–732, 1989.
2. Applegate WB: Hypertension. In Hazzard WR, Blass JP, Ettinger WH, et al (eds): Principles of Geriatric Medicine and Gerontology, 4th ed. New York, McGraw-Hill, 1998, pp 713–720.
3. DeGowan EL, DeGowan RL: Bedside Diagnostic Examination. London, Macmillan, 1969, pp 379–382.
4. Drugs for hypertension. Med Lett 41:23–28, 1999.
5. Klag MJ, Whelton PK, Randall BL, et al: Blood pressure and end-stage renal disease in men. N Engl J Med 334:13–18, 1996.
6. Pahor M, Guralnik JM, Corti MC, et al: Long-term survival and use of antihypertensive medications in older persons. J Am Geriatr Soc 43:1191–1197, 1995.
7. Preston RA, Materson BJ, Reda DJ, et al: Age-race subgroup compared with renin profile as predictors of blood pressure response to antihypertensive therapy. Department of Veterans Affairs Cooperative Study Group on Antihypertensive Agents. JAMA 280:1168–1172, 1998.
8. SHEP Cooperative Research Group: Prevention of stroke by antihypertensive drug treatment in older persons with isolated systolic hypertension. Final results of the Systolic Hypertension in the Elderly Program (SHEP). JAMA 265:3255–3264, 1991.
9. The sixth report of the Joint National Committee on Prevention, Detection, Evaluation, and Treatment of High Blood Pressure. Arch Intern Med 157:2413–2446, 1997.

21. DENTAL CARE

Roy S. Feldman, D.D.S., DMSc, and Mary Ann Forciea, M.D.

1. Why is oral health particularly important for the elderly?

The mouth and oral cavity serve a variety of critical functions in people of all ages:
- Entry of food into the gastrointestinal tract
- Implementation of speech and communication (verbal and nonverbal)
- Maintenance of identity and self-esteem with facial appearance

In addition, examination of the mouth and oral cavity can provide critical information about the presence of systemic disease.

Elderly patients are at a much higher risk than younger patients for tooth loss, dental caries, gingival and periodontal disease, and oral cancers. This increased risk is due not only to increased "wear-and-tear" on the teeth and gingiva over a lifetime, but also to lower standards for dental care and less access to care during the youth and maturity of patients who are now elderly.

2. How should the primary care provider ask patients about their oral health?

The following is a synopsis of screening questions useful in the history. Occasionally family caregivers may have to provide supplementary information.
- Do you have pain in your teeth, gums, or tongue?
- Do you experience bleeding from your gums?
- Is your mouth continually dry?
- Do you have sores in your mouth or on your tongue?
- Do you have loose, missing, or broken teeth?
- Do you have difficulty biting, chewing, or swallowing?
- Do you think you have halitosis?
- Do you have an altered sense of taste?
- If you wear dentures, do you have problems with any of the following:

  Fit?   Sores on palate or gums under dentures?

  Stability during chewing?   Impaction of food under dentures?
- How do you take care of your oral hygiene?

3. What constitutes a reasonable screening examination of the oral cavity for the primary care provider?

Primary care providers should always ask patients to remove prostheses before the examination. Tongue blades and gauze pads may be used to assist in exposing the structures of the oral cavity for examination. Palpation with gloved fingers is necessary to probe for induration. Examination with a flashlight increases the yield of discovered lesions. The following structures and associated lesions should receive special attention:

Structure	Lesion
Extraoral	
Skeletal structure	Misalignment of jaw, symmetry
Neck	Lymph node enlargement or pain, salivary gland size and consistency
Ears	Sensitivity to pain, congestion behind tympanic membrane
Temporomandibular joint	Tenderness, crepitus
Paranasal sinuses	Pain, reduced transillumination
Breath	Halitosis

Intraoral

Lips and mouth	Ulcers, swelling, redness, cracking lesions
Buccal mucosa	Tenderness, discoloration, induration
Tongue (dorsal and ventral)	Color, coating lesions, tremor
Palate	Symmetry, discolorations, lesions
Oropharynx	Color, masses, exudates, gag reflex
Gingiva	Color, bleeding, hypertrophy, exudates, food impaction
Teeth	Caries, root exposure
Prostheses	Fractures, retention, stability

4. When is a referral to a dentist appropriate?

Ettinger has developed the following useful list:

General	Tooth-related	Denture-related
Unexplained pain	Visible decay	Loose
Infection unresponsive to treatment	Loose or mobile teeth	Missing denture teeth
Persistent problems with mastication	Persistent bleeding	Palatal or gingival
Persistent halitosis		lesion under
Visible or palpable lesions		dentures

5. How should good oral hygiene be maintained?

Many older patients retain many of their own teeth. Brushing regularly with a toothpaste containing fluoride remains critical, even late in life. Dental floss should continue to be used to remove plaque and food from between teeth. Fluorides, present for decades in dentifrices, gels, and pastes, are now available in rinses, which may be excellent additions to the daily routine of people at risk for root surface caries. Acidulated sodium fluoride and stannous fluoride may be applied either within prostheses that are constructed as overdentures and maintain roots of teeth for support or to exposed roots with finger, brush, or cotton swab. Additional products are marketed without flavoring as mild dentifrices for sore and sensitive mouths and gums.

Geriatric patients should use mouth rinses with caution. Many contain relatively high alcohol concentrations (up to 25%), and most have been derived from the dental equivalent of herbal therapy, often at levels capable of promoting sensitivity and irritation in frail mouths. Chlorhexidine is most frequently prescribed at monthly intervals but should not be scheduled as a maintenance therapy for periodontal disease. Oral care is required on a regular basis, including plaque control and elimination of etiologic factors by prophylaxis (tooth-cleaning), scaling (scraping of calculus from tooth roots, often below the gingiva), and root planing (smoothing of the root to facilitate plaque removal). Extensive data document the efficacy of these therapies in controlling disease.

6. How should patients care for their dentures?

Dentures should be cleansed daily, much like the natural dentition. Perhaps twice a day, the dentures may be washed or scrubbed with any cleaning solution, even toothpaste. Most importantly, dentures must be cleaned on both surfaces. Removing the denture at night is advised, because the mouth is most comfortable when the dentures are not worn overnight. A soak is not necessary; 100% humidity (e.g., wrapped in a wet paper towel) is sufficient. If a soak is chosen, the solution may include a commercial cleanser, dilute vinegar, or even bleach at 1:10 dilution.

7. What methods of control may be useful in geriatric periodontal patients?

Control of periodontitis by mechanical (removal of etiologic agents by scaling) and antimicrobial therapies is effective at slowing or arresting progression of tissue loss about the teeth. Localized drug delivery systems may hold the key to maintenance therapy in geriatric patients. The combination of mechanical therapy and insertion of plastic fibers or chips containing the tetracyclines, to which many periodontal pathogenic bacteria are susceptible, may prove successful in decreasing these infections over time in special populations. Even in the absence of supportive care, these technqiues have shown significant reduction in disease recurrence after treatment and may provide an alternative to personnel-intensive mechanical therapy, which is often difficult to achieve in long-term care populations. The use of chlorhexidine mouthwash (Peridex or Dental-Guard) for antimicrobial effect in the management of gingivitis may well assist antifungal therapy.

Gingival inflammation, postoperative healing, and oral ulcerative diseases may improve with antimicrobials. However, no chemical agents have been shown to benefit periodontitis, which is an infection within periodontal tissues and presumably beyond the therapeutic efficacy of mouthwashes and rinses. Attempts to infuse inflamed tissues with these agents have failed to demonstrate efficacy in clinical trials.

8. When should oral candidiasis be suspected?

Oral candidiasis is frequently detected as a white pseudomembranous slough that is easily wiped off the mucosa to reveal an erythematous base. Pain may be a feature, leading to the term **denture-sore mouth**. Oral candidal infection does not lead to the formation of pockets of infection around teeth roots or result in loosening of the teeth.

9. List the risk factors for oral candidiasis.

Nutritional deficiencies	Immune deficiencies (e.g., AIDS, malignancy)
Antibiotic therapy	Ill-fitting or worn dental prostheses
Chemotherapy	Xerostomia
Steroid therapy	

10. What are the common clinical manifestations of oral candidiasis?

- Acute atrophic candidiasis (antibiotic-sore mouth)
- Angular cheilitis (perlèche)
- Chronic atrophic candidiasis (denture-sore mouth)
- Pseudomembranous candidiasis (thrush)

11. Are pharmacotherapeutic agents helpful in managing candidal infection?

Therapy directed at the candidal infection, either local and topical or systemic, also requires decontamination of dental prostheses, which otherwise will reseed the oral cavity. Dental prostheses are washed, scrubbed, and maintained in either commercial antifungal agents or dilute bleach or vinegar solutions. The dentures are then rinsed before they are replaced into the mouth.

Antifungal agents most useful in oral regimens include:
- Nystatin suspension ("swish and swallow")
- Clotrimazole troches (useful for chronic administration)
- Ketoconazole suspension (prepared as 200 mg/day for up to 2 weeks)
- Fluconazole (most applications require a single daily dose, but it is expensive)

Topical cream application is not recommended for oral candidiasis or angular cheilitis.

12. What is xerostomia? How is it treated?

Xerostomia ("dry mouth") may be a sign or symptom as well as a clinical diagnosis of decreased or absent salivary production and secretion. Salivary glycoproteins, prominent in two distinct molecular weights, may be responsible for symptoms of dryness when salivary production is apparently normal. Conversely, clinicians are familiar with elders who fail to recognize severe salivary deficiency. Other symptoms that help to identify the cause include dysphagia, dysgeusia, burning mouth or tongue, and difficulty in phonation. Observation of diminished salivary flow rate or complaints of chronic dry mouth sensation are not sufficient diagnostic criteria; rather, combinations of these factors provide clinically important indications.

Xerostomia affects the ability to chew, presumably at the inception of the swallow. Accordingly, patients may avoid certain foods, especially chewy and crunchy foods, in favor of drier, sticky, and presumably sweeter alternatives. This pattern may lead to or perpetuate nutritional imbalances as well as dental pathology.

Pharmacologic aids in the management of xerostomia include salivary substitutes and salivary stimulants. Salivary substitutes may aid mastication in that the mucosa may allow the food bolus to be positioned for mastication and prevent sequestration of stagnant food in the cheek, a condition that mimics the rodent buccal cheek pouch. An added benefit is the inclusion of fluoride in some substitutes. Unfortunately, salivary stimulation with sugared candies is a frequent self-medication favored by elders, many of whom have exposed cervical (root) areas of the teeth. In this fragile and sensitive environment, such a practice precipitates caries. Salivary stimulation may be successful as long as residual salivary gland tissue remains after radiation therapy, infection, or surgical ablation. Of interest is the recent introduction of systemic pilocarpine to the armamentarium.

Simple stimulation by chewing gums or sugarless lemon drops is an appropriate first-line prescription. Unflavored stimulants are currently marketed for patients with hypersensitivity to flavoring because of mucositis or ulcerations. The prevalence of xerostomia among certain patient populations may compromise nutrition, medication compliance, social function, and activities of daily living. A successful secretagogue may become the standard of care. Although we do not know the prevalence of xerostomia in different populations, we are well aware of the sequelae of dental caries, pain, and loss of function.

13. Can anything be done about halitosis?

Halitosis is probably not strongly associated with xerostomia, but underlying periodontal disease, poor oral hygiene, or dental abscess may be significant. Such problems may also be associated with the frequency of "morning breath" and the complaint of xerostomia in the morning. Halitosis is the most frequently reported temporal complaint, and the differences in stimulated salivary flow and minor salivary gland output are pronounced between complainers and noncomplainers. Oral hygiene measures, including removal of residual keratin and accretions on the tongue, are best directed at morning accumulations, along with hydration and salivary stimulation.

14. Denture-wearing patients frequently use adhesive to retain the prosthesis. Are adhesives effective? What special care is involved?

Denture adhesives, such as powders, creams, and pastes, are least favored on both coasts of the United States but have broader acceptance in the middle of the country. They have little acceptance from the dental community. Moreover, denture wearers seem to use adhesives without correlation to denture quality or fit. Many patients believe that adhesives increase retention or resistance to lateral displacement and improve denture function. The adhesives should be removed at each cleaning and the dentures kept in 100% humidity for the period of sleep. Dental prostheses should be removed each evening for healing of the oral mucosa, which is prone to ulceration. Because dentures worn around the clock are associated with increased atrophy of the maxillary and mandibular ridges, all dentures should be removed to retard loss of alveolar (bony) ridges. Dentures should be maintained in 100% humidity; immersion in liquid is unnecessary.

BIBLIOGRAPHY

1. Berkey DB, Shay K: General dental care for the elderly. Clin Geriatr Med 8:579–597, 1992.
2. Ettinger RL: The unique oral health needs of an aging population. Dent Clin North Am 41:633–649, 1997.
3. Feldman RS, Kapur KK, Alman JE, Chauncey HH: Aging and mastication: Changes in performance and in the swallowing threshold with natural dentition. J Am Geriatr Soc 28:97–103, 1980.
4. Loesche WJ, Bromberg J, Terpenning MS, et al: Xerostomia, xerogenic medications and food avoidances in selected geriatric groups. J Am Geriatr Soc 43:401–407, 1995.
5. McGrath C, Raman B: The importance of oral health to older people's quality of life. Gerodontology 16:59–63, 1999.
6. Schmidt A, Lemback H, Feldman RS: Dental health factors in long term care environments. In Ellen RP (ed): Periodontal Care for Older Adults. Toronto, Canadian Scholars' Press, 1991, pp 48–59.
7. Williams RC: Periodontal disease. N Engl J Med 322:373–377, 1990.

22. PREVENTING ADVERSE DRUG REACTIONS

Katherine Waltman, Pharm. D., and Sandeep Wadhwa, M.D., M.B.A.

1. When should an adverse drug reaction (ADR) be suspected?

Whenever an elderly patient has an unexpected change in function, an ADR should be considered and should prompt a careful evaluation of drug therapy (e.g., recent medication additions, deletions, or changes in dosing times). A functional change may involve the physical, cognitive, affective, or virtually any other domain of function. A change in mental status or behavior may be caused by prescription or over-the-counter (OTC) sedatives, antihistamines, nonsteroidal anti-inflammatory drugs (NSAIDs), or H_2-blockers. Similarly, a gait disorder caused by parkinsonism may be precipitated by an antipsychotic drug.

A chronically taken drug also may lead to a change in function if a new drug or changing physiology increases the drug's plasma concentration or sensitivity to its effect. For example, phenytoin-induced ataxia may be prompted by addition of one of the many drugs (e.g., cimetidine, isoniazid) that may increase phenytoin levels. Whenever a new medication is prescribed, a careful review should be made of concomitant drugs and diseases, with attention to potential interactions or synergies that may lead to an ADR.

2. Why are elderly patients more susceptible to ADRs?

As many as 30% of elderly outpatients have suffered ADRs. ADRs may play a role in causing 10–17% of hospital admissions for elderly patients. On average, elderly patients use 30% of all medications, although they account for only about 12% of the total population. Age is clearly associated with increasing numbers of both chronic and acute illnesses. These illnesses often require the utilization of multiple health care providers. The use of multiple drugs (polypharmacy) and multiple providers increases the likelihood of ADRs. Adherence to a medication regimen also becomes more challenging. In addition, age-related changes in pharmacokinetics, pharmacodynamics, and homeostatic mechanisms make elderly patients more vulnerable to unwanted drug effects.

3. When should nondrug therapy be considered?

Many acute and chronic illnesses require drug therapy for optimal management. However, nondrug approaches always should be considered initially. Too often physicians feel a pressure to close an ambulatory visit with the writing of a prescription. Often we misjudge a patient's concern about symptoms as a desire for a medication when in reality the concern is for reassurance or merely attention. Many patients respond more positively to receiving a nondrug prescription. For example, a daily-walk recommendation is taken more seriously by patients when written on a prescription form. Nonpharmacologic interventions, such as exercise, weight reduction, and smoking cessation, have been shown to be extremely effective in the elderly in addressing several major chronic conditions, such as diabetes, hypertension, and ischemic heart disease.

The urge to prescribe should never circumvent a careful work-up and the identification of a safer nondrug approach. This consideration is particularly important for patients with symptoms or behavior that may warrant a psychotropic drug. A patient with insomnia may be using caffeine or some other stimulant late in the day, have unrealistic expectations of the sleep cycle, or have an inadequately treated medical illness that causes pain or anxiety. Patients with dementia-related behavior may respond better to environmental modifications than to antipsychotic or neuroleptic agents.

4. What is the difference between pharmacokinetics and pharmacodynamics?

The route a drug takes may be divided simplistically into five steps:

1. Ingestion and absorption
2. Distribution
3. Effect at receptors and ultimate physiologic or pharmacodynamic effect
4. Metabolic transformation
5. Final elimination

Pharmacokinetics refers to what the body does to the drug through the processes of absorption, distribution, metabolism, and elimination. The **half-life** ($t\frac{1}{2}$) describes the amount of time it takes for the drug concentration to fall by one-half after uptake into the body. The **volume of distribution** (Vd) describes the theoretical volume of tissue or body fluids that serves as a reservoir for the drug. **Clearance** (Cl) characterizes the number of milliliters of plasma per unit of time that is cleared (by whatever mechanism) of a drug. These pharmacokinetic parameters bear straightforward, arithmetic relationships. The $t\frac{1}{2}$ of a drug is proportional to the Vd of the drug divided by Cl. Thus, if the Vd of a drug increases with age and the Cl decreases, the $t\frac{1}{2}$ may increase substantially.

Pharmacodynamics describes what the drug does to the body. Ultimately, it is the pharmacodynamic or physiologic effect that allows a drug either to be effective or to have an unwanted or adverse effect. In some cases the intended pharmacodynamic effect may yield an unwanted effect (see question 6). Aging and disease may alter the pharmacokinetics and pharmacodynamics of a drug and thus make ADRs more likely.

5. Describe the age-related pharmacokinetic changes that contribute to ADRs.

Pharmacokinetic Changes with Aging

	PHYSIOLOGIC CHANGES	CLINICAL SIGNIFICANCE
Absorption	Higher gastric pH Decreased small bowel surface area	Not clinically significant
Distribution	Reduced total body water	Higher concentration for water-soluble drugs
	Reduced muscle mass, increased body fat	Increased distribution and longer half-life for fat-soluble drugs
	Lower serum albumin	Increased free fraction in plasma of protein-bound acidic drugs
Metabolism	Decreased phase 1 hepatic metabolism Reduced hepatic mass	Decreased first-pass metabolism Decreased rate of biotransformation
Elimination	Decreased renal plasma flow and glomerular filtration	Decreased renal elimination of drugs and metabolites

Adapted from Vestal RE: Aging and pharmacokinetics: Impact of altered physiology in the elderly. In Physiology and Cell Biology of Aging, vol 8. New York, Raven Press, 1979, p 198.

6. What age-related pharmacodynamic differences contribute to ADRs?

Pharmacodynamic differences in drug effects associated with aging are much less understood than pharmacokinetic differences. Older patients are generally more sensitive to the doses or plasma levels of a number of medications considered appropriate for younger patients, such as sedatives and narcotic analgesics. Lower doses or plasma levels of these drugs may give the desired effect, whereas "usual" doses or levels may cause toxicity. Serum concentrations appropriate for the young may cause ADRs in the elderly. Only for rare drugs, such as the beta-adrenergic antagonists and agonists, do older patients have less sensitivity. Examples of drugs with age-related increased sensitivity include benzodiazepines (sedation), opiates (increased analgesia), and warfarin (increased anticoagulant effect).

7. Which classes of drugs are most likely to cause ADRs in the elderly?

Any drug may cause an ADR, and drugs used frequently in the elderly population are most often implicated in ADRs. The greater the number of drugs that a patient takes, the greater the risk for experiencing an ADR. Surveys of older people living in the community show that analgesic and cardiovascular medications are used by at least one-third. Patients taking multiple medications (≥ 5 drugs/day) most often report ADRs associated with cardiovascular or central nervous system drugs. Gastrointestinal agents, central nervous system agents, and endocrine/metabolic drugs reportedly are used by about 10% of older people. In addition, 30–65% of older people report using OTC analgesics, and 11–25% report using OTC gastrointestinal drugs. Studies of hospitalized patients find that analgesics, sedatives, and antipsychotics account for nearly 50% of preventable ADRs in this setting.

8. Give examples of drugs that generally are considered inappropriate in the elderly.

Drugs that cause potent anticholinergic side effects (e.g., dry mouth, blurred vision, urinary retention, confusion), excessive sedation, and orthostatic hypotension generally are avoided in the elderly, especially when alternatives exist that have a more benign side-effect profile and provide equal or superior efficacy.

DRUG OR DRUG CLASS	ADR/COMMENT	POSSIBLE ALTERNATIVE(S)
Antidepressants Amitriptyline Doxepin	Potent anticholinergics, strong sedatives	Selective serotonin reuptake inhibitors, nortriptyline, desipramine
Trimethobenzamide (antiemetic)	Extrapyramidal symptoms, confusion, ? efficacy	Prochlorperazine (short-term), lorazepam
Antihistamines Chlorpheniramine Diphenhydramine Hydroxyzine	Potent anticholinergics	Cetirizine, loratadine (allergy symptoms); cough/cold preparations without antihistamine
Antiplatelet agents Dipyridamole Ticlopidine	Orthostasis Neutropenia	Aspirin, clopidogrel
Antispasmodics (GI) Dicyclomine Hyoscyamine	Anticholinergic effects, ? efficacy	
Antispasmodics/relaxants Carisoprodol Cyclobenzaprine Methocarbamol Oxybutynin	Anticholinergic effects, sedation, weakness, ? efficacy	Baclofen
Barbiturates	Confusion, sedation, addiction	Lorazepam, oxazepam, temazepam
Benzodiazepines Chlordiazepoxide Diazepam Flurazepam	Prolonged sedation, falls/ fractures, long t½	Lorazepam, oxazepam, temazepam
Cardiovascular drugs Disopyramide	Heart failure, anticholinergic effects	Procainamide, amiodarone
Methyldopa	Depression	Diuretic, beta blocker, other antihypertensives
Reserpine	Depression, sedation, impotence, orthostasis	*See* methyldopa

Table continued on following page

DRUG OR DRUG CLASS	ADR/COMMENT	POSSIBLE ALTERNATIVE(S)
Indomethacin	Central nervous system effects	Acetaminophen (pain), ibuprofen, nabumetone
Narcotic analgesics		
Meperidine	Tremor, seizures	Acetaminophen, codeine, morphine
Pentazocine	Confusion, hallucinations	
Propoxyphene	Sedation, constipation, efficacy similar to acetaminophen	
Chlorpropamide (sulfonylurea)	Syndrome of inappropriate secretion of antidiuretic hormone, long t1/2, hypoglycemia	Glyburide, glipizide, repaglinide

Adapted from Beers MH: Explicit criteria for determining potentially inappropriate medication use by the elderly: An update. Arch Intern Med 157:1531–1536, 1997.

9. Give examples of pharmacodynamic drug–disease interactions that should be considered to avoid ADRs in the elderly.

DISEASE	DRUG(S)	POTENTIAL ADR(S)
Chronic obstructive pulmonary disease	Beta blockers	Bronchospasm, worsened respiration
Benign prostatic hypertrophy	Anticholinergics, bladder relaxants, narcotics	Urinary retention, obstruction
Constipation	Anticholinergics, calcium channel blockers, narcotics	Obstruction, impaction
Dementia	Anticholinergics, psychotropics	Confusion, delirium
Diabetes	Diuretics, steroids	Hyperglycemia
Hypertension	Amphetamines, NSAIDs	Blood pressure elevation
Peptic ulcer disease	Aspirin, NSAIDs, anticoagulants	Hemorrhage

10. Identify pharmacodynamic drug–drug interactions that may cause ADRs in the elderly.

DRUG COMBINATIONS	POTENTIAL ADR(S)
Anticholinergics, sedatives, anxiolytics, antidepressants, H_2-blockers	Impaired cognition, delirium, memory deficits
Antipsychotics, metoclopramide, sedatives, prochlorperazine	Decreased mobility, gait disorders, postural instability, movement disorders
Gentamicin, furosemide, vancomycin	Ototoxicity, nephrotoxicity

11. List examples of cytochrome P450 drug–drug interactions that may cause ADRs in the elderly.

The concentrations of drugs that are metabolized by (or substrates for) the hepatic cytochrome P450 (cyt P450) system may be altered by cyt P450 enzyme inhibitors or inducers. Inhibitors raise the level of the substrate drug as a consequence of impaired or inhibited hepatic metabolism. Increased levels of the substrate drug increase the patient's risk for an ADR. Alternatively, inducers may increase the metabolism of the substrate drug, which may result in subtherapeutic levels or response.

Examples of Enzyme Inhibitor Interactions

SUBSTRATE DRUG/ (CYTP450 ISOEZYME)	ENZYME INHIBITORS	POTENTIAL ADR(S)
Alprazolam (cytP3A4)	Cimetidine Erythromycin Fluconazole Grapefruit juice	Sedation, falls, fractures
Cisapride* (cytP3A4)	See alprazolam inhibitors	Torsade de pointes, fatal arrhythmias
Phenytoin (cytP2C9)	Amiodarone Fluconazole	Ataxia, falls, slurred speech
Theophylline (cytP1A2)	Cimetidine Ciprofloxacin Erythromycin	Arrhythmias, insomnia, nausea, vomiting
Warfarin (cytP2C9) (cytP1A2)	Amiodarone Cimetidine Fluvoxamine	Bleeding

* Always review drug interactions before initiating cisapride; several drugs may increase the risk of fatal arrhythmia.

Examples of Enzyme Inducer Interactions

SUBSTRATE DRUG(S)/CYTP450 ISOENZYME	ENZYME INDUCER(S)
Warfarin, theophylline (cytP1A2)	Rifampin, cigarette smoke, barbiturates
Cyclosporine (cytP3A4)	Rifampin, barbiturates, phenytoin, carbamazepine

12. Which commonly used drugs require plasma level monitoring to help prevent ADRs?

Aminoglycosides Phenobarbital Quinidine
Carbamazepine Phenytoin Theophylline
Digoxin Procainamide Valproic acid

Assessment of drug concentration must not replace careful assessment of the intended and unwanted pharmacodynamic effects. For example, a theophylline level of 12 µg/ml may be subtherapeutic in a young asthmatic patient but may cause anorexia and weight loss in a frail elderly patient. In addition, most assays of drug concentrations quantitate total drug, which includes both protein-bound and active unbound fractions. For a drug that is highly protein-bound, such as phenytoin, a "normal" total concentration in a frail hypoalbuminemic patient may result in an increased free fraction with possible toxicity. Thus, drug concentration monitoring may serve as a guide to avoid gross overdosage, but it must not be used as a substitute for thoughtful evaluation of the individual patient.

13. How do herbal supplements contribute to ADRs in the elderly?

Scant literature addresses the use of herbal therapies in the elderly. Elderly patients with cancer or Alzheimer's disease may turn to herbal therapies. In recent years many companies have developed herbal products and advertisements that often are aimed at the geriatric population. Use and acceptability of herbal agents are likely to increase. It is, therefore, important to inquire and be knowledgeable about the use of herbal products to assess the potential for drug interactions and adverse effects. For example, an elderly patient may take St. John's wort to improve mood without realizing that it may interact with a prescribed antidepressant, putting the patient at risk for serotonin syndrome. The use of *Ginkgo biloba* with aspirin, NSAIDs, or anticoagulants may increase the risk for bleeding complications. Likewise, an elderly patient taking the herb ma huang (ephedra) for respiratory problems may experience uncontrolled hypertension or insomnia. These scenarios typify the need for careful assessment of use, side effects, drug interactions, and efficacy. Practitioners also should inform elderly patients that these "supplements" are not regulated as medications and, therefore, may differ in content from batch to batch.

14. How can I get my elderly patients to adhere to their drug regimens?

- Understand the patient's drug history in detail.
- Use the "brown bag" approach at each ambulatory visit (patients are instructed to bring all bottles and packages of prescriptions, OTC medications, home remedies, and herbal preparations that they are taking).
- Give permission for the patient to relate exactly how drugs are taken.
- Probe for the patient's opinion about problems and adverse effects.
- Educate the patient about the relative importance of each medication.
- Assess the patient's level of literacy and visual function.
- Provide both verbal and written (large-type) instruction.
- Use family, visiting nurses, pharmacists, and home health providers as allies to encourage adherence.
- Simplify drug regimens, and avoid polypharmacy.
- Use once- or twice-daily dosage forms.
- Eliminate drugs with no indication or benefit.
- Use the least number of drugs to manage the maximal number of conditions.
- Avoid adding medication(s) to treat an ADR of another medication.
- Easy-open bottles, pill boxes, medication calendars, blister packaging, and alarm reminders are useful devices to promote adherence.
- Pay attention to cost if this is a concern to the patient.

BIBLIOGRAPHY

1. Bates DW, Cullen DJ, Laird N, et al: Incidence of adverse drug events and potential adverse drug events: Implications for prevention. JAMA 274:29–34, 1995.
2. Beers MH: Explicit criteria for determining potentially inappropriate medication use by the elderly: An update. Arch Intern Med 157:1531–1536, 1997.
3. Carlson JE: Perils of polypharmacy: 10 steps to prudent prescribing. Geriatrics 51:26–35, 1996.
4. Chrischilles EA, Foley DJ, Wallace RB, et al: Use of medications by persons 65 and over: Data from the established populations for epidemiologic studies of the elderly. J Gerontol 47: M137–M144, 1992.
5. Chutka DS, Evans JM, Fleming KC, Mikkelson KG: Drug prescribing for elderly patients. Mayo Clin Proc 70:685–693, 1995.
6. Hanlon JT, Schmader KE, Koronkowski MJ, et al: Adverse drug events in high risk older outpatients. J Am Geriatr Soc 45:945–948, 1997.
7. Lazarou J, Pomeranz BH, Corey PN: Incidence of adverse drug reactions in hospitalized patients. JAMA 279:1200–1205, 1998.

23. THE OLDER DRIVER

Sheila Pasupathy and Risa Lavizzo-Mourey, M.D., M.B.A.

1. Is driving an important issue among older adults?

The ability to drive defines independence and provides a sense of self-esteem for many older adults. Suggesting that it is unsafe to drive is a major threat to their sense of control in everyday life. On a pragmatic level, driving represents the sole means of transportation for many seniors. Studies in 1994 show that 88% of older Americans rely on a private automobile for most of their transportation needs. The trend to "gray in place" represents the desire of older adults to remain in rural or suburban communities where mass transit is not easily accessible.

Driving cessation often leads to decreased quality of life because people lose the ability to participate freely in social opportunities, visit family, go to the grocery store, or engage in essential activities independently. The resulting increase in loneliness and isolation may adversely affect health and well-being. Hardest hit are couples in cohorts over the age of 80. Women of this generation often never learned to drive and depend completely on their husbands for mobility. Unfortunately, many older people do not have a strong network of support or access to appropriate social/community supports to maintain independent living. Thus, research in this area generally focuses on two objectives: (1) to identify and rehabilitate people with impairments to prolong driving independence and (2) to identify and create viable driving alternatives for people who need to compensate for mobility loss.

2. What are the costs of poor driver safety among the elderly?

Studies by the National Highway Traffic Administration show that the number of traffic fatalities is on the rise for older cohorts.

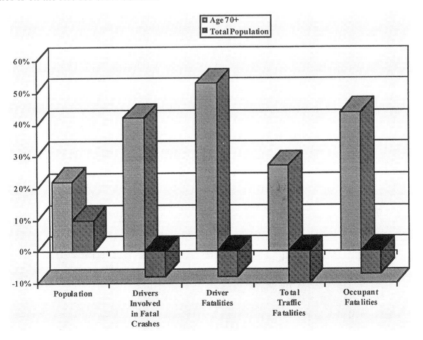

Percent Change, 1987–1997. Source: National Highway Traffic Safety Administration.

Although older adults drive substantially less than younger drivers, they incur a disproportionate number of crashes per mile driven. In addition, older driver safety problems are exacerbated by increasing fragility. Older drivers suffer higher rates of injury and fatality in a crash than any other age group. These statistics illustrate the seriousness of driving risk for the elderly—a trend that must be reversed in the face of a burgeoning senior population.

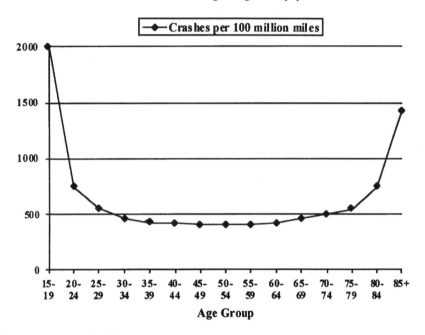

Source: Addressing the Safety Issues Related to Younger and Older Drivers. A: A Report to Congress, January 19,1993, on the Research Agenda of the National Highway Traffic Safety Administration.

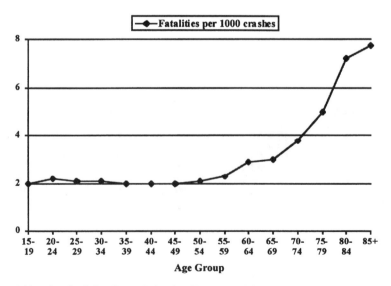

Source: Addressing the Safety Issues Related to Younger and Older Drivers. A: A Report to Congress, January 19,1993, on the Research Agenda of the National Highway Traffic Safety Administration.

3. **The ability to drive depends on which functions?**
Driving is a highly integrative task that depends on psychomotor, cognitive, and sensoriperceptual functions. Specifically, vehicle operation requires the interaction of sustained visual attention, adequate speed of mental processing, timely and accurate responses, and adequate sensory motor control.

4. **Does normal aging have an impact on driving skills?**
Normal aging results in a number of basic functional changes that affect driving skills. Fortunately, evidence indicates that older drivers exhibit good judgment by adjusting their driving practices to accommodate declining function.

FUNCTION	AGE-RELATED CHANGES	DRIVING-RELATED IMPAIRMENTS
Psychomotor	Decreased number and size of muscle fibers Decreased responsiveness to electrical stimulation Decreased myosin adenosine triphosphatase activity Degradation of joints and tendons	Reductions in musculoskeletal function result in: • Slowing • Deteriorated strength • Reduced dexterity and coordination • Increased reaction time
Sensoriperceptual	Decreased visual acuity Drop in peripheral field vision Decreased retinal illuminance Increased light scattering Reduced amplitude of accommodation—presbyopia Loss of retinal photoreceptors Loss of retinal ganglion cells as well as other age-related cortical changes	Changes in optical and visual function result in: • Decreased night visual acuity • Decreased resistance to glare • Decreased contrast sensitivity • Increased dark-adaptation time interval

5. **What medical conditions affect driving ability?**
Studies show that certain medical conditions, prevalent in older adults, increase crash risk:
Seizure disorders. People afflicted with epileptic seizures may experience loss of motor function and/or total loss of consciousness. Every U.S. state has varying restrictions against driving for people with epilepsy.
Stroke. Presenting symptoms of stroke include motor, sensory, and cognitive deficits—all essential for safe driving. Recommendations from the American Medical Association suggest that changes of higher cerebral functions in association with cerebrovascular accidents should be an indication to stop driving.
Diabetes. Hyperglycemia may result in symptoms of fatigue and sluggishness. In addition, chronic complications of diabetes such as macroangiopathy, microangiopathy, and diabetic retinopathy may have a detrimental impact on driving.
Cardiovascular disease. Many conditions classified under cardiovascular disease impair driving ability. For instance, sick sinus syndrome causes lethargy, weakness, light-headedness, dizziness, and episodes of near-syncope or actual loss of consciousness.
Arthritis. Arthritis may generate pain causing unconscious hesitancy and total restriction of motion, which can greatly affect braking, turning, and gripping the wheel.
Dementia. Dementia, depending on severity, affects cognitive functions necessary for competent driving. Loss of cognitive function affects judgment, memory, and attention.
Parkinson's disease. Parkinson's disease is characterized by resting tremor, pill rolling of the fingers, forward flexion of the trunk, and muscle rigidity and weakness. These motor impairments affect overall vehicle control.

6. How do eye problems affect driving ability?

According to the Framingham Eye Study, the four leading causes of vision impairment among older adults are age-related macular degeneration, cataract, glaucoma, and diabetic retinopathy. Driving involves the simultaneous use of central and peripheral vision. Thus, the effects of these conditions critically affect crash risk.

CONDITION	EFFECT ON VISION
Age-related macular degeneration	Distortion and/or loss of central vision
Cataract	Loss of vision acuity, contrast sensitivity Increased sensitivity to glare, nearsightedness
Glaucoma	Gradual loss of peripheral vision Eventual damage to central vision
Diabetic retinopathy	Gradual development of severe blurred vision–macular edema Potential loss of vision via retinal detachment

7. Which medications can affect the ability to drive safely?

Any medication has the potential to affect driving ability profoundly. The following groups of medications are especially risky:

MEDICATION	POTENTIAL EFFECT ON DRIVING ABILITY
Benzodiazepines	Impaired vision, attention, information processing, memory, motor coordination, ability to perform combined skills task, and driving under controlled conditions
Antidepressants	Impaired attention, memory, motor coordination, and open road driving
Opioid analgesics	Impaired vision, attention, and motor coordination Sedation
Antihistamines	Sedation Impaired coordination, simulated driving, and open road driving
Hypoglycemics*	Impaired cognition, memory, vision, information processing, and motor control

* A threat only if hypoglycemia is induced.

8. What is the physician's role in evaluating driver safety?

Physicians have a duty to protect their patients' lives. Thus, when a patient's health impairs the ability to drive, physicians have a duty to recommend limitations or cessation if driving poses a threat to the patient. The good news is that many elders self-regulate—they limit their driving based on their own limitations. Unfortunately, some are not fully aware of their limitations and continue to drive under unsafe conditions. To distinguish safe drivers from unsafe drivers, physicians should include an assessment of driving skills in the normal evaluation of the geriatric patient. Evaluating driving competency is a particular challenge for physicians faced with resolving the conflict between an elderly patient's quality of life and public safety. Unnecessary limitations on driving ability may have a detrimental effect on the patient's well-being, whereas failure to recommend driving cessation when it is appropriate may lead to a crash that harms the patient and/or others. Therefore, a physician must take care in assessing and making judgments about driving performance and must be prepared to discuss recommendations with patients and their families.

9. How is driving safety evaluated?

Criteria for determining who is at risk for crashes have not been validated, but questions related to driving can serve as triggers for further evaluation. A preliminary screen in a simple yes/no form may assess the following:

• Driving frequency and distances
• Driving patterns (e.g., freeway vs. local roads, day vs. night driving)
• Changes in driving patterns in the past year
• Use of medications known to impair driving
• Presence of driving-impairing medical conditions
• Condition of driving-related functions
• Number of accidents

Based on the initial screen, physicians must be prepared to question and examine further patients whose responses indicate potential risk. This next level of assessment should attempt to elucidate problem areas and uncover additional medical conditions through basic examinations. Examples of tests that may be used include:

• Mini-Mental State Exam for dementia
• Neurologic exam and gait and balance test for Parkinson's disease
• Snellen eye chart for vision
• Cervical spine, hip, and knee mobility test for arthritis

If the presence of a driving-impairing condition is confirmed, the physician must perform another level of assessment to determine severity of illness. At this point, the physician may need to gather more information about the nature of the uncovered condition, or he/she may refer the patient to other professionals who can better determine whether the condition poses a threat to driving ability. Referral to an occupational therapist for a formal driving screening is recommended. Driving screenings at best simulate driving with video and at the least probe specific cognitive and motor skills required during driving for comparison with age-appropriate norms. Poor performance on a driving screen may be enough to convince an unsafe driver to stop. Many states have legislation requiring physicians to report disabled patients to the registry of motor vehicles, even if they are unable to drive only temporarily. If reported by a physician, a patient must participate in a more complete medical evaluation.

10. Which medical conditions are physicians obligated to report to the Department of Transportation?

Almost all states have established regulations regarding drivers with impairments. The Department of Transportation states that physician reporting is a highly effective mechanism for identifying medically impaired drivers. Over 40,000 reports are submitted each year, of which 72% signify impairments that are significant enough to merit temporary or permanent recall of driving privilege. Policies vary from state to state and may be obtained through the Bureau of Driver Licensing. Pennsylvania's reporting requirements include the following:

• A person with visual acuity of less than 20/100 combined vision with best correction may not be qualified to drive. Other vision policies restrict driving to daylight hours and certain areas.
• A person with a seizure disorder shall not be qualified to drive unless the person has been free from seizure for at least 6 months from the date of the last seizure, with or without medication. Waivers of the freedom-from-seizure requirement may be made on recommendation by a physician under specific conditions.
• A person with any of the following conditions shall not be qualified to drive:
  1. Unstable or brittle diabetes or hypoglycemia, unless the patient has been free from any related syncopal attack for at least 6 months.
  2. Cerebral vascular insufficiency or cardiovascular disease, which, for the preceding 6 months, has resulted in either (1) syncopal attacks or loss of consciousness or (2) vertigo, paralysis, or loss of qualifying visual fields.
  3. Periodic episodes of loss of consciousness that are of unknown etiology or not otherwise categorized, unless the person has been free from such episodes for the year immediately preceding.
• Providers may make recommendations to restrict driving if the patient has a condition that, in the opinion of the provider, is likely to impair the ability to drive safely.

11. What options are available to rehabilitate drivers at risk for crashes?

Many older adults who are forced to limit or stop driving based on functional impairments are often not aware of retraining options that allow them to get behind the wheel safely once more. Several options are available:

1. Occupational therapists have developed comprehensive programs that not only assess a patient's capacity to drive but also analyze deficits that may improve through training. For example, an occupational therapist may design an exercise program to increase physical strength, endurance, and mobility if a physical condition hampers driving. Such programs are comprehensive and give patients a chance to become mobile again.

2. Specialized adaptive equipment may be used to compensate for functional limitations. Many older adults without cognitive deficits respond well to such implements. For example, people who do not have adequate strength in their legs may benefit from hand controls that facilitate use of gas and brake pedals. Other commonly prescribed equipment compensates for reduced range of motion, reaction time, dexterity, and peripheral vision.

3. Several organizations offer driver training programs that cover a variety of issues, including new safety rules and common traffic problems associated with age. Such programs are usually 4–8 hour courses and are sponsored by associations such as the National Safety Council, the American Automobile Association, and the American Association of Retired Persons. New pilot projects have been launched by companies such as General Motors. These courses have limitations in improving driving ability because they do not address the debilitating effects of medical conditions in conjunction with normal aging and generally do not impart skills training to overcome functional impairments.

BIBLIOGRAPHY

1. Johansson K, Lundberg C: The 1994 International Consensus Conference on Dementia and Driving: A brief report. Alzheimer Dis Assoc Disord 11:62–69, 1997.
2. Morgan R, King D: The older driver—a review. Postgrad Med J 71:525–528, 1995.
3. Owsley C, Ball K, McGwin G, et al: Visual processing impairment and risk of motor vehicle crash among older adults. JAMA 279:1083–1088, 1998.
4. Owsley C, Stalvey B, Wells J, Sloan M: Older drivers and cataract: Driving habits and crash risk. J Gerontol 54:M203–M211, 1999.
5. Retchin S (ed): Medical Considerations in the Older Driver. Clinics in Geriatric Medicine, vol. 9. Philadelphia, W.B. Saunders, 1993.
6. Wallace R: Cognitive change, medical illness and crash risk among older drivers: An epidemiological consideration. Alzheimer Dis Assoc Disord 11:31–37, 1997.

IV. Conditions Requiring Special Consideration

24. ASSESSING FUNCTION

Keith M. Robinson, M.D.

1. What is functional assessment?

Functional assessment is the measurement of a patient's performance of the survival skills required to negotiate everyday life. Traditionally, it has focused on those skills that relate to basic physical and cognitive functions:

Self-care
    Activities of daily living
    Instrumental activities of daily living
    Mobility/balance
    Comprehension/communication

These skills generally can be thought of as those required to function safely within one's household and effectively in the local community.

Functional Survival Skills

	SELF-CARE	MOBILITY	COMMUNICATION
Household	Eating/drinking	Bed moblity	Hearing
	Bathing/grooming	Transfers. e.g., bed to chair, chair to	Vision
	Dressing	toilet, chair to shower seat	Orientation
	Toileting	Ambulation with or without an	Attention
	Bowel/bladder control	assistive device, level vs. non-	Memory
	Sexuality	level surfaces (e.g., stairs)	Language (talking,
	Cooking	Balance	gesturing)
	Laundry	Wheelchair ambulation and parts	Spatial perception
	Housekeeping	management	Organization
	Taking medications		Problem-solving
Community	Prevocational and	Nonlevel surface ambulation, with	Using telephones
	vocational skills	or without an assistive device	Writing/typing/word
	Shopping	(e.g., curbs, ramps, uneven terrain)	processing
	Banking	Community wheelchair ambulation	Supervising others
	Managing financial	(manual vs. motorized)	in self-care and
	and legal affairs	Driving	mobility needs
		Using public transportation, e.g.,	
		bus, taxi, wheelchair, van	

2. Is functional assessment different in older people?

More functional disability is observed during normal aging. Community surveys of older Americans have documented that:

- 25% have difficulty performing heavy housework
- 20% have difficulty walking
- 10% have difficulty bathing, managing money, and using the telephone
- 5% have difficulty dressing, using the toilet, and eating

The elderly residing in long-term care institutions experience even more disabilities:
- 70% require assistance with toileting and transfers from bed to chair
- 50% have bowel or bladder incontinence
- 40% require assistance when eating

3. How is functional ability assessed?

The individual must be observed in relation to his or her environment. A comprehensive survey includes essential physical and cognitive functioning, the physical environment of the patient, the socioeconomic situation of the patient, and the patient's wishes concerning quality of life.

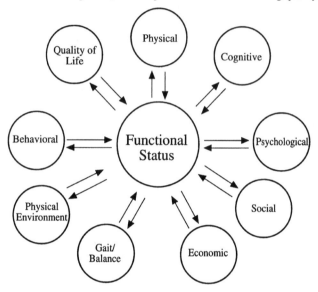

Comprehensive geriatric functional assessment.

The use of **measurement tools** to assess function has advantages and disadvantages. These tools attempt to quantify behavior and can be useful in documenting changes that occur with progressive illness or treatment, yet there are limitations to a quantitative approach. If the instrument relies on self-reports, validity is often in question. When behaviors are reduced to a numerical score, nuances that may be crucial to performance may be missed. These behaviors often are important to observe since they can be the target of specific rehabilitation interventions aimed toward optimizing function.

In **clinical practice**, functional assessment measurement tools can be used to guide a more qualitative approach for assessing function in the outpatient office or at the bedside. A quick survey of the major aspects of comprehensive functional assessment can be integrated into the traditional medical history and physical examination. Patients typically present to clinicians with **functional complaints** (e.g., falling, forgetting). The differential diagnostic approach to medical problem-solving is also quite effective in organizing functional complaints into a hierarchy of etiologies regarding impaired anatomy and physiology. The clinician must come full circle and consider the identified disease(s) and anatomic or physiologic impairment(s) more explicitly within the context of the patient's everyday life and his or her physical and socioeconomic environment. Practical solutions then may emerge for enhancing patient function with such an approach.

4. Who should do what parts in a comprehensive assessment of an older adult?

Comprehensive functional assessment is time- and labor-intensive. The physician usually is neither trained nor expected to perform such an evaluation alone or at one point in time. However, the physician is expected to be familiar with critical areas of everyday life and the contextual forces that define the lives of older patients. The physician must orchestrate the assessment by involving specific key personnel who can assist in providing this information. Further, the physician must synthesize this information so that medical decisions can be based on it. The table presents a possible division of labor among specialists who can be consulted to participate in the comprehensive functional assessment of the older adult. Many of these consultants are nonmedical rehabilitation specialists. Often, consultation with one of them or a physiatrist, who is an expert in functional assessment and functionally oriented treatments, can be useful for facilitating the functional assessment and appropriate treatment interventions aimed to enhance or stabilize function of their older patients.

Nonmedical Specialists Who Participate in Geriatric Functional Assessment

Physical therapist—Basic mobility skills including bed mobility, transfers, wheelchair mobility; ambulation; assistive devices for ambulation including canes, walkers, and wheelchairs; spasticity management with therapeutic exercises; sensory facilitation of motor control; gait training, including training with orthotic and prosthetic devices of the lower limb.

Occupational therapist—Daily living skills including feeding, grooming, toileting, dressing, and homemaking; fine motor skills of the hand and upper limbs, including splinting (orthotics) and wheelchair accessories; cognitive remediation, especially memory and visuoperception; driving evaluation.

Speech/swallowing therapist—Cognitive remediation related to communication, especially in attention, memory, language comprehension, conceptual organization, language production (including nonverbal technologies); swallowing as it relates to oral-motor and pharyngeal function, aspiration precautions, and oral feeding with different food consistencies.

Neuropsychologist—Formal, in-depth, and quantitative evaluation of cognitive and intellectual function; translation of the cognitive profile of intellectual strengths and weaknesses into a behaviorally based set of strategies subsequently used by therapists, nurses, family members, and other care providers.

Behavioral psychologist—Explicit design of behavioral management strategies and programs (often in concert with medications) aimed at optimizing communication for patients having difficulty with self-monitoring, aggression, poor initiation, and other behaviors that disrupt rehabilitation treatments and social interactions.

Counseling psychologist—Psychotherapeutic treatment (often in concert with medications) of loss reactions, depression, and other affective disorders observed during recovery and sometimes disruptive to participation in therapeutic programs.

Recreation therapist—Evaluation and remediation of motor and cognitive function in both individual and group nondidactic settings while focusing on participation in leisure activities.

Case manager—Orchestrates appropriate medical, surgical, rehabilitation, and social services depending on the recovery trajectory, treatment priorities, health insurance, and financial resources.

Social worker—Clarifies social support system, its ability to provide safe and stable emotional support, residential sites, personal care, and transportation; clarifies eligibility and coverage of health and welfare services and health insurance plans; mobilizes resources for coverage of essential health and rehabilitation services with informal and formal care providers acting in complementary roles; often defines the discharge plan; provides emotional support for patients and their social support system members.

Nurse—Assists and supervises the patient in using cognitive and functional skills learned in therapies; patient education of medication schedules and self-monitoring of medical problems, such as diabetes, seizure disorders, skin care, bowel and bladder training programs; facilitates coping with loss and adaptation to illness.

Nutritionist—Collaborates with physicians, nurses, and therapists to establish caloric and nutritional needs during recovery; makes recommendations for nutritional support depending on the most reliable means of entry of food (oral, enteral, parenteral) and dietary advancement.

Prosthetist/orthotist—Assesses need for, and fabricates body part replacements in, amputees (prosthesis); assesses need for and fabricates devices that facilitate motor control and conserve energy consumption during mobility (orthotics), especially of lower limbs.

Discharge planner/clinical resource manager—A nurse or social worker who operationalizes the discharge plan to ensure continuity of care and to facilitate expedient hospital discharge; usually confined to arranging home services but sometimes includes outpatient services.

5. Can the traditional physical exam be changed to include a better assessment of functional status?

The traditional medical approach to data collection (history and physical examination) and differential diagnosis deconstructs the individual into a conglomeration of impaired anatomic and physiologic functions and organ systems. The power of this approach must be appreciated for making causal connections that may help to understand an individual patient's disability and handicap. Further, these organ-specific indicators become essential for measuring efficacy of medical and surgical treatments. Yet, these provide incomplete measurements of function.

The World Health Organization model becomes useful for considering function at several levels and then directs us how to extend medical data collection and problem-solving to enhance measurement of function. **Impairment** defines function at the organ system level and is measured by such indicators as pulmonary function tests and cardiac ejection fraction. **Disability** defines function of the individual in the form described under question 1. **Handicap** defines function of the individual in relation to social roles, such as work and interpersonal aspects of living. This conceptual approach seems intuitive and common-sensical, but data collection beyond the level of impairment too often is forgotten during evaluation of older adults.

As defined in question 1, a survey of survival skill performance is recommended to improve traditional medical history-taking. Similarly, the traditional physical exam provides limited data from which the clinician can extrapolate the functioning of the person in his or her immediate environment. For example, the presence of spastic and weak limbs during the elementary neurologic exam provides limited data for predicting ability to transfer and walk. But direct observation of the patient performing these activities in the office or at the bedside may provide further data to predict his or her abilities. By asking care providers and key members of a patient's social support system in the home, community, or work environments to verify the patient's self-reports and your observations of the patient's functional performance, you can gain a broader view of the functional status within his or her larger community.

6. How does mental status affect the evaluation of functional abilities?

The successful performance of most functional activities requires that basic cognitive domains (attention, memory) and higher-level cognitive domains (language, visuoperception, executive functioning) be relatively intact. The Mini-Mental Status Examination (MMSE) is a widely used screening tool. It is, however, a poor predictor of function. When comprehensive evaluation of functional abilities is required and the MMSE is abnormal, formal cognitive testing should be requested. (See Chapter 3.)

7. How are gait, balance, and falling risk evaluated in the older adult?

Risk Factors for Falling

Lower limb impairment	Generalized weakness
Visual impairment	Environmental hazards
Previous stroke	Orthostatic hypotension
Parkinson's disease	Benzodiazepine use
Barbiturate use	Antihypertensive agents/diuretics

The basic cardiopulmonary and elementary neurologic examinations provide limited information for assessing gait, balance, and falling risk. Observing the simulated or actual performance of transfers and ambulation during the physical assessment becomes essential. A baseline heart rate, blood pressure, and respiratory rate should always be compared to the response immediately after a transfer and/or ambulation trial, and then during the recovery period after these activities are performed in the office or at the bedside. This informal clinical exercise-tolerance test can provide input regarding overall level of endurance and ability to conserve energy during movement.

A directed gait evaluation as well must be performed. To do this, a basic understanding of the normal gait cycle is necessary. Additionally, observation of the patient transferring between different surfaces that are at different heights (e.g., soft mattress to low bedside chair or commode) can be useful to assess falling risk during this aspect of basic mobility. (See Chapter 34.)

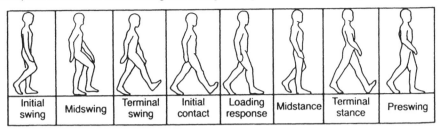

| Initial swing | Midswing | Terminal swing | Initial contact | Loading response | Midstance | Terminal stance | Preswing |

The gait cycle.

8. Describe a simple test for evaluating mobility and falling risk.

A useful instrument for assessing mobility and falling risk in the elderly is the modified **"get up and go" test**. This test is done in ambulatory patients only. One practice run is allowed. The physician makes qualitative observations about each aspect of the mobility trial:

1. The patient should sit comfortably in a straight-backed, high-seat chair with arm rests.
2. Ask the patient to rise from the chair (with or without an assistive device, as is his or her usual manner of ambulation).
3. Ask the patient to stand still momentarily (10 sec) with eyes open (with or without an assistive device, as is his/her usual manner).
4. Ask the patient to stand still momentarily (10 sec) with eyes closed (again with or without an assistive device). You may need to guard the patient from falling.
5. Ask the patient to walk approximately 50 ft forward (with or without a device and/or assistance as appropriate, preferably toward a wall).
6. Ask the patient to turn around at the end of 50 ft.
7. Ask the patient to walk back to the chair, another 50 ft, to the original destination.
8. Ask the patient to sit down when he/she reaches the chair.

Another useful clinical screening tool involves three maneuvers easily performed in an outpatient setting: (1) tandem standing for three seconds; (2) standing up from a seated position with arms crossed over the chest, 5 times within 30 seconds; and (3) a timed walking trial out and back for a standardized distance, including turning, without stumbling or falling. If any of these maneuvers cannot be performed, the patient is at high risk for falling. The time that it takes during the walking trial over a standardized distance can be followed prospectively.

9. When are assistive devices such as canes or wheelchairs useful?

Before you recommend a specific assistive device, the weight-bearing status of the legs must be established (e.g., by the orthopedic surgeon in a patient recovering from joint replacement surgery or by the vascular surgeon in someone recovering from a vascular bypass procedure in the legs).

- Ambulation in parallel bars in physical therapy and with a walker or crutches requires full weight-bearing by both arms and at least 50% to full weight-bearing by one leg. Use of crutches requires better dynamic standing balance than use of a walker.
- Use of a walker with wheels is appropriate when weight-bearing by all four extremities is permitted and when dynamic standing balance is compromised (e.g., in a patient with a parkinsonian gait with retropulsion).
- Ambulation with a hemi-cane, quad cane, or straight cane requires full weight-bearing by the arm in which the cane is held and in the leg on the same side, and at least 50% to full weight-bearing on the other leg that is to be unloaded. Ambulation with a cane requires good dynamic standing balance. The patient should hold the cane in the hand/arm opposite the impaired leg.

In all assistive devices, the level of hand placement (i.e., cane/walker height from the floor) is generally at the level of the greater trochanter of the hip. This position allows for approximately

20–30° of elbow flexion and the most efficient length-tension cocontraction relationship of the elbow flexors and extensors during use of the assistive device.

10. Why is an environmental evaluation important during the functional assessment of an older adult?

The environment in which a person lives should be evaluated to reduce physical barriers that prevent the elderly patient from living safely in his or her home. The presence of stairs on entry or inside the household may limit someone with ambulatory dysfunction to a homebound status or to one floor of their household, temporarily or permanently. If a patient ultimately proves unable to ambulate on stairs, ramping for community access, motorized wheelchairs or scooters for longer-distance ambulation, and stair-lifts or stair-glides may be considered. These are expensive and often not reimbursable by health insurance payers. Older adults with limited incomes usually cannot afford such items.

Setting up a safe, convenient, limited environment becomes acceptable to some disabled older adults when they are confined to one floor of their household:

1. Placement of essential items within reach in the kitchen can facilitate control and energy conservation during meal preparation.

2. In homes without accessible bathrooms, kitchen sinks can be adapted and bedside commodes can be used for bathing and toileting.

3. In homes with accessible bathrooms, inexpensive insurance-reimbursable equipment, such as long-handled reachers and sponges, hand-held showers, tub/shower seats, toilet/shower bars, and raised toilet seats, can be easily installed.

4. Expensive equipment, such as hydraulically controlled tub chair lifts, will require fastidious medical documentation to justify insurance reimbursement.

5. Hospital beds with electrical controls to raise the head of the bed may help with out-of-bed transfers and re-positioning while in bed to prevent skin breakdown.

6. Lifeline systems (not insurance reimbursable) may be useful to those who live alone and are at high risk for falling.

7. Memory cueing systems in the form of signs and log books can help the forgetful person in performing specific activities, such as turning off the stove or lights.

Home care agencies provide physical and occupational therapists who can perform home-environment assessments and make recommendations for medically necessary equipment to reduce physical barriers and optimize functional control in one's home.

11. Why is an evaluation of the social and economic context important during the functional assessment of the older adult?

The social support system surrounding the elderly patient is the major determinant for whether an elderly person can live at home again after hospitalization. Medicare reimbursement for skilled nursing or therapy services is generous but incomplete, typically limiting home health care/homemaker sessions to 9 hours over a 7-day week. This may be satisfactory for some patients, but many older people require ongoing supervision to compensate for cognitive deficits, physical assistance to perform regular toilet or commode transfers, and community-based transportation to attend outpatient visits, shop, and bank.

All possible resources must be explored in the informal care network surrounding older patients to maintain them in their own homes. The economic resources of the patient, including personal income and health insurance benefits, determine the consuming power of the older adult who requires purchase of formal services and durable medical equipment to be maintained in his/her own home. Yet, many middle-class American elderly, who are beneficiaries of Social Security and Medicare as well as secondary forms of health insurance, and who have good pension plans, cannot afford to live at home and pay for part-time or full-time home care services when necessary.

12. Is relocation to a planned community for the elderly a reliable option?

Many planned communities are being developed in this country that promise lifetime supervision and care regardless of intensity of need. However, these are expensive to buy into and are considered either risky investments or a compromise in control for some elderly people who have experienced immigration, a major economic depression, and several world wars. Some local communities have active, government-supported Agencies on Aging (AOA) that can subsidize the purchase of home-care services for income-limited disabled older adults, but medical and functional justification must be argued and waiting-lists can be long. Consultation with the social work department of the hospital or of a long-term care facility is the best strategy for implementing these recommendations.

13. What is deconditioning?

Deconditioning is a syndrome of negative anatomic and physiologic effects resulting from inactivity, bedrest, and sedentary lifestyle. With therapeutic exercise programs that primarily aim to increase cardiopulmonary endurance and muscle strength and endurance, these effects are reversible. Bedrest and inactivity can be viewed as sometimes necessary treatments in acutely ill people, but with undesirable side effects, i.e., the deconditioning syndrome.

The Deconditioning Syndrome: Effects of Inactivity and Bedrest

Musculoskeletal
 Joint contractures
  Arthrogenic
  Soft tissue contracture
  Myogenic contracture
 Muscle weakness and atrophy
 Decreased coordination
 Osteoporosis

Integument
 Skin atrophy
 Pressure sores

Cardiovascular
 Orthostatic hypotension
 Increased resting heart rate
 Elevated systolic blood pressure
 Reduced stroke volume
 Decline in cardiac output
 Stasis of blood flow
 Increased coagulability

Endocrine/Metabolic
 Carbohydrate intolerance
 Increase in serum parathyroid hormone
 Decreased androgen level and
  spermatogenesis
 Increased daily nitrogen loss
 Negative calcium balance
 Decreased Na, K

Genitourinary
 Increased incidence of bladder/renal stones,
  UTI, and difficulty in voiding
 Incomplete bladder emptying

Respiratory
 Diminished tidal volumes, minute volumes,
  and maximal breathing capacity
 Reduction in vital capacity and functional
  reserve capacity
 Increased respiratory rate
 Uneven distribution of secretions, difficulty
  in clearance of secretions
 Impaired coughing mechanism/reduced
  bronchial ciliary activity

Gastrointestinal
 Loss of appetite
 Atrophy of intestinal mucosa and glands
 Slower rate of absorption
 Distaste for protein-rich foods
 Constipation
 Inhibition of peristalsis

Neural
 Sensory deprivation
 Impaired balance and coordination
 Confusion and disorientation
 Anxiety and depression
 Decreased intellectual capacity

14. How are the functional consequences of deconditioning evaluated?

The assessment of the functional consequences of deconditioning focuses on cardiopulmonary endurance and on muscle strength and endurance. The length of time of required bedrest should be established, as well as the level of activity prior to bedrest. The less active a person is before necessary bedrest, and the longer the period of inactivity, the more deconditioned and the longer it will take for this person to remobilize to an acceptable activity level during recovery.

The **cardiopulmonary effects** of deconditioning are fairly evident on physical examination during informal exercise tolerance testing as the reversal of cardiopulmonary conditioning or training effects: orthostatic hypotension, resting tachycardia (at least 90 bpm), abrupt increase in heart rate and respiratory rate (and sometimes systolic blood pressure) in response to minimal activity, and prolonged time to re-achieve baseline heart rate and blood pressure after discontinuing exercise. During one-trial manual **muscle testing**, strength and active range of motion may be interpreted as normal. Poor muscle endurance will be observed, however, only during repetitive (e.g., 10-trial) antigravity movements. Soft-tissue contractures (especially shoulders and heel cords) may be evident only at end-range.

Poor cardiopulmonary fitness, muscle endurance, and weakness from inactivity may not necessarily be manifest without observing the patient trying to rise from a supine position, arising from a chair, reaching overhead, or standing/weight-shifting in place for 20–30 seconds. A pattern of proximal weakness often is observed during deconditioning, since the larger muscle groups of the shoulder and hip girdles are more demanding of oxygen during antigravity movements.

15. Can deconditioning be avoided in these severely ill patients?

The effects of deconditioning can be disastrous for an older adult. Simple bedside therapeutic exercises, initiated even in the intensive care unit during the acute phase of illness and recovery, can alleviate inactivity effects:

> Clearance out of bed to a chair for upright (not reclined or semireclined) sitting and progressive sitting protocols
> Bathroom privileges to a bedside commode
> Progressive gentle strengthening, endurance, and range of motion exercises and ventilatory muscle exercises
> Ankle pumps to facilitate lower limb venous return
> Bedside sitting, standing and weight-shifting activities
> Progressive daily ambulation trials

Many of these therapeutic exercises can be supervised by nursing staff after consultation with physical and occupational therapists.

BIBLIOGRAPHY

1. Applegate WB, Blass JP, Williams TF: Instruments for the functional assessment of older patients. N Engl J Med 322:1201–1214, 1990.
2. Fleming KC, Evans JM, Weber DC, Chutka DS: Practical functional assessment of elderly persons: A primary-care approach. Mayo Clinic Proc 70:890–910, 1995.
3. Graafmans WC, Ooms ME, Hofstee HMA, et al: Falls in the elderly: A prosective study of risk factors and risk profiles. Am J Epidemiol 143:1129–1136, 1996.
4. Guralnik JM, Ferrucci L, Simonsick EM, Salive ME: Lower extremity function in persons over the age of 70 years as a predictor of subsequent disability. N Engl J Med 332:556–561, 1995.
5. Mathias S, Nayak US, Isaacs B: Balance in elderly patients: The "get-up and go" test. Arch Phys Med Rehabil 67:387–389, 1986.
6. Sandel ME, Robinson KM, Goldberg G, et al: Neurorehabilitation. In Cruz J (ed): Neurologic and Neurosurgical Emergencies. Philadelphia, W.B. Saunders, 1998, pp 503–546.
7. Seeman TE, Charpentier PA, Berkman LF, et al: Predicting changes in physical performance in a high-functioning elderly cohort: MacArthur studies of successful aging. J Gerontol 49:M97–M108, 1994.
8. Siebens H: Deconditioning. In Kemp B, Brummel-Smith K, Rarnsdell JW (eds): Geriatric Rehabilitation. Boston, Little, Brown, 1990, pp 177–191.

25. PERIOPERATIVE MANAGEMENT

Jerry Johnson, M.D., and Harold Mignott, M.D.

1. Does chronologic age affect the risk for adverse postoperative events?

Although many studies show that older patients have a higher mortality rate than younger patients, chronologic age is not the major predictor of postoperative outcome when other factors are considered. The most important predictors of postoperative morbidity and mortality in the elderly are the urgency of the procedure and the presence of coexisting illness, particularly cardiac and pulmonary disease. Many studies of postoperative outcomes in the elderly combine patients undergoing elective and emergency surgeries as well as low-risk patients with few coexisting diseases and patients with multiple coexisting diseases. Chronologic age should not be viewed as an independent risk factor for postoperative complications, and surgery should not be denied solely on the basis of age.

2. Why is it important to understand preoperative assessment in the elderly?

Preoperative assessment in older patients is important because of the high probability that older patients will require surgery and because of the increased risk of morbidity and mortality in the elderly. Surgical rates are 55% higher in patients over age 65, and 40% of admissions of older patients to general hospitals are for surgical services. Older patients account for 75% of all postoperative deaths.

Although the trend in studies of perioperative outcomes in the elderly is toward a decreasing mortality rate, postoperative mortality is higher among elderly than among younger adults. The surgical mortality rate of patients over age 65 undergoing cardiac revascularization procedures is about 5% compared with 1% in younger adults. Typical postoperative mortality rates of older patients undergoing major intraabdominal surgery range from 3–5%, about twice that of persons under age 65.

3. How does the type of surgical procedure affect perioperative outcomes?

Surgeries that involve the thoracic or abdominal cavities confer the greatest postoperative risk. Low-risk surgeries, with mortality rates substantially < 1%, include cataract surgery, hernia repair, and transurethral resection of the prostate. On the other hand, cardiac and peripheral vascular procedures such as abdominal aortic aneurysm repair confer the highest risk, ranging from 3–10% on average. Emergency surgery (surgery occurring within 24 hours of admission to the hospital) doubles to quadruples the risk of mortality for any given procedure.

4. What is the role of the general medical or geriatric medical consultant in evaluating a patient during the preoperative period?

The often-used concept of "clearing" the patient for surgery is misleading in that one cannot provide absolute assurance that no adverse events will occur in patients undergoing surgery in any age group. The goals of the preoperative assessment are to identify risk factors, to quantify the magnitude of the risk factors (if possible), and to offer recommendations to correct factors that are correctable.

5. What chronic problems should be considered in the evaluation of older patients?

In addition to acute medical problems (i.e., cardiac or pulmonary disorders and infections), the consultant also should screen for the presence of chronic problems:

Preexisting dementia predisposes to delirium, which may then lead to a cycle of dehydration, malnutrition, deconditioning, and acute infections. However, studies have not evaluated dementia as an independent risk factor.

Depression predisposes to dehydration and deconditioning.

Malnutrition or undernutrition has been shown in several studies to be associated with significantly higher mortality (among patients with > 20% weight loss preoperatively). However, whether nutritional supplements in the preoperative phase improve surgical outcome is highly controversial. Most experts agree that delaying surgery to provide preoperative nutrition is not warranted except, possibly, for the severely malnourished.

Parkinsonism can lead to deconditioning, falls, and prolonged recovery.

Prostate disease can lead to urinary retention and subsequent infections.

All of above chronic disorders carry the risk of predisposing the patient to the development of pressure ulcers.

6. Does decreased mobility or exercise tolerance affect the postoperative outcome?

Decreased mobility or exercise tolerance is an important nonspecific predictor in the elderly, because of its association not only with adverse cardiac outcomes but also with mortality in general. In one study comparing active vs. inactive patients for surgical complications, active was defined as able to leave home by one's own efforts at least twice weekly. All complications, including life-threatening complications, were more frequent in the inactive patients. Another study indicates that the inability to exercise sufficiently (i.e., to attain a heart rate of 100 bpm) is predictive of postoperative cardiac ischemic events.

7. What information should be sought by the medical history?

The frequency of multiple comorbidities in elderly patients necessitates a comprehensive history and physical examination. The **cardiac history** should attempt to identify the past evidence of coronary artery disease or congestive heart failure. A myocardial infarction in the previous 6 months, active congestive heart failure, and unstable angina confer substantial risk of postoperative cardiac complications. With the exception of extreme levels, chronic hypertension does not increase the risk of postoperative complications. However, evidence of recent fluctuations in blood pressure or new-onset hypertension may indicate instability during the procedure. The **pulmonary history** should attempt to identify the presence of chronic obstructive pulmonary disease or asthma.

A past history of **thromboembolic events** involving the lower extremities or pulmonary emboli is a substantial risk factor for postoperative thromboembolic events. These complications are seen most frequently in **orthopedic surgery of the knee and hip** and in pelvic or intra-abdominal surgery for malignant conditions. About 40–60% of patients undergoing hip fracture repair sustain deep venous thrombosis, and 20% experience at least one pulmonary embolus.

8. What information can be obtained by the physical examination?

The **cardiac exam** should aim to detect the presence of active heart failure or a cardiac murmur, particularly aortic stenosis, the most common valvular disease in the elderly. The physician should listen carefully for an S_3 heart sound and examine the patient for an increased jugulovenous pulse. Bradycardia, tachycardia, and irregularities suggesting ectopic beats can be detected by physical examination. The pulses should be examined carefully, and any evidence of edema should be recorded. The physician should take note of decreased breath sounds, which may suggest chronic obstructive pulmonary disease, rales, or bronchospasms, which may suggest pulmonary disease or heart failure.

The **neuropsychiatric exam** is aimed at determining whether the patient has cognitive impairment, acute or chronic depression, evidence of Parkinson's disease, or focal weakness. The patient should be observed ambulating for evidence of potential deconditioning and gait instability, which may be exacerbated during the postoperative period.

9. Which preoperative indexes are useful in predicting postoperative complications?

Anesthesiologists have long used **Dripps' Physical Status Scale**, which classifies patients in five groups from class I (healthy persons) to class V (patients who are moribund and not expected to survive 24 hours with or without the operation). This scale, although useful in predicting the postoperative complications in patients in the extreme classes, does less well as a predictor in classes II, III, and IV. More importantly, it gives no insight into correctable factors.

The **cardiac risk index (CRI)**, a predictor of postoperative cardiac outcomes in noncardiac surgery, is the best known predictive tool. Nine independent risk factors of adverse cardiac outcomes have been identified and assigned points as follows:

VARIABLE	ASSIGNED POINTS
Third heart sound (S_3)	11
Elevated jugulovenous pressure	11
Myocardial infarction in past 6 months	10
EKG shows > 5 premature ventricular contractions per minute	7
EKG shows premature atrial contractions or any rhythm other than sinus	7
Age > 70 years	5
Emergency procedure	4
Intrathoracic, intraabdominal, or aortic surgery	3
Poor general status: metabolic or bedridden	3

These nine factors are used to classify patients into four categories of risk as follows:

CLASS	POINT TOTAL	NO OR MINOR COMPLICATIONS (%)	LIFE-THREATENING COMPLICATIONS(%)	CARDIAC DEATH (%)
I	0–5	99	0.7	0.2
II	6–12	93	5	2
III	13–25	86	11	2
IV	> 26	22	22	56

Rather than memorize the point system, bear in mind that patients over age 70 who undergo an intraabdominal, intrathoracic, or aortic procedure and who have any of the first five factors above have a total of 13 points, sufficient to place them in one of the two highest risk categories by this scale. Detsky modified the CRI, adding points for unstable angina, pulmonary edema, and class II or III status by the Canadian Cardiovascular Society Scale for angina. Eagle derived a third, simpler cardiac index (discussed in question 11) in patients undergoing vascular surgery. High scores on the CRI or Detsky indexes are greater than 12 or 15 points, and a high score on the Eagle index is greater than 3 criteria. Multiple studies have indicated that low-risk categories in these clinical indexes tend to underestimate the risk of cardiac complications in patients undergoing peripheral vascular procedures.

10. Which routine preoperative tests should be obtained?

The purpose of preoperative testing is to uncover diseases and problems unrecognized by the history and physical examination or to confirm the diagnosis suspected by the history and examination. Routine tests that should be obtained in all elderly patients include the following:
- Fasting glucose: screens for diabetes
- Complete blood count: may indicate the presence of infection or anemia
- Electrolytes, blood urea nitrogen, and creatinine: may indicate the risk of arrhythmias
- Chest radiograph: screens for occult pulmonary disease
- EKG—detects ischemia or arrhythmias

11. When are noninvasive cardiac tests indicated?

Because of the concern about postoperative ischemic events, **thallium testing**, most often with dipyridamole, has become almost a routine procedure before all surgery in the elderly in some medical centers (15–90%). Such a routine approach is not indicated. Because patients at low risk require no intervention and patients at high risk are known candidates for revascularization, imaging studies are most useful for patients at intermediate risk. As defined by Eagle and colleagues, intermediate risks can be identified by Q waves on the resting EKG, history of ventricular ectopy requiring treatment, diabetes, and known angina. A complex guideline from the American College of Cardiology/American Heart Association (ACC/AHA) combines the type of procedure (i.e., vascular procedures are high-risk procedures), exercise capacity, prior evidence of coronary disease, and other clinical indicators, such as diabetes, into an algorithm that determines whether screening tests should be obtained. The American College of Physicians has created a similar but less complex guideline. Most importantly, experts agree that preoperative cardiac imaging to lower the risk of surgery should be obtained only in patients in whom a prophylactic cardiac surgical intervention is indicated, regardless of the preoperative context.

An **echocardiogram** may be useful in persons in whom a systolic murmur is suspicious for aortic stenosis. Measures of left ventricular ejection fraction are useful in quantifying risks in patients undergoing cardiac procedures. For noncardiac procedures, such studies are not indicated in the preoperative period in asymptomatic patients. Holter monitoring and exercise testing are not consistently useful in asymptomatic patients.

12. When is invasive monitoring required?

Right-heart catheterization is indicated in patients undergoing major vascular procedures and in patients with active heart failure, significant aortic stenosis, unstable angina, or recent myocardial infarction. Under other circumstances, right-heart catheterization adds marginal information to that which can be obtained by a careful and thorough history and physical examination and testing described above.

13. When are pulmonary function tests indicated?

All procedures do not confer an increased risk of pulmonary complications. Thus, age > 65 or 70 is not an absolute indication for pulmonary function testing. All patients undergoing lung resection should undergo pulmonary function testing first. Patients undergoing incisions of the upper abdomen or thorax probably should undergo pulmonary function testing, especially if the following factors are present: cough, known chronic obstructive pulmonary disease, cigarette smoking, dyspnea, or other known pulmonary disease. On the other hand, orthopedic procedures and procedures of the lower abdomen confer minimal risk of pulmonary compromise; thus, pulmonary function tests are not indicated in asymptomatic patients.

Because body size and age affect pulmonary function tests, and because there is a paucity of data about normal pulmonary function tests in people over age 75, the most appropriate cutoffs to apply in the elderly as predictors of respiratory complications are uncertain. Furthermore, most studies of pulmonary risks have enrolled people with known lung disease, particularly chronic obstructive pulmonary disease. These data may not apply to the elderly in general. Nevertheless, the data suggest the following cutoffs as predictors of significant respiratory complications:

- PCO_2 > 45 mmHg
- FEV_1 < 2 L (particularly < 1 L)
- Maximal ventilatory volume < 50% predicted

14. What specific preoperative recommendations are useful?

General recommendations. Cessation of smoking is helpful, but must be undertaken at least 2 weeks before surgery. Training in coughing and deep breathing should be undertaken before surgery. If chronic obstructive pulmonary disease is present, aggressive use of bronchodilators should be implemented both pre- and postoperatively. Of course, any pulmonary infections must be treated before the operation.

Thromboembolism. Prophylaxis of thromboembolic events is based on the type of procedure and the patient's level of risk. In many cases, low–molecular-weight heparin (LMWH), low-dose unfractionated heparin, and warfarin are effective in lowering the risk of thromboembolus. LMWH requires no monitoring and has a lower incidence of thrombocytopenia than unfractionated heparin, but it is more expensive. In general, when started preoperatively, once-daily LMWH is effective, but when it is started postoperatively, twice-daily dosing is superior. Warfarin has the disadvantage of requiring extensive monitoring. Hirudin, a polypeptide derived from leeches that directly inactivates thrombin, is an expensive alternative that may cause fewer bleeding complications than LMWH. Minidose warfarin (1 mg) daily and aspirin are consistently ineffective compared with alternatives. Pneumatic compression stockings, although more effective than placebo, are less effective than other options.

For **high-risk general surgery patients** and for most nonorthopedic surgery, low-dose unfractionated heparin and LMWH are comparable. Patients undergoing surgery because of an intraabdominal or pelvic malignancy should receive low-dose heparin begun on the day of surgery. In the elderly, a dose of 5,000–7,500 units every 12 hours is usually adequate. LMWH with or without intermittent pneumatic compression is also effective.

Among **high-risk orthopedic surgery patients**, the recommendations vary with the type of procedure. Patients undergoing **hip replacement** have three options. LMWH and warfarin produce comparable reductions in thromboemboli. In a direct comparison, LMWH was superior to warfarin, but meta-analyses have found them comparable or found that that LMWH has a small advantage. Both are more effective than low-dose unfractionated heparin. The dose of LMWH varies with the compound. Results are comparable among the agents tested if they are used twice daily starting postoperatively (12–24 hr) or once daily starting preoperatively (8–12 hr). Warfarin should be initiated on the evening before surgery at 10 mg and adjusted subsequently to maintain the international normalized ratio (INR) in the 2.0–3.0 range. In one study, hirudin was superior to LMWH when used in a fixed dose twice daily, beginning 30 minutes preoperatively. Patients undergoing repair of a **hip fracture** also have three options, but which agent is optimal is unclear. In a meta-analysis, low-dose unfractionated heparin was comparable to LMWH. Low-dose warfarin (prothrombin time 1.5 times control) confers a reduction in deep vein thrombosis comparable to heparin, although the one study that directly compared warfarin and LMWH found LMWH slightly more effective. In patients undergoing **total knee replacement**, LMWH is superior to warfarin but must be begun 12 hours postoperatively to prevent bleeding complications. Minidose warfarin (1 mg) and aspirin are much less effective than the other alternatives for any of the three types of orthopedic surgery.

Pneumatic compression stockings should be used in patients undergoing **neurosurgery**.

Cardiac medications. In patients at risk of postoperative ischemia, antianginal medications should be maximized. Antihypertensive therapy, particularly with a beta blocker or alpha$_2$ blocker (e.g., clonidine), should be continued at the preoperative dose up to and including the day of surgery. Heart failure and clinically significant arrhythmias (most commonly atrial fibrillation) should be controlled before surgery. Patients with coronary artery disease or who are at risk of coronary artery disease should be treated with a beta blocker to lower the heart rate to 55–60 beats per minute before and up to 7 days after surgery.

Coronary artery revascularization. Prophylactic coronary artery bypass surgery for the sole purpose of preventing a perioperative event is unwarranted. No randomized clinical trials have tested the hypothesis that prophylactic coronary artery bypass grafting or angioplasty in the preoperative period is warranted, and the morbidity and mortality of the prophylactic coronary procedure must be considered in comparing the risks of revascularization with the risks of no revascularization. In general, the physician should perform a revascularization procedure only if it would be performed in the absence of the surgical procedure.

15. How should pain be prevented and controlled during the perioperative period?

Pain is one of the major components of a wide range of neural, endocrine, metabolic, immunologic, and inflammatory changes that constitute the stress response to surgery. Recent evidence has shown that surgical trauma induces processes of nervous system sensitization that contribute to and enhance postoperative pain and leads to chronic pain, providing a rational basis for proactive, preoperative analgesic strategies. The precipitous rise in catecholamines and corticosteroids postoperatively elevates the risk of a cardiac ischemic event. Pain after operation is the most important factor responsible for regional impairment of ventilation. Abdominal pain activates a spinal reflex arc with sympathetic hyperactivity that inhibits intestinal propulsive activity. Finally, elderly patients are more sensitive to the effects of analgesia and sedatives, making them more sensitive to the adverse consequences of the high doses of analgesics required once pain is fully developed.

The optimal form of pain treatment is applied pre-, intra-, and postoperatively to preempt the establishment of pain hypersensitivity both during and after surgery. Systemic opioid analgesia given on demand postoperatively is often poorly effective and should not be used as the mainstay of treatment. Practitioners have several options to manage pain effectively, beginning preoperatively. NSAIDs, such as diclofenac (75 mg over 30–120 minutes) or ketorolac (10–30 mg), can be initiated 1 hour preoperatively. Morphine, 5–10 mg preoperatively, can be given intravenously. Tramadol, which can be given orally, intramuscularly, or intravenously, may offer an advantage over standard opioids. Finally, many types of intraoperative regional blocks are effective but require skilled personnel.

Once pain has developed, many techniques have been used with varying degrees of success. Preoperative analgesics should be continued on a routine schedule. Patient-controlled analgesia allows patients to self-administer small boluses of an opioid, but patients must be mentally capable of managing the process. Intraoperative regional blocks can be continued postoperatively.

16. What should be the focus of postoperative care?

In the postoperative period, continuation of monitoring and treatment of risk factors uncovered during the preoperative care are most important. The most important factors at this point are ischemic heart disease, heart failure, arrhythmias, thromboemboli, respiratory complications, delirium, and general deconditioning. The patient should be monitored for the development of heart failure, angina or myocardial infarction, and arrhythmias. An EKG on days 1 and 2 identifies 96% of postoperative myocardial infarctions. About one-half of patients with known coronary artery disease develop frequent or nonsustained ventricular tachycardia that does not require aggressive monitoring unless accompanied by a myocardial infarction. Continued monitoring and prevention of deep venous thrombosis with anticoagulants are essential until the patient is mobile. Judicious use of analgesics is vital, but sometimes they must be discontinued because of delirium. Exercise is important for general reconditioning as well as prevention of thromboemboli. An individualized exercise program under the direction of a physical therapist is warranted in most patients.

BIBLIOGRAPHY

1. Dalen J, Hirsh J: Fourth American College of Chest Physicians Consensus Conference on Antithrombotic Therapy. Chest 108(Suppl):225S–522S, 1995.
2. Eagle KA, Brundage BH, Chaitman BR, et al: Guidelines for perioperative cardiovascular evaluation for noncardiac surgery. Report of the American College of Cardiology-American Heart Association Task Force on Practice Guidelines. J Am Coll Cardiol 27:910–948, 1996.
3. Eagle KA, Coley M, Newell JB, et al: Combining clinical and thallium data optimizes pre-operative assessment of cardiac risk before major vascular surgery. Ann Intern Med 110:859–886, 1989.
4. Johnson J: Surgical principles in the aged. In Gallo J, Busby-Whitehead J, Rabins P, et al (eds): Reichel's Care of the Elderly: Clinical Aspects of Aging. Philadelphia, Lippincott-Williams & Wilkins, 1999, pp 536–542.
5. Mangano D, Goldman L: Preoperative assessment of patients with known or suspected coronary disease. N Engl J Med 333:1750–1757, 1995.
6. Mangano D, Layung E, Wallace A, Tateo I: Effect of atenolol on mortality and cardiovascular morbidity after non-cardiac surgery. N Engl J Med 335:1713–1720, 1996.
7. Morrison RS: The medical consultant's role in caring for patients with hip fracture. Ann Intern Med 128:1010–1020, 1998.
8. Richardson J, Bresland K: The management of postsurgical pain in the elderly population. Drugs Aging 13:17–31, 1998.
9. Weitz J: Low-molecular-weight heparins. N Engl J Med 337:688–697, 1997.
10. Zibrak JD, O'Donnell CK, Morton K: Indications for pulmonary function testing. Ann Intern Med 112:763, 1990.

26. ADVANCE DIRECTIVES

Joel E. Streim, M.D.

1. What is an advance directive?

A written document, completed by a competent person, that aims to guide health care decisions in the event that the person should become unable to communicate medical preferences or participate in medical decision-making.

2. What are the three different types of advance directives?

Instruction directives indicate the types of treatment or treatment approaches that the person would want in various clinical situations. These typically focus on life-sustaining treatments, though they may also concern less critical treatments. This type of directive may be made informally, through oral instructions given to family members, friends, or caregivers, or formally in a written "living will."

Proxy directives designate someone whom the person wants to make health care decisions on his or her behalf if he or she becomes unable to do so. This is sometimes referred to as a durable power of attorney for health care decisions.

A **values history** may also contain advance directives. This may be a written, audiotaped, or videotaped personal discussion of the person's values and goals. It provides an opportunity to make known one's specific values, beliefs, and attitudes regarding life, longevity, quality of life, suffering, the dying process, and death.

3. Explain what is meant by "durable" power of attorney.

When a patient who is still competent designates a proxy decision-maker for health care matters, the patient continues to make autonomous decisions (i.e., without involvement of the proxy) as long as he or she remains competent. Decisions are not made by proxy until the patient becomes incapacitated, at which time the power of attorney "springs" into effect. (For this reason, "durable" power of attorney is sometimes called "springing" power of attorney.) From that point forward, the incapacitated person (whose judgment may now be impaired) cannot rescind the proxy appointment; hence, the power of attorney is said to be durable.

4. What does federal law require of patients regarding advance directives?

The Patient Self-Determination Act was passed by Congress as part of the Omnibus Budget Reconciliation Act of 1990 and became federal law in December 1991 (U.S. Public Law 101-508). Under this law, at the time of admission to an acute care hospital or nursing home that participates in Medicare or Medicaid programs, the admitting facility is required:

1. To ask patients if they have executed an advance directive
2. To furnish them with information about advance directives
3. To inform them of their rights under the law to execute such directives if they wish
4. To inform them of their rights to accept or refuse any form of medical treatment

All patients are thereby given the opportunity to make their preferences for future treatment known to their health care providers. However, patients are not required to draft directives or state their treatment preferences, and their eligibility for admission or treatment is not affected by their having or not having an advance directive.

5. Who should be responsible for discussing advance directives with elderly patients?

Although the staff in a hospital or nursing home admissions office may ask patients about their advance directives to comply with federal law, discussions regarding patient values and treatment preferences are probably best accomplished in the context of an ongoing primary care practitioner–patient relationship, as well as between the patient and trusted family members or friends who might later serve as proxy decision-makers.

6. Are patients who are old and frail likely to become upset when a health care provider asks them to consider hopeless situations or terminal illness?

Most patients who are in the late stages of life, including those who are near death, are relieved when someone asks about their concerns regarding the end of life. Most of them also appreciate the opportunity to express their preferences for how their health care is to be managed. The relatively few patients who are anxious about such matters will decline to discuss them or may be so highly defensive that they deny such discussions are applicable to them personally.

7. How should the discussion about advance directives be focused?

While there are no established standards for these discussions, some attempts to develop guidelines in recent years have emphasized the need for patients to communicate a set of life values, even more than choices about specific treatments. This is because it is impossible for patients to anticipate all of the possible future illness and treatment situations, coupled with the presumption that a surrogate or proxy decision-maker will be better able to make a decision that reflects what the patient would have chosen for him or herself if that surrogate is well-informed about the patient's overall values. It is not expected that such discussions will be completed in one session. Getting to know a patient's values is a process that occurs over a series of visits and ideally in the context of an ongoing relationship.

Health care providers must appreciate the ways in which religious beliefs, ethnic background, and family values influence health care directives and decisions. It is important to inquire about the patient's cultural and family background and belief system, so that resultant health care choices can be respected and supported even when based on values that differ from those of the provider. Inclusion of close family members or friends in discussions of values and health care preferences is especially helpful, because they are often in the best position to appreciate nuances of the patient's culture and beliefs, to accept those important factors that serve as the foundation for the patient's directives, and to support the patient's choices regarding future health care.

8. Are health care providers and facilities legally bound to follow all advance directives contained in living wills?

No. Not all states have laws that recognize living wills. For those states that now have living will statutes, most only recognize directives that apply to situations in which a person becomes hopelessly or terminally ill; these states stipulate that patients' directives can be implemented only in conformity with existing laws, including those dealing with suicide and euthanasia. When a patient's living will addresses clinical conditions that are not hopeless or imminently terminal, or when their directives call for health care options that would violate state or federal law, health care providers and facilities are not legally bound to follow the directives.

Even in situations that do not entail conflict with the law, health care providers sometimes find that a patient's advance directive is in conflict with the provider's personal or professional values. When this occurs, the health care provider or facility has the option of transferring the patient to the care of a provider or facility that can better abide by the patient's wishes.

9. In what situations are advance directives unlikely to be followed by health professionals and family members?

Conflicts may be more likely to arise when the patient's advance directive applies to a condition in which it is the patient's wish that a specific life-sustaining intervention be withheld or, if already in place when such a condition arises, withdrawn. Although many health care professionals, clergy, and families are able to accept a directive to withhold or withdraw a life-sustaining intervention, others regard such a directive as a form of assisted suicide, passive euthanasia, or even murder. Some find it especially objectionable to withdraw a life-sustaining intervention that is already in place because of the belief that it gives them a more "active" role in bringing about the patient's death. Sometimes the acceptability of withholding or withdrawing a life-sustaining measure is determined by whether available treatment for the condition is considered futile or offers reasonable hope of meaningful benefit.

In such scenarios, whether or not treatment is considered futile, there is often disagreement about whether the patient's advance directive should be followed. Although such disagreements are sometimes brought before hospital ethics committees or adjudicated by the courts, most cases are resolved by discussion among health care professionals, clergy, family members, and friends who care for the patient.

10. Is there a legal standard for competency to execute an advance directive?

No. While there are legal standards for testamentary capacity and competency to manage one's affairs, there are no specific guidelines for competency to execute an advance directive. All adults are presumed competent to state their treatment preferences and execute an advance directive under the Patient Self-Determination Act, unless a plenary guardian of the person has been appointed under state law.

11. What happens if cognitive impairment prevents an older adult from establishing an advance directive?

Only a small minority of elderly patients with cognitive impairment are ever brought to court and adjudicated incompetent. After a person has been adjudicated incapacitated or incompetent, under most state laws he or she cannot execute valid advance directives in his or her own behalf. The court-appointed guardian of the person then is empowered to make subsequent health care decisions in the patient's behalf. However, if the patient established a power of attorney for health care matters *before* becoming incapacitated, that power of attorney springs into effect at the time the patient is found on *clinical* grounds to be incapacitated. In such cases, a legal determination of incapacity is usually not necessary.

The remainder of cognitively impaired elders retain their full legal rights to issue advance directives in their own behalf. In some cases, they continue to establish advance directives with insufficient comprehension of what they are choosing, or at the other extreme, clinicians or family members may prematurely usurp their right to make their own decisions. In other cases, when clinicians and family members believe that a patient is losing the cognitive capacity to make such decisions, they informally begin to assist in the decision-making process. Patients with some preserved cognitive function may be allowed to continue to participate in that decision-making process, expressing values and preferences that are then taken into consideration as health care providers and family members make final decisions. As cognitive impairment worsens to the point where the patient is no longer able to understand, deliberate, or communicate anything meaningful about future health care choices, an informal decision-maker is designated. Thus, even in the absence of a legally appointed decision-maker, decisions regarding future health care choices are still made, with the patient fully autonomous, partially included, or fully excluded from the process. The law does not dictate how this should be properly accomplished when patients have less than full decision-making capacity.

12. How should the clinician determine a patient's cognitive capacity to create an advance directive?

In the case of clear and total incapacity (e.g., a persistent vegetative state or coma), it is obvious that the patient cannot formulate advance directives, and there is even no legal obligation to inform the patient of their right to do so. However, in all other cases, on admission to hospitals and nursing homes, patients are required by law to be informed of their right to formulate advance directives and are presumed legally competent to establish such directives. This stands in contrast to epidemiologic estimates that approximately 6 million people in the United States have significant cognitive impairment that renders them clinically incapable of making their own health care decisions. However, no formal clinical standards exist for determining when a patient's cognitive impairment precludes them from being capable of formulating an advance directive or, conversely, when the situation safely permits a cognitively impaired patient to participate in this process.

Nevertheless, during discussions regarding the patient's rights and options in formulating advance directives, clinicians have opportunities to appraise the capacity of patients to:

1. Maintain a stable set of values and goals
2. Comprehend the relevant information
3. Reason and deliberate about their choices
4. Appreciate the situation and its possible outcomes
5. Communicate their choices

When the patient's responses during the informing process give the clinician reason to question the patient's decision-making capacity, it is still left to the clinician to judge how best to balance preservation of the patient's right to make autonomous decisions with the obligation of the clinician to protect a vulnerable patient from making flawed decisions that do not truly reflect the patient's values and goals. Many ethicists and legal scholars have suggested that in determining capacity to formulate advance directives, it is preferable for the clinician to err on the side of promoting patient autonomy. However, this debate about **autonomy** vs. **beneficence** is not yet resolved.

13. What is the role of ethics committees in disputes about the patient's ability to participate in the formulation of advance directives?

In many situations, clinicians and family members are able to reach a consensus or agreement regarding the extent to which a patient can participate in the formulation of advance directives. However, when a disagreement cannot be resolved among those who share responsibility for the care of the patient, an ethics committee may play a helpful role, and this approach is generally preferable to resorting to remedies through the legal system. Most hospital ethics committees do not render binding decisions but rather serve in a consultative capacity. They focus the goals of the deliberation, clarify the facts of the case, identify values in conflict, and make recommendations for dealing with conflicts to facilitate decision-making. Unfortunately, for patients residing in the community or in long-term care facilities, the availability of ethics committees is limited.

14. Should elderly patients with mild to moderate cognitive impairment be advised to formulate a durable power of attorney even if they are incapable of making a living will?

Yes. Some elderly patients who are already cognitively impaired at the time they choose to formulate an advance directive may not have the capacity to make a living will, but they may still be capable of appointing a health care proxy and should be given the opportunity to do so for legal, ethical, and pragmatic reasons. This important step can avert the need to petition for legal guardianship at a later date when the patient is totally incapacitated. In most states, appointment of a health care proxy is much simpler, less costly, and less time-consuming than establishing a guardianship.

15. What standards or guidelines exist for surrogate decision-making by persons appointed as proxies or guardians?

There are two main ethical standards by which surrogates can make health care decisions on behalf of incapacitated patients. The preferred standard is **substituted judgment**. This directs the surrogate to choose what he or she believes the patient would have chosen. If the surrogate decision-maker has no knowledge of what the patient would want in a given situation, then the surrogate can follow the **best interest principle**. This directs the surrogate to make the choice that is most likely to serve the best interests of the patient. When surrogates are faced with difficult decisions and unclear parameters on which to base their decisions, they can appeal for advice from health care professionals, attorneys, and hospital ethics committees. In some communities, guardianship advisory services have recently been developed.

BIBLIOGRAPHY

1. Fazel S, Hope T, Jacoby R: Assessment of competence to complete advance directives: Validation of a patient centered approach. BMJ 318:493–497, 1999.
2. Gerety MB, Chiodo LK, Kanten DN, et al: Medical treatment preferences of nursing home residents: Relationship to function and concordance with surrogate decision-makers. J Am Geriatr Soc 41:953–960, 1993.
3. Grossberg GT: Advance directives, competency evaluation, and surrogate management in elderly patients. Am J Geriatr Psychiatry 6(2 Suppl 1):579–584, 1998.
4. Kern SR: Issues of competency in the aged. Psychiatr Ann 17:336–339, 1987.
5. Lee DL, Swinburne AJ, Fedullo AJ, Wahl GW: Withdrawing care: Experience in a medical intensive care unit. JAMA 271:1358–1361, 1994.
6. Omnibus Budget Reconciliation Act, 1990. U.S. Public Law 101-508, sect 4206 and 4751.
7. Ott BB: Advance directives: The emerging body of research. Am J Crit Care 8:514–519, 1999.
8. President's Commission for the Study of Ethical Problems in Medicine and Biomedical and Behavioral Research: Making Health Care Decisions, vol 1. Washington, D.C., Government Printing Office, 1982.
9. Rich BA: Advance directives: The next generation. J Legal Med 19:63–97, 1998.
10. Singer PA, Siegler M: Advancing the cause of advance directives. Arch Intern Med 152:22–24, 1992.
11. Tulsky JA, Fischer GS, Rose MR, Arnold RM: Opening the black box: How do physicians communicate about advance directives? Ann Intern Med 129:441–449, 1998.

27. PALLIATIVE CARE

Janet Abrahm, M.D.

1. What are the major types of pain? How do they present?

There are three main types of pain: somatic, visceral, and neuropathic. **Somatic pain**, such as postoperative pain or pain from bony metastases, arises from cutaneous or deep tissues. The pain is usually very well-localized and is dull or aching in character.

Visceral pain, arising from organ infiltration, compression, or stretching, is poorly localized, deep, squeezing, and pressure-like. It may be referred to cutaneous sites, such as the diaphragmatic pain that is felt in the shoulder region. When it is acute, there is often associated nausea, vomiting, or sweating. Patients with an acute myocardial infarction, cholecystitis, bowel obstruction, or liver enlargement due to tumor infiltration present with visceral pain.

Neuropathic pain arises from traumatic or ischemic injury to the peripheral or central nervous systems or from nerve infiltration, compression, or other damage. The pain is usually severe, burning, or vise-like, but is occasionally shooting, like an electric shock. Patients with diabetic or alcoholic neuropathy or herpes zoster have neuropathic pain, as do patients with spinal cord compression.

Pain complaints also may arise in people who have no anatomic lesions. The pain complaint may be the only manner in which the patient is able to express nonspecific feelings of distress caused by anxiety, financial problems, anger, loneliness, depression, or grief over poor health or lost relatives. Because these concerns may exacerbate any concomitant painful sensations, alleviating them can treat the cause of the distress and thereby significantly decrease the need for pain medications.

2. What are the components of an adequate pain assessment?

Effective pain management requires repeated, comprehensive assessment of the patient's pain(s). Although the elderly experience pain to the same degree as younger patients, they often under-report their pain, ascribing it to normal changes expected with aging. Scales that quantify patient reports of pain are valid, reliable, and reproducible. They should be used, much as a blood sugar determination is used in diabetes, to monitor the efficacy of therapy. Cognitively impaired patients may not be able to recall and compare pain levels before and after therapy has been introduced, but they can reliably report their pain at any given time. Repeated assessments, therefore, will accurately reflect the adequacy of the pain control.

If, for example, you are using a scale of 0 (no pain) to 10 (the worst pain imaginable), the change in the rating 1 hour after pain medication is given will indicate how to adjust the medication. The physician must determine both the intensity of the pain and the functional distress caused by the pain (e.g., is it interfering with the patient's ability to eat, sleep, interact with others, move, walk, or talk or with the patient's emotions or concentration). The goal is to lower the pain to a level acceptable to the patient.

3. How does chronic pain differ in its manifestations from acute pain?

Patients in chronic pain do not present the common autonomic manifestations of acute pain (i.e., tachycardia, elevated blood pressure, sweating, or facial grimacing). Such patients will often be quiet and withdrawn, manifesting little spontaneous movement; they can be depressed or irritable and will complain of discomfort if moved. When their pain is relieved, however, they often become mobile and engaged and involved with other people.

4. What common nonpharmacologic methods are effective for pain control?

Hypnosis: Simple hypnotic techniques to minimize patient anxiety and pain include rehearsing the planned test or procedure, distraction techniques (e.g., listening to music), and dissociation (e.g., daydreaming or imagining to be somewhere else). Even without formal hypnotic induction, the words used by the practitioner to describe procedures are very important. Using the phrase "You will feel something; everyone feels this a little differently" in place of "This is going to hurt a lot!" gives the patient permission to alter the sensation and also may diminish the experience of pain. Other cognitive therapies, such as relaxation training or psychological or spiritual counseling, are also helpful.

Hyperstimulation analgesia: Ice massage, using a paper cup filled with ice, is a form of hyperstimulation analgesia that is particularly well-accepted by elderly patients with cancer pain. **Acupuncture** can be helpful for patients with osteoarthritis or neuropathic pain. It is the intensity, not the precise site, of the mechanical stimulation that induces the anesthesia. This anesthesia is not simply due to placebo effect. **Transcutaneous electrical nerve stimulation** (TENS) devices using electrical hyperstimulation are indicated for patients with dermatomal pain, such as postherpetic neuralgia or radiculopathy from spinal cord compression. For optimal effect, a physiatrist or physical therapist familiar with the device should train the patient in its use.

Other: For arthritis pain, **dry heat** or **hydrotherapy** often is used, as is **physical therapy**, which maximizes function and minimizes disability. **Orthotic devices** or prostheses to reduce joint loading and minimize abnormal stresses can limit pain as well as progression of joint damage. Removing fluid from the joint also can provide relief. In certain patients with extensive deformities, synovectomy, joint replacement, or **other surgeries** are indicated for pain relief. **Trigger point injection** can provide relief for many patients with myofascial or certain neuropathic pain syndromes (e.g., post-thoracotomy pain).

5. How are the nonpharmacologic and pharmacologic therapies used for different types of pain?

Pain Regimens for Geriatric Patients

SEVERITY	FREQUENCY	TYPE	AGENTS
Mild	Intermittent	Somatic, visceral	Acetaminophen, COX-2 "selective" NSAID Nonacetylated salicylates (aspirin, NSAIDs)* Trigger point injection Nonpharmacologic means (hypnosis, ice massage, wet or dry heat) Orthotic devices
Moderate	Intermittent	Somatic, visceral	Combination agent (ASA, acetaminophen/NSAID with codeine, oxycodone, hydrocodone) Tramadol Acupuncture Hypnosis
	Intermittent or continuous	Neuropathic	Combination agent Tricyclic antidepressant or anticonvulsant Steroids, capsaicin TENS, hypnosis Peripheral nerve, ganglion block, lysis
Severe	Intermittent	Somatic, visceral, neuropathic	Strong, short-acting opioids Tricyclic antidepressants Nonacetylated salicylates or acetaminophen
	Continuous	Somatic, visceral, neuropathic	Substitute a sustained-release or long-acting opioid for the short-acting opioid† in the regimen for severe, intermittent Steroids Peripheral, central nerve ablation

* Significant toxicities at therapeutic doses in geriatric patients. ASA = acetylsalicylic acid; NSAIDs = nonsteroidal anti-inflammatory drugs.

† Short-acting: oxycodone (alone), Dilaudid (hydromorphone), immediate-release morphine, transmucosal fentanyl.

6. Which patients would benefit from nonopioid analgesics?

Nonopioid analgesics (aspirin, acetaminophen, NSAIDs) should be given to patients with **mild pain**, especially of somatic or visceral type. Acetaminophen or nonacetylated salicylates, such as salicylic acid and choline magnesium salicylate, cause less toxicity and therefore should be the first-line agents for elderly patients. Selective inhibitors of COX-2 (e.g., celecoxib, meloxicam) also may cause less gastrointestinal toxicity and inhibition of platelet function than the nonselective agents that inhibit both COX-1 and COX-2. They may be preferred for patients who have developed serious side effects from a nonselective NSAID or who have other contraindications. It is important to prescribe an adequate dose of the drug at regular intervals, switching to another nonopioid analgesic only when maximal doses of the first are ineffective. The limited metabolism of salicylates can, however, lead to salicylate toxicity if the patient takes the pills more often than recommended. The nonopioid analgesics should be continued in patients with moderate pain when opioid analgesics are added, as they will potentiate the pain-relieving effect of the opioid.

Tramadol is a nonopioid that binds opiate receptors and is effective for mild to moderate pain. Starting dose is 50 mg 4 times/day; patients > 75 with normal renal/hepatic function should not exceed 300 mg/day.

7. What drugs are particularly helpful for patients with bone pain?

The nonopioid analgesics are especially useful in patients with bone pain. Effective new agents for patients with bone pain caused by cancer include the bisphosphonates (e.g., pamidronate), strontium-89, and samarium-153-lexidronan. The treatment of low back pain of nonmalignant origin requires a combination of pharmacologic, nonpharmacologic, rehabilitative, psychological, and occasionally surgical and anesthetic strategies.

8. What problems may occur in elderly patients using NSAIDs?

Renal insufficiency, peptic ulcer disease, bleeding diatheses, and exacerbation of fluid retention in patients with cirrhosis or congestive heart failure. Renal function should be assessed 1 or 2 weeks after initiation of the NSAID.

9. What agents are helpful for patients with neuropathic pain?

Tricyclic antidepressants (amitriptyline, nortriptyline), anticonvulsants (phenytoin, carbamazepine, gabapentin), capsaicin, and steroids are nonopioid analgesics with particular efficacy in relieving moderate or severe neuropathic pain.

Postherpetic neuralgia, which occurs in 1–2% of geriatric patients each year, is not very responsive to opioid medications. Although it is very effectively treated in younger patients with amitriptyline, nortriptyline (Pamelor) is better tolerated in the elderly because it has fewer anticholinergic side effects. Dosing begins at 50 mg at bedtime. Serum levels comparable to those required for antidepressant effect usually are required. Topical capsaicin (0.075%), TENS devices, and nerve block or lysis are also useful.

Trigeminal neuralgia, which occurs mostly in geriatric patients, responds to the anticonvulsant carbamazepine (Tegretol) or baclofen. Tegretol is started at 100 mg twice daily, with careful monitoring for decreases in the white blood cell count. Doses need to be increased very slowly, as tolerated and needed to a target of ≤ 1400 mg/day. Baclofen doses increase from 5 mg 3 times/day to as high as 50 mg 3 times/day, if needed.

10. How can compliance with an opioid prescription be ensured?

Opioid analgesics are the mainstay of therapy for patients with moderate to severe pain of any type, whether of malignant or nonmalignant origin. Education of the patient and family is often required to dispel the misconceptions about opioid therapy. The fear of addiction is a common cause of inadequate dispensing of opioids and a barrier to their acceptance by patients. The physician can increase compliance by providing a full explanation of the differences between addiction and physical dependence, along with reassurance that patients with malignancies who take opioids do not become addicts. Patients also may fear that if they take narcotic medications for moderate pain, these agents will no longer be effective if more severe pain occurs. A functional goal of therapy, such as returning to a favorite hobby or reinstituting normal activities of everyday life, may enable the patient and family to accept the opioid.

11. Which opioid medications should be used in elderly patients?

A wide variety of medications are available for use by the oral, transmucosal, rectal, transdermal, or parenteral route. These include the short-acting agents codeine, hydrocodone, oxycodone, hydromorphone, and morphine and the longer-acting agents methadone, transdermal fentanyl, and morphine or oxycodone in sustained-release preparations. Oxycodone or hydrocodone (5 mg/pill) are the opioids in the combination agents with acetylsalicylic acid, acetaminophen, and NSAIDs.

The choice of agent should be dictated by the frequency and type of the pain being treated. **Intermittent, moderate to severe pain** lasting hours to several days is amenable to oral short-acting (3–4 hr) analgesics with appropriate potency. **Severe pain** of relatively constant intensity should be treated with oral long-acting oxycodone or morphine preparations (given every 8–12 hrs) or fentanyl, absorbed through a transdermal patch (renewed every 72 hours). Meperidine is the least useful narcotic for patients with long-lasting moderate to severe pain. It provides pain relief for only about 1–2 hours, and its metabolite can cause seizures. Because of its long half-life, methadone is problematic in elderly patients.

Combinations of a nonopioid analgesic along with an opioid (e.g., Percodan) are very useful, even for patients with moderate somatic or visceral pain of nonmalignant origin. Patients with pain of bony origin, such as severe osteoarthritis or rheumatoid arthritis, are ideal candidates for these agents.

12. How is physical dependence different from addiction?

In a patient with physical dependence, "Physiologic adaptation of the body to the presence of opioid is required to maintain the same level of analgesia," whereas in addiction (psychological dependence), there is a "pattern of compulsive drug use characterized by a continual craving for an opioid and the need to use the opioid for effects other than pain relief."[11]

Fewer than 1% of people who use opioids for pain become addicted to them. They may continue to need them to keep their pain at a tolerable level and may even develop a physiologic dependence, but they will not start stealing TV sets. They will not begin to crave the drugs or seek them to "get high."

13. What other routes are available for patients who cannot take opioids orally?

Opioids: Analgesic Equivalents

	PARENTERAL (MG)	ORAL (MG)	RECTAL (MG)
Morphine	10	30	30
Oxycodone	—	20	N/A
Hydromorphone	1.5	7.5	5
Meperidine*	75	300	N/A

* Chronic use may cause seizures.

Opioids can be given transmucosally, rectally, transdermally, or via subcutaneous, intravenous, or spinal infusions. For patients with severe pain, intravenous drug delivery using a **patient-controlled analgesia system** may be required.

Rectal opioids in short-acting formulations (morphine, oxymorphone, and hydromorphone) have about the same potency and half-life as orally administered agents and therefore have to be given frequently. Sustained-release morphine preparations have the same potency and half-life when administered rectally as they do orally, but they are not approved for rectal use. Patients switched from oral or rectal to parenteral routes of the same medication, or who are given another opioid because they have unacceptable side effects from the first, must have the dose altered accordingly to avoid overdose or undertreatment.

A **transdermal fentanyl system** continuously delivers fentanyl from its reservoir into the skin, achieving a relatively constant plasma fentanyl concentration at 14–20 hours after the initial patch is placed. New patches are placed every 72 hours. Rescue medication (10% of the total 24-hour dose) must be provided, especially during the first 48 hours of use of the patch. This patch is not recommended for patients who need immediate pain relief. Oral transmucosal fentanyl is designed to provide fast (i.e., in 15 minutes) relief of intermittent, severe pain, such as that which occurs during a decubitus dressing change or with moving a patient with bone metastasis. Elderly patients or those with respiratory insufficiency usually require lower doses. Because drug remains in the skin reservoir after the patch is removed, in overdose, naloxone infusion may be required until the drug is eliminated from the skin depot.

14. How is a patient converted from oral or parenteral morphine to a transdermal fentanyl patch?

The table provides information on converting dosages. For example, a patient who has been receiving 90 mg of sustained-release morphine every 12 hours should be given a 75-μg fentanyl patch ($90 \times 2 = 180$ mg morphine daily—151–210 mg oral morphine on the table—corresponding to a 75-μg fentanyl patch). A patient on a morphine drip of 2 mg/hr should be started on 50 μg of fentanyl (2 mg/hr × 24 hrs = 48 mg parenteral morphine daily—31–50 mg parenteral morphine—corresponding to 50 μg of fentanyl).

Dosage Conversions

FENTANYL (μg/hr)	MORPHINE (mg/day)	
	PARENTERAL	ORAL
25	10–30	30–90
50	31–50	91–150
75	51–70	151–210
100	71–90	211–270
125	91–110	271–330
150	111–130	331–390

15. In addition to NSAIDs, which medications can add to the pain-relieving effect of the opioids and thereby minimize the dose needed?

Low doses of tricyclic antidepressants (TCAs, such as nortriptyline, 50 mg given at bedtime) are well-tolerated and are effective within 2–3 days. Although nortryptiline has the fewest anticholinergic side effects of the TCA class, it should not be given to patients with known glaucoma, urinary retention, or first-degree heart block. Side effects (usually associated with amitriptyline) may include autonomic effects, which can be mild (dry mouth, constipation) or more severe (postural hypotension, glaucoma, or urinary retention).

16. How should the constipation and sedation associated with opioids be managed?

Laxatives must be given routinely, not on an as-needed basis, to patients treated with any opioids. Bowel irritants such as Senokot or resins such as lactulose are the most effective agents. Docusate is not effective, and fiber only exacerbates the problem.

Benzodiazepines, barbiturates, and chloral hydrate are not recommended as sleep medications for patients receiving opioids, because they produce excessive daytime sedation. The TCA nortriptyline is preferred as a sleep medication: low doses (e.g., 50 mg) potentiate pain relief, have few anticholinergic side effects, and produce moderate sedation. When possible, medications that produce sedation as a side effect (e.g., cimetidine or diphenhydramine) should be discontinued.

Sedation or confusion induced by opioids may resolve if a different opioid is used. Use the opioid equianalgesic table and decrease the equianalgesic dose of the new agent to allow for incomplete cross-tolerance. If this is ineffective, dextroamphetamine (2.5–7.5 mg orally) or methylphenidate (Ritalin, 10 mg orally with breakfast) will decrease sedation. Doses can be slowly escalated as needed. The amphetamine can be important in helping patients be as alert and pain-free as possible for an important event, such as a child's wedding or an important anniversary. Methylphenidate is contraindicated in patients with cardiac disease, as serious arrhythmias may occur. Patients may also become overstimulated or anxious and develop insomnia, paranoia, or confusion. Paradoxically, however, many elderly patients with depression respond well to similar doses of methylphenidate, with increased appetite and a better sense of well-being.

Naloxone reverses opioid-induced respiratory and CNS depression, but caution should be exercised before administering naloxone to a patient chronically receiving opioids: severe withdrawal may be precipitated. In such patients, rather than administering the usual 0.4-mg/ml dose, dilute the 0.4 mg of naloxone into 10 ml of saline, and give only enough to reverse respiratory depression, not enough to awaken the patient.

17. Define and describe the term *terminal sedation*.

Rare patients who are within days to weeks of death and who have distressing symptoms that cannot be controlled in any other way may require sedation to unconsciousness. This practice is called "terminal sedation." Expert palliative care, psychiatric, and pastoral care consultation should be obtained. If they are unable to provide sufficient relief, the primary physician should next consult extensively with the family and patient and obtain their informed consent to the sedation. Hospital admission for terminal sedation is not required if adequate personnel can be provided in the home or long-term care facility. Under the physician's direction and close nursing monitoring, phenobarbital as a suppository (120–200 mg every 12–24 hr) or intravenously (130 mg every 30 min), lorazepam infusion (0.5–1 mg/hour), or midazolam infusions (0.5–1.5 mg/hr, increased as needed) will induce sedation adequate to relieve the symptoms. Parenteral or enteral feedings and hydration usually are not provided but can be if required to fulfill the goals of the patient.[3]

18. Discuss the special problems presented by opioids and adjuvants in the elderly.

Pharmacokinetics both of opioids and psychotropic adjuvant medications are altered in the elderly. Elderly patients (age 70–89) have decreased opioid clearance, which leads to a prolonged duration of effect. Effective doses are one-half to one-quarter of those needed in younger patients. Long-acting agents such as methadone, sustained-release oxycodone or morphine, or fentanyl patches should be used with caution in the frail elderly, as the drug may accumulate and cause excessive toxicity. Drugs with short half-lives are preferred, and initial doses should be half those used with younger patients. The acute urinary retention due to opioids (especially in patients with prostatic hypertrophy) and hypotension and tachycardia caused by TCAs can be more frequent and of more clinical severity in this population.

19. What are the special problems of pain control in patients with dementia?

Little is known about the problem of giving pain medications to elderly patients with dementia. However, patients with AIDS dementia have been found to be much more sensitive to the adverse side effects of opioids. Sedation and confusion have been especially troublesome but have responded to psychostimulants such as methylphenidate or to antipsychotics such as haloperidol without diminution of the pain relief. It may be reasonable, therefore, to add psychostimulants or antipsychotic agents in appropriate elderly demented patients who develop these side effects from the opioids used to control their pain. Whenever possible, nonpharmacologic therapies, such as relaxation, hypnosis, or other cognitive therapies, should be used.

20. How can hospice contribute to the pain management of elderly patients?

Hospice is a philosophy of care that seeks to provide maximum comfort and quality of life for terminally ill patients and their families without prolonging or shortening the duration of life remaining. Medicare and most HMOs offer hospice plans. Patients with cancer or nonmalignant conditions whose physicians certify that they have a life expectancy of 6 months or less are eligible for hospice. A do-not-resuscitate (DNR) order is not always required.

Joint Commission on Accreditation of Healthcare Organizations–certified hospices provide teams of multidisciplinary professionals and volunteers who help families and other caregivers manage the problems of dying patients in their homes or in nursing homes. The team includes a nurse, social worker, chaplain, and physician; homemakers, home health aides, and volunteers are also available if needed. All medications, laboratory tests, oxygen, ambulance transport, medical supplies, and medical equipment needed for comfort care are provided through the Medicare hospice benefit. Hospice also offers in-hospital care for patients who require it and respite care for families who need up to 5 days of relief from their caregiving duties. Bereavement services are provided for the survivors for at least one year following the patient's death.

Working with the patient's primary health care provider (i.e., physician, nurse practitioner, or physician assistant) hospice teams thus address the physical, psychological, social, and spiritual/existential causes of distress in terminally ill patients. Hospice personnel also serve as resources for other home care providers in managing difficult pain problems or other areas of distress such as dyspnea or delirium. Many hospices offer home care services for patients with skilled care needs who are terminally ill but do not wish to elect the hospice benefit; patients and families served by such home care services often have the same nursing and home health aide personnel and durable medical equipment suppliers as are provided in hospice. If they later decide to elect the hospice service, they thus have maximum continuity of care.

21. What are the common mistakes and misperceptions in treating pain in the elderly?

1. Failure to use a quantitative pain scale and assess pain routinely and the assumption that cognitively impaired patients cannot give accurate pain assessments.

2. Use of NSAIDs in patients with significant risk of toxicity in an effort to avoid opioid use. NSAIDs should be used with caution, if at all, in elderly patients with a history of gastrointestinal intolerance or bleeding, renal insufficiency, hypertension, congestive heart failure, or cirrhosis.

3. Failure to prescribe opioids for patients whose pain levels are moderate or severe, whether the pain is of malignant or nonmalignant origin.

4. Failure to provide an aggressive routine laxative regimen to prevent opioid-induced constipation.

5. Failure to discontinue medications that contribute to sedation and thereby limit tolerable opioid dose.

BIBLIOGRAPHY

1. AGS Clinical Practice Committee: Management of cancer pain in older patients. J Am Geriatr Soc 45:1273–1276, 1997.
2. AGS Panel on Chronic Pain in Older Persons: The management of chronic pain in older persons. J Am Geriatr Soc 46:635–651, 1998.
3. Cherny NI, Coyle N, Foley KM: Guidelines in the care of the dying cancer patient. Hematol Oncol Clin North Am 10:261–286, 1996.
4. Donner B, Zenz M, Tryba M, Strumpf M: Direct conversion from oral morphine to transdermal fentanyl: A multicenter study in patients with cancer pain. Pain 64:527–534, 1996.
5. Eisenberg E, Berkey CS, Carr DB, et al: Efficacy and safety of nonsteroidal antiinflammatory drugs for cancer pain: A meta-analysis. J Clin Oncol 12:2756–2765, 1994.
6. Ferrell BA: Pain evaluation and management in the nursing home. Ann Intern Med 123:681–687, 1995.
7. Ferrell BR, Ferrell BA (eds): Pain in the Elderly. Seattle, IASP Press, 1996.
8. Ferrell BR: Patient education and nondrug interventions. In Ferrell BR, Ferrell BA (eds): Pain in the Elderly. Seattle, IASP Press, 1996, p 35.

9. Forman WB: Opioid analgesic drugs in the elderly. Clin Geriatr Med 12:489–500, 1996.
10. Gloth FM: Concerns with chronic analgesic therapy in elderly patients. Am J Med 101(Suppl 1A):19S–24S, 1996.
11. Jacox A, Carr DB, Payne R, et al: Management of Cancer Pain: Clinical Practice Guideline No 9. Washington, DC, UPHS, AHCPR, 1994, AHCPR publication 94-0592.
12. Kost RG, Straus SE: Postherpetic neuralgia—pathogenesis, treatment, and prevention. N Engl J Med 335:32–42, 1996.
13. Levy MH: Pharmacologic treatment of cancer pain. N Engl J Med 335:1124–1132, 1996.
14. Lipman AG: Analgesic drugs for neuropathic and sympathetically maintained pain. Clin Geriatr Med 12:501–515, 1996.
15. Parmelee PA: Pain in cognitively impaired older persons. Clin Geriatr Med 12:473–487, 1996.
16. Portenoy RK: Adjuvant analgesics in pain management. In Doyle D, Hanks G, MacDonald N (eds): Oxford Textbook of Palliative Medicine, 2nd ed. New York, Oxford University Press, 1997, p 361.

28. EARLY DETECTION OF ELDER ABUSE, NEGLECT, AND EXPLOITATION

Elizabeth Capezuti, Ph.D., R.N.

1. What constitutes elder abuse and neglect?

- **Physical abuse** is the infliction of bodily injury and may be manifested by lacerations, fractures, soft-tissue trauma, burns, or bruises.
- **Sexual abuse** is any form of intimate sexual activity without consent. This includes sexual activity with those unable to give adequate consent, such as those with dementia or the older mentally retarded person.
- **Emotional or psychological abuse** is the infliction of mental anguish, such as intimidation by yelling, insulting, threatening, or silence.
- **Financial exploitation** is the misuse of an older person's funds or assets without his or her explicit knowledge or consent. It may take many forms, such as the withdrawal of small amounts of money from banking accounts or the overcharging for grocery shopping or housekeeping by persons providing these services.
- **Caregiver neglect** is the malicious neglect by a caregiver of an older person's needs, whether for retaliation, disinterest, or financial incentives. Examples include inadequate provision of nutrition and the misuse of medications, such as oversedation with tranquilizers.
- **Self-neglect** is disregard of one's personal well-being and home environment.

2. What is the significance of elder mistreatment?

Elder mistreatment is associated with significantly decreased survival after controlling for other factors associated with increased mortality. One to 2 million older Americans are mistreated annually. To date, there has been only one population-based survey conducted, which found a prevalence of 32/1000 older persons. According to the National Elder Abuse Incidence Study, there were approximately a half million new cases of elder mistreatment in 1996.

3. What causes elder abuse?

Physical abuse and financial exploitation are usually due to the psychopathology of the perpetrator and have little to do with the older person's characteristics. Perpetrators (family members or nonrelatives) are more likely to abuse alcohol or drugs, to be mentally ill, and/or to be financially dependent on the older person.

Neglect of an older individual due to lack of information or resources, usually referred to as "passive neglect," is not considered mistreatment. It often is seen when the caregivers have their own physical or mental handicaps. Adult children may be developmentally disabled or mentally ill or may be elderly themselves and, as a result, unable to provide sufficient care. Passive caregiver neglect may be rectified by providing education and community supports.

Active caregiver neglect, which implies malicious intent, has not been demonstrated to be due to the stress and burdens of providing care to an older person. These caregivers also are likely to have substance abuse issues, have serious untreated mental illness, or be financially dependent on the older person. Caregivers who are socially isolated and lack social supports (family, friends, or community-based services) or those with a history of violence, such as spousal abuse, also have been implicated.

Victims and perpetrators of any type of mistreatment are found in all socioeconomic groups.

4. What leads to self-neglect?

The exact cause of self-neglect is often difficult to determine. In some cases, there appears to be a mental health problem, such as chronic schizophrenia, depression, or dementia. In other cases, the older person demonstrates no deficits in cognitive functioning but is fearful of "outsiders." These older persons may be reclusive, suspicious, and territorial. The key to successful intervention with this type of elder is to establish a trusting relationship that allows the older person to feel in control. This is usually best handled by case managers in private or county social service agencies, who can provide long-term follow-up.

5. **Discuss the role of mental status assessment in the evaluation of elder mistreatment.**
   Mental status assessment, especially cognitive functioning, is an essential component of the evaluation; it is necessary to determine if the person is able to make a decision to remain in an abusive relationship with a perpetrator or remain in a self-neglecting situation. Furthermore, new onset of confusion has been found to be a significant risk factor for elder mistreatment. Accusations of abuse should be assessed within the context of other psychiatric symptoms, such as delusions and hallucinations, which may or may not lend credence to the allegations. Displays of paranoia or anxiety in the presence of the suspected perpetrator may be related to fear, thus leading to inquiries of other family members or friends to provide further information about the relationship. The older person presenting with new onset of disorientation, confusion, or extreme lethargy may be the victim of oversedation. Depression can be the cause of self-neglect or may indicate resignation to an abusive situation.

6. **What are the physical findings of physical abuse?**
   Physical abuse should be considered when investigating the underlying cause of any injury. Identification of physical abuse, however, is often complicated by normal age changes that may mimic trauma. In senile purpura, even gentle handling of an older person's skin may result in bruising because of capillary fragility. Bilateral **bruises** of the upper arms, however, are more likely to result from forcibly holding, grabbing, or shaking a person. **Fractures, dislocations, and sprains** need to be explored within the context of other suspicious signs and symptoms of abuse. **Imprint injuries** (bruises that retain the shape of the object, such as a belt buckle, hand, or iron) are strong physical indicators of abuse. A person physically restrained may have **rope burns** or marks on the ankles or wrists. **Burns** in an unusual location, such as cigarette burns on the back, are highly significant. **Spotty absence of hair**, contrary to the typical temporal pattern of balding in aging men, may be due to vigorous hair-pulling.

7. **List the chief indicators of neglect.**
   - Malnutrition
   - Dehydration
   - Pressure ulcers
   - Contractures
   - Oversedation
   - Poor hygiene
   - Urine burn excoriations
   - Manifestations of inadequately treated medical problems (i.e., unfilled prescriptions and recurrent urinary tract infections)

   One indicator alone cannot confirm a diagnosis of mistreatment, but a suspicious history with a recurrent presentation of signs should raise the clinician's suspicions of mistreatment. Many signs of neglect also can be attributed to common age-related health problems. For example, malnutrition may be explained as the older person's lack of appetite, just as poor personal hygiene may be attributed to one's refusal to be bathed. Therefore, care must be exercised not to be overly accusatory and threaten your relationship with the caregiver.

8. **What should be emphasized in interviewing possible victims and perpetrators of mistreatment?**
   The interview should proceed from the least threatening questions to a more directed inquiry. The history of a presenting physical injury needs to be evaluated for **inconsistencies** and the following questions should be addressed:
   - Could the injury actually have occurred in the manner in which the suspected abuser or victim has explained?
   - Is the individual bed-bound and seeking treatment for several fractures?
   - Did the person "fall down the stairs" and present with bilateral upper arm bruising?

If possible, interview the victim separately from the caregiver. However, do not always expect to get a different story than the suspected abuser's story, because the victim may have been coached or threatened before being brought in for treatment.

When evaluating an injury or signs of deteriorating health (e.g., malnutrition, dehydration, multiple pressure sores), the **index of suspicion** is raised when the elderly individual is taken to an emergency department or family physician located far from home. This occurs when the family or caregiver believes the staff in the local emergency department or the physician has become suspicious of the home situation. It also is suspect when someone other than the primary caregiver brings the person to the physician's office or emergency department and knows little of the older person's health status, medications, and so forth. The inability to answer questions may be a way to block the physician's probing of the cause of an injury or of inadequate care. Any individual who is brought in for treatment late in the illness process or who repeatedly needs treatment despite a previously well-thought-out discharge plan should be evaluated for needed in-home supports or breakdown of a current home care system.

9. **What type of situations should alert the clinician to the possibility of financial exploitation?**

If a cognitively intact individual is unaware of his or her own financial situation or there is an apparent discrepancy between financial resources and lifestyle, the clinician may want to probe further or to refer to a social worker. In the latter instance, be aware that lifestyle preferences and income may be incongruent, particularly as some individuals may not be willing to spend money on necessary services. On the other hand, some individuals in the early stages of dementia often will lose the ability to manage their money. Without intervention in these situations, bills may go unpaid, Social Security checks uncashed, and available money squandered.

10. **What resources are available for intervention?**

Currently, every state has an adult protective services (APS) system, which, in addition to investigating suspected cases (usually with a home visit), provides special services for the victims of mistreatment. Provisions for emergency shelter, home care, food, and transportation, as well as legal counsel and evaluations by health care providers, may be provided, depending on each state's funding of APS. The amount of involuntary intervention by protective service workers also depends on individual state laws.

Geriatric and geropsychiatric programs in hospitals and outpatient offices are familiar with the problems of elder mistreatment. If such specialized services are not available, hospital social work departments, local area agencies on aging, and visiting nurses associations can provide coordination and referral services.

Many police departments and district attorney's offices have special domestic violence units to handle cases of abuse or neglect.

11. **Are physicians mandated to report suspected elder mistreatment?**

In 42 states and the District of Columbia physicians are required to report suspected mistreatment of elders residing in the community to APS. With few exceptions, the mistreatment need only be suspected, not fully substantiated. Many mandatory and voluntary reporting statutes grant immunity from civil and criminal liability to those who report in good faith. States without mandatory reporting laws (as of 1999) include Colorado, Illinois, New York, New Jersey, North Dakota, Pennsylvania, South Dakota, and Wisconsin. The primary functions of physicians in suspected cases referred to APS are to document the physical findings and to provide a judgment about the older person's decision-making capacity.

The Joint Commission on the Accreditation of Health Care Organizations requires hospital emergency departments to provide personnel training in the detection and management of the problem. Moreover, emergency departments must develop protocols to deal with cases of mistreatment that address the collection of evidence, the documentation of examinations, and the treatment provided. A current list of community agencies for referral for services should also be readily available. These agencies can provide both immediate and long-term support for victims of elder mistreatment.

12. How does institutional mistreatment differ from mistreatment that occurs in the community?

The various types and manifestations of mistreatment are the same, but the location and responsibility of the perpetrator are chief differences. Institutional mistreatment can occur in hospitals, nursing homes, or board-and-care facilities. The perpetrator may be an individual staff member who physically or sexually abuses a patient, or the perpetrator may be an institutional milieu that discourages the appropriate provision of care. For example, the patients may be physically restrained instead of ambulated because of inadequate staffing levels, thus leading to problems associated with immobility such as contractures and pressure ulcers. Most states require mandatory reporting of physical abuse and financial exploitation to the state health department; several also mandate the reporting of institutional neglect.

Reporting of suspicions of institutional mistreatment should be made to the state ombudsman. The Older Americans Act of 1976 mandated that each state establish ombudsman programs to investigate allegations of mistreatment in nursing homes.

BIBLIOGRAPHY

1. American Medical Association: Diagnostic and Treatment Guidelines on Elder Abuse and Neglect. Chicago, IL, American Medical Association, 1992.
2. Capezuti E, Brush B, Lawson WT: Reporting elder mistreatment. J Gerontol Nurs 23:24–32, 1997.
3. Lachs MS, Pillemer K: Current concepts: Abuse and neglect of elderly persons. N Engl J Med 332:437–443, 1995.
4. Lachs MS, Williams CS, O'Brien S, et al: Older adults: An 11-year longitudinal study of adult protective service use. Arch Intern Med 156:449–453, 1996.
5. Lachs MS, Williams CS, O'Brien S, et al: Risk factors for reported elder abuse and neglect: A nine-year observational cohort study. Gerontologist 37:469–474, 1997.
6. Lachs MS, Williams CS, O'Brien S, et al: The mortality of elder mistreatment. JAMA 280:428–432, 1998.

29. WOMEN'S HEALTH ISSUES

Michelle Battistini, M.D.

1. What are the most common complaints that cause an older woman to see a gynecologist?

Other than a routine exam, the most common reasons an aging woman visits a gynecologist are symptoms related to pelvic relaxation, vaginal discharge, vaginal bleeding, vulvar irritation or pruritus, and urinary incontinence. With increasing frequency, regardless of the primary reason for their visit, many women and their referring physicians have concerns and questions about hormone replacement therapy.

2. What is pelvic relaxation? How is it diagnosed?

Pelvic relaxation is the loss of normal and adequate supportive tissues along the vaginal canal, resulting in prolapse or herniation of pelvic structures into the vagina. The loss of support may occur universally or at specific sites along the length of the vagina.

The diagnosis of pelvic relaxation and the specific site of prolapse is made during physical examination with the patient in the dorsal lithotomy position or standing upright. If the examination is limited to the lithotomy position, a more accurate diagnosis is made by having the patient strain; this is accomplished by asking her to cough hard or to perform a Valsalva maneuver.

Pelvic Support Structures

STRUCTURE	NATURE	COMPONENTS	FUNCTION

Pelvic diaphragm	Muscular	Levator ani
		  Pubococcygeus
		  Puborectalis
		  Iliococcygeus
			Control of urination
			Maintenance of fecal
			  continence
			Support of abdominal and
			  pelvic viscera
			Integral role in birth process

Urogenital diaphragm	Muscular and fascial	Ischiocavernosus
		Bulbocavernosus
		Deep transverse
		Perineal
			Supports external urethra
			Contains external urethral
			  sphincter
			Maintains position of bladder
			  neck
			Supports vaginal introitus
			Contains neurovascular
			  supply to pudendum and
			  clitoris

Endopelvic fascia	Thickened retro-peritoneal fascia	Pubocervical fascia—
		  anterior
		Mackenrodt's ligament
		  (cardinal ligament)—
		  lateral and superior
		Uterosacral ligaments—
		  posterior
			Periurethral and visceral
			  support
			Base of broad ligament
			
			Cul de sac support

3. How are disorders of pelvic relaxation classified?

The site of relaxation determines which organ will prolapse and the classification of the disorder.

Classification of Pelvic Relaxation Disorders

LOCATION OF ANATOMIC DEFECT	PROLAPSED ORGAN	DISORDER
Anterior vaginal segment	Urethra/bladder	Cystourethrocele Cystocele
Superior vaginal segment	Cervix/uterus/vaginal cuff	Cervical/uterine/vaginal vault prolapse
	Cul de sac	Culdocele, enterocele*
Posterior vaginal segment	Rectum	Rectocele
	Perineum	Perineal laceration

* Enteroceles may involve posterior segment as well.

4. What causes pelvic relaxation?

Usually multiple factors contribute to the weakening of pelvic support structures, including the following:

- Vaginal delivery
- Estrogen deficiency
- Sexual activity
- Chronic occupational stress
- Stress secondary to gravity
- Obesity
- Chronic cough
- Chronic constipation
- Surgical or acute trauma
- Neurologic disorders
- Congenital abnormalities
- Prior pelvic surgery

5. What symptoms are associated with pelvic relaxation?

Pelvic relaxation may be asymptomatic and detected only on physical examination. When women present with symptoms, the symptoms may be generalized or related to the specific organ that is prolapsed. Examples include:

- Vaginal fullness or pressure
- Pelvic pressure
- Backache
- Inability to empty bladder
- Difficulty with voiding
- Coital dysfunction
- Urinary incontinence
- Protrusion of organ outside vagina
- Difficulty with defecation
- Anal incontinence for flatus or stool
- Vaginal discharge or bleeding

Often women complain of feeling as though (1) they are "sitting on a ball"; (2) something is protruding from the vagina; or (3) they have a sensation of vaginal pressure, fullness, or fatigue.

Urethroceles (see table in question 3) are frequently associated with urinary incontinence.

Pure cystoceles may cause difficulty with bladder emptying; patients report having to reduce the cystocele manually or to assume various positions to void adequately. Incomplete bladder emptying may predispose to urinary tract infections and related symptoms.

Rectoceles may be associated with incomplete defecation and a sensation of rectal fullness; patients may report the need to split the vagina or perineum to defecate completely.

Perineal defects may cause anal incontinence of flatus and feces.

Complete prolapse of any of these structures may lead to surface irritation with resultant vaginal discharge or surface ulceration with vaginal bleeding. The severity of symptoms frequently, but not always, varies directly with the severity or degree of prolapse, which is determined at the time of physical examination.

6. Describe the system for grading the severity of pelvic relaxation disorders.

No universal system for grading these disorders is yet available. Below is a summary of commonly used terminology. Each area of weakness is defined and graded according to its maximal descent. Alternatively, a description of the defect can be used; for example, the cervix descends 2 cm beyond the introitus.

Pelvic Relaxation Disorders—Classification of Severity

EXTENT OF DESCENT	GRADE	SEVERITY	DEGREE
Normal position	Grade 0	Normal	Normal
Halfway to hymen	Grade 1	Mild	First-degree descensus
To hymen	Grade 2	Moderate	Second-degree descensus
Halfway past hymen	Grade 3	Moderately severe	Procidentia
Maximum descensus	Grade 4	Severe	Procidentia

7. What treatments are available for pelvic relaxation?

Pelvic relaxation can be treated with both surgical and nonsurgical therapeutic options. **Nonsurgical interventions** do not restore anatomic integrity to the pelvic structures; they are designed to relieve symptoms and prevent worsening of the condition. Nonoperative interventions strengthen muscular and fascial support structures, support herniated organs, and avoid exacerbating factors; they include the use of Kegel exercises, estrogen therapy, vaginal pessaries, and stool softeners.

Surgical intervention includes procedures that are reparative or palliative. **Reparative surgical procedures** are designed to restore anatomic integrity to pelvic structures; they are site-specific and can be accomplished through an abdominal, vaginal, or combined approach. When a reparative option is chosen, a thorough preoperative evaluation of pelvic support structures is imperative. All sites of relaxation are repaired at the time of surgery to avoid recurrence. In addition, the preoperative and postoperative use of nonsurgical strategies to strengthen support tissues enhances the success of the repair and reduces the risk of recurrence. **Palliative procedures**, generally designed to obliterate the vaginal lumen, are performed less commonly today. They are usually reserved for the elderly patient who is no longer sexually active and has persistent or recurrent symptoms after other treatment options have been tried. The choice of treatment is based on several factors, including severity of symptoms, degree of prolapse, medical condition and preference of the patient, and success of prior conservative interventions. Age alone should not be considered a contraindication to surgical therapy.

Treatment of Pelvic Relaxation Disorders

NONSURGICAL MANAGEMENT	SURGICAL MANAGEMENT
Strengthen pelvic musculature: Kegel exercises, vaginal cones, biofeedback, electrostimulation	**Reparative procedures:** repair of all identifiable defects Anterior defect: anterior colporrhaphy, periurethral suspension
Strengthen nonmuscular support: estrogen therapy, topical or as replacement therapy	Superior defect: hysterectomy, vaginal vault suspension (abdominal or vaginal approach), enterocele repair
Mechanical support: vaginal pessary use	Posterior defect: posterior colporrhaphy, perineoplasty
Avoid exacerbating factors: limit increases in intraabdominal pressure (e.g., avoid heavy lifting); stool softeners, high-fiber diets; review and adjust medications	**Palliative procedures:** obliteration of vaginal canal Anterior defect: colpocleisis with or without incontinence repair, hysterectomy Superior defect: colpocleisis, cervical amputation (Manchester-Fothergill procedure) Posterior defect: colpocleisis

8. What are vaginal pessaries? How are they used?

Vaginal supportive pessaries have been used for many years in the treatment of pelvic relaxation. The 17 different types of pessaries vary in shape and size, depending on their proposed purpose. They are composed of inert materials such as Lucite and rubber; most modern pessaries are made of silicone. Pessaries can be used as a temporary treatment for symptomatic relief in women who are waiting for surgery or as permanent treatment in women who are poor surgical risks or choose a nonsurgical option. The most common pessaries used for treatment include:

- Ring, with and without support
- Gelhorn
- Doughnut
- Schaatz
- Gehrung

Pessaries require precision fitting by an individual experienced in their use. Poor sizing can cause obstruction of the urinary outflow tract and erosion of the vaginal epithelium with resultant ulceration. Patients should be instructed to report any difficulty with urination, foul vaginal discharge, or vaginal bleeding. Topical estrogen cream is prescribed before pessary fitting to rejuvenate the vaginal walls. This treatment is continued intermittently (1–2 nights/week) while the pessary is in place. Pessary hygiene includes periodic removal and cleansing of the pessary (every 2–6 months). Patients can be instructed in pessary care, but often they come to the office.

9. What are Kegel exercises? How are they done?

Kegel exercises were introduced in the middle of the 20th century by Dr. Kegel as a treatment primarily for urinary stress incontinence. They are designed to strengthen the pubococcygeus muscle (PCM). Because the PCM plays a major role in pelvic support, Kegel exercises also may be used in the treatment of pelvic relaxation. Patients are instructed to contract the PCM, hold for 3–10 seconds and then relax for 3 seconds. They do so for 20 minutes, 3 times/day, repeating the exercise from 100–300 times. To assist the patient in identifying the correct muscle, different techniques are used. Patients can be told to tighten the muscle that holds gas in the rectum or to stop their urine in midstream and feel the muscle used to do so. Often it is useful to teach Kegel exercises during the pelvic exam. Slight pressure is applied to the muscle through the vaginal wall; the patient is then instructed to squeeze the fingers. Perineometers, vaginal cones, and biofeedback devices are used to facilitate the proper exercise technique.

10. What is menopause?

Many women need to define their position along the spectrum of declining ovarian function. Frequently they ask questions such as "Am I through with menopause?", "Am I in the menopause?", or even "Just what is menopause?"

Menopause is permanent cessation of menstruation, which marks the loss of ovarian endocrine activity seen during the reproductive years. The median age of menopause in North America is 51.5 years, with a normal range of 48–55 years. The hallmark of menopause is loss of ovarian production of estradiol, the potent estrogen of the reproductive years. Ovarian production of androstenedione is also reduced. Production of testosterone is the same or slightly increased because of stromal stimulation by elevated levels of the gonadotropins, follicle-stimulating hormone (FSH) and luteinizing hormone (LH). However, serum testosterone levels fall due to the reduced level of androstenedione precursor. Although there is essentially no ovarian production of estrogen after menopause, circulating levels of estrogen are variable and can be significant, primarily in the form of estrone, a less potent form. Estrone and, to a lesser extent, estradiol are formed from the peripheral conversion of androstenedione and testosterone, primarily in adipose tissue.

The years of waning ovarian function prior to menopause are often referred to as the **transition**. This period of fluctuating ovarian function is manifested by cycle irregularities and various symptoms related to fluctuations in hormone levels. **Perimenopause** refers to the few years immediately before and after cessation of menses. The term **climacteric** is often used to describe the years from the transition through menopause and into the postmenopausal period. How a woman experiences menopause and the years thereafter is as varied as life itself and depends on the complex interplay of hormonal, physical, and psychosocial factors.

HORMONE	SERUM LEVELS POSTMENOPAUSE	SERUM LEVELS PREMENOPAUSE
Estradiol	5–40 pg/ml	20–600 pg/ml
Estrone	5–40 pg/ml	15–200 pg/ml
Androstenedione	20–50 ng/dl	100–150 ng/dl
Testosterone	10–40 ng/dl	20–80 ng/dl

11. What are the symptoms of menopause?

The most common acute symptom of menopause, the hot flush or flash, is related to vaso-motor instability secondary to reduced estrogen levels in the thermoregulatory centers in the brain. Hot flushes are experienced by 85% of menopausal women and are the most common reason for seeking treatment. Flushes tend to occur more commonly at night and may cause significant sleep disturbance. Hot flushes can be precipitated by environmental factors such as stress, alcohol, hot foods, and warm weather. They frequently worsen with tamoxifen therapy. For most women, the frequency and severity of flushes tend to decrease and subside within the first 3–5 years after menopause; in up to one-third of women, however, they may persist longer. Vaginal changes secondary to reduced estrogen levels include decreased lubrication and loss of elasticity, frequently leading to symptoms of dryness, dyspareunia, pruritus, and atrophic vaginitis. Urinary symptoms of urgency, frequency, and worsening of incontinence reflect the estrogen receptivity of the bladder and urethra.

12. What is the role of estrogen replacement therapy (ERT) after menopause?

Estrogen receptors are found in virtually every organ system throughout the body. Symptoms and medical consequences represent the end-organ response to reduced estrogen levels characteristic of menopause. ERT is indicated for treatment of symptoms and prevention of the long-term medical consequences of reduced estrogen levels. The consequences of the hormonal events of menopause occur in a woman who is also aging. It is important, yet sometimes difficult, to differentiate for women and their families which changes are related to aging, which to the hormonal effects of menopause, and which to a combination of both. Other effects of ERT include maintenance of skin turgor, decreased joint pain, an increased sense of well-being, and improvement in some aspects of memory and cognition. Reductions in tooth loss and development of macular degeneration of the retina have been described with estrogen use.

13. What are the indications for ERT?

Indications for Hormone Replacement Therapy

SYMPTOM CONTROL	MEDICAL BENEFITS
Vasomotor instability—hot flushes	Prevention of osteoporosis
Sleep disturbances	Reduction of cardiovascular risk
Dyspareunia, vaginal dryness, atrophic vaginitis	? Amelioration of Alzheimer's dementia
Urinary urgency, frequency	? Reduction of colon cancer risk
Urinary stress incontinence	

The two major, well-documented medical benefits of ERT are osteoporosis prevention and reduction of cardiovascular risk. ERT initiated shortly after the menopause prevents the accelerated bone loss that occurs during the first 5–7 postmenopausal years. Long-term use is associated with a 50% reduction in fracture risk. ERT in the elderly, even when initiated long after menopause, has been shown to reduce the risk of hip fracture. Estrogen is currently one of the pharmacologic agents used in both prevention and treatment of osteoporosis.

Perhaps the most significant effect of ERT from an individual and public health perspective is its effect on the reduction of cardiovascular morbidity and mortality. The incidence of fatal and nonfatal myocardial infarction is reduced by 50% with ERT. Analysis of data released from the Nurses Health Study revealed no alteration in the reduction of cardiac events with the addition of a progestin. In addition, at the time of cardiac catheterization users of ERT appear to have a lower incidence of significant stenosis and improved long-term survival (98% vs. 69%) at 10 years compared with nonusers. Preliminary data suggest that ERT may play a role in the prevention and progression of Alzheimer's dementia. Definitive documentation of this effect is an area of active research. ERT may reduce the risk of development of colon cancer, but this also awaits further documentation.

14. Should hormone replacement therapy be prescribed for risk reduction in women with known coronary artery disease?

To date, only one randomized, placebo-controlled trial, the HERS trial (Heart and Estrogen/Progestin Replacement Study), has looked at the role of continuous combined hormone replacement therapy in women with known coronary artery disease. This 4-year study failed to reveal a beneficial effect. It is believed that hormone replacement therapy should not be newly prescribed in women with established disease. However, because there appeared to be a trend toward decreased risk after years 3 and 4, women already on hormone replacement therapy who are diagnosed with coronary artery disease can be continued on therapy. Results of ongoing trials will further define the benefits of hormone replacement therapy in the future.

15. Describe the mechanisms by which estrogen achieves its beneficial effects.

Reduction of bone loss	Antiresorptive action on osteoclasts in bone
	Increased efficiency of calcium absorption in GI tract
	Decreased renal calcium excretion
Reduction of cardiovascular risk	Improved lipid profile
	Decreased total cholesterol
	Increased high-density lipoprotein (HDL) cholesterol
	Decreased low-density lipoprotein (LDL) cholesterol
	Increase in coronary blood flow
	Antioxidant–antiatherogenic effect

Results of one large clinical trial that evaluated the effect of ERT on cardiovascular risk factors (the PEPI trial) revealed that the addition of progestin did not eliminate the beneficial effect of estrogen on lipid and fibrinogen levels.

16. Does ERT cause cancer?

One of the most common reasons for avoidance of ERT after menopause is fear of cancer. It has been well documented that the use of unopposed estrogen in women with an intact uterus increases the risk for endometrial hyperplasia and endometrial cancer by a factor of 2–10. Risk increases with dose and duration of use. For this reason, it is standard to add a progestational agent, for at least 12–14 days a month, to the replacement regimen (PERT) in women who have not undergone hysterectomy. Use of PERT according to this standard has been shown to eliminate the increase in risk of endometrial cancer and hyperplasia. The PERT regimen may be considered in women without a uterus who have a history of severe endometriosis, because endometrial carcinoma originating in endometriotic implants and recurrence of endometriosis have been reported.

Unfortunately, the effect of ERT and PERT on breast cancer risk is less clearly defined. Current reports continue to yield conflicting results. Short-term use ($\leq$ 5 years) of either ERT or PERT is not associated with an increased relative risk of breast cancer. Past use, regardless of duration, does not seem to increase risk. Still in question is the possibility of a small-to-moderate increase in risk among older women who are current users of long duration (> 10 years).

However, the current recommendation is that the benefits of ERT/PERT continue to outweigh the risks in light of the substantial benefits in terms of cardiovascular and osteoporotic disease. The lowest possible dose to accrue the greatest benefit should be used. No association has been proved between ovarian cancer and hormone replacement therapy (HRT).

17. Describe the standard regimens for HRT.

Standard Regimens for Hormone Replacement Therapy

REGIMEN	ESTROGEN	PROGESTIN	ADVANTAGES	DISADVANTAGES
Unopposed	Days 1–25 Every day	None	Maximal established benefit No progestin side effects	High incidence of endometrial hyperplasia Increased risk for endometrial cancer Requires annual biopsy if uterus present
Cyclic combined	Days 1–25	10–14 days Days 16–25 or 13–25	Oldest standard regimen Adequate endometrial protection	Cyclic menstrual-like bleeding Recurrence of symptoms on off days Premenstrual-like symptoms
Sequential	Every day	10–14 days/month (duration is dose-dependent) Days 1–10 or 14 Last 10–14 days	Adequate endometrial protection No hormone-free days, less hormonal fluctuation, less symptom recurrence	Progestin withdrawal bleeding Premenstrual-like symptoms
Continuous combined (most popular current regimen)	Every day	Every day	Eliminates cyclic bleeding Reduces cyclic premenstrual side effects, including migraine headaches Easy regimen to use	Irregular bleeding Long-term endometrial protection yet to be established
Periodic progestin	Every day	Weekdays (weekends off)	No cyclic and less irregular bleeding Less progestin exposure, reduced side effects	Long-term endometrial protection yet to be established Complicated regimen to use
		Quarterly (14 days every 3 months)	Less progestin exposure, reduced side effects	Withdrawal bleeding heavier than monthly episodes Long-term endometrial protection yet to be established

18. What are the standard doses of estrogen? Of progestins?

Standard Doses of Estrogen

ESTROGEN	BRAND NAME	DOSE
Conjugated equine estrogens	Premarin	0.625 mg
Estropipate	Ogen	0.625–1.25 mg
Micronized estradiol	Estrace	0.5, 1.0 mg
Transdermal 17-estradiol	Estraderm, Climara, Alora	0.05, 0.1 mg
	Vivelle	0.0375, 0.05, 0.1 mg
Estropipate	Ortho-est	0.625–1.25 mg
Esterified estrogen with methyltestosterone	Estratest	1.25/2.5 mg
	Estratest H.S.	0.625/1.25 mg
Esterified estrogen	Estratab	0.3, 0.625–1.25 mg

Standard Doses of Progestins

PROGESTIN	BRAND NAME	DOSE
Medroxyprogesterone acetate	Provera Cycrin Amen	Cyclic/sequential: 5–10 mg Continuous: 2.5, 5.0 mg Periodic: 10 mg × 14 days
Micronized progesterone	Prometrium	Cyclic/sequential: 200 mg Continuous: 100–200 mg
Norethindrone	Micronor Norlutin Nor-QD	Cyclic/sequential: 2.5–5.0 Continuous: 0.35–2.1
Norethindrone acetate	Aygestin Norlutate	Cyclic/sequential: 5–10 mg Continuous: 1 mg
D/L-norgestrel	Ovrette	Cyclic/sequential: 0.075 mg

19. Does HRT cause hypertension or strokes?

No. This common misperception is based on the association of early high-dose oral contraceptives with an increased risk of hypertension and cardiovascular disease. ERT and PERT are not associated with an increased risk of hypertension, nor is well-controlled hypertension a contraindication to HRT. Because a small number of women may develop an idiosyncratic elevation of blood pressure, routine blood pressure monitoring is advocated. An increased risk of cerebrovascular events with the use of HRT has not been identified. In fact, long-term use appears to be associated with an overall reduction in mortality attributable to cardiovascular disease.

20. Can a woman with a history of thromboembolic disease use HRT?

The standard regimens used in HRT do not adversely affect coagulation factors and until recently were not thought to be associated with an increased risk of thromboembolic events. However, a 2–4-fold increase in the risk of venous thromboembolic events has been described in recent studies. HRT is not contraindicated in women with a remote history of thrombosis associated with trauma. In women with conditions associated with an increased risk of thromboembolism, a previous episode, a positive family history, morbid obesity, or immobilization, the use of HRT should be based on individual risk/benefit analysis and counseling. In women with symptoms of or at increased risk of cardiovascular disease or osteoporosis, it may be appropriate to offer HRT after adequate counseling. The incidence and absolute risk remain low. Acute thromboembolic disease is a contraindication to HRT.

21. When is HRT contraindicated?

Absolute contraindications
Unexplained vaginal bleeding
Acute liver disease
Impaired liver function, acute or chronic
Recent vascular thrombosis
Carcinoma of breast (except in certain circumstances)
Carcinoma of the endometrium (with some exceptions)
Diagnosis of hypercoagulable state

Relative contraindications
Seizure disorders
High triglyceride levels
Migraine headaches (with exceptions)
Atraumatic thrombophlebitis
Current gallbladder disease
Increased risk of thromboembolic events

After appropriate diagnosis and management of vaginal bleeding, HRT can be considered according to standard indications and contraindications. Liver dysfunction, whether acute or chronic, may result in unacceptably high levels of estrogen due to altered liver metabolism. HRT is generally contraindicated in patients with a history of an estrogen-sensitive neoplasm, most commonly breast or endometrial cancer. In certain circumstances, however, such patients may use HRT after extensive counseling about risk and benefit. These decisions need to be made individually. HRT has been used in patients with a history of stage I, low-grade adeno-carcinoma of the uterus with no demonstrable increase in risk of recurrence. Limited case series involving survivors of breast cancer have reported no negative impact on recurrence or survival, but such reports cannot serve as a basis for generalized use of HRT in this popula-tion. In conditions listed as relative contraindications, risk may or may not outweigh the ben-efits of HRT, and decisions need to be made individually. In addition, adjustments of dose or route of administration may limit risk (e.g., transdermal as opposed to oral route in patients with cholelithiasis).

The risk of recurrent thromboembolic episodes associated with the use of HRT in women with hypercoagulable disorders has not been defined. Until this risk is defined clearly, nonhor-monal interventions should be considered first-line therapies for symptom management and med-ical benefits associated with HRT.

22. What are the most common side effects of HRT?
The most common complaints are usually related to the addition of a progestational agent. Many of these side effects can be managed with improved patient education or by changing the progestational agent, dosage, or route of administration. **Resumption of menstrual-like bleed-ing** with the use of cyclic PERT is one of the most common reasons for discontinuance. Bleeding normally occurs near or at completion of the course of progestin administration. Use of a continuous course of progestin usually eliminates these cycles. Although 50% of patients may experience irregular bleeding on initiation of a continuous regimen, 60–70% achieve amenorrhea within 1 year.

Women may complain of **premenstrual-like symptoms**—such as depression, irritability, breast tenderness, and bloating—with cyclic administration of a progestational agent. Options include a lower dose for a longer duration, substitution of a continuous regimen, or changing the progestational agent. Recently, the use of medroxyprogesterone acetate, 10 mg for 14 days every 3 months, has been suggested as an alternative. This regimen appears to provide ade-quate endometrial protection, although the periodic bleeding episodes are somewhat heavier than with monthly administration. European authors report success with use of a progestin-re-leasing IUD, which offers endometrial protection while limiting side effects. Unopposed ERT can be considered when all other measures fail to relieve progestational side effects, but such patients must undergo annual endometrial biopsy for detection and treatment of endometrial hyperplasia.

Breast symptoms, such as fullness, tenderness, or increase in size, are commonly noted with initiation of HRT. Patient education and reassurance often alleviate the anxiety associated with these changes. Breast symptoms typically subside with continued use.

Exacerbation of migraine headaches may occur with cyclic regimens but frequently sub-sides with initiation of a continuous regimen. Often, changing the estrogen or route of adminis-tration may resolve these and other less common complaints.

Although women on HRT often complain of **weight gain**, significant changes in weight have not been consistently noted; patients should be counseled about exercise and nutrition.

23. What are the indications for evaluation of the endometrium other than unopposed ERT?
Routine endometrial biopsy before initiation of HRT is no longer indicated. With combined regimens the risk of endometrial hyperplasia and carcinoma is reduced to that of the general pop-ulation. Therefore, evaluation of the endometrium is indicated in women with an abnormal bleed-ing pattern. Withdrawal bleeding earlier than day 10 of 14 of the progestational agent in a sequential regimen typically is considered abnormal, as is bleeding at other times in the "cycle." The more difficult determination is the definition of abnormal bleeding with a continuous regi-men. Persistent prolonged bleeding or heavy bleeding is usually considered an indication for

evaluation of the endometrium—either by going directly to biopsy or by measuring the thickness of the endometrial stripe with endovaginal ultrasonography. If ultrasonography is used initially, biopsy is recommended when the endometrial stripe is greater than 5 mm in thickness, nonhomogeneous in appearance, or incompletely visualized.

24. Should all women take HRT?

The debate continues as to whether menopause is an endocrinopathy warranting treatment in all appropriate women or a normal life stage warranting treatment only for specific indications. Statistics show that most postmenopausal women choose not to take HRT. HRT should be encouraged for women with unwanted symptoms or at increased risk for osteoporosis or cardiovascular disease. Women without contraindications who choose HRT should be supported in their decision. All women should receive counseling about proper nutrition, adequate calcium intake, regular exercise, and routine preventive health care.

25. Is vaginal bleeding after menopause a sign of serious disease?

In women not receiving HRT, all postmenopausal bleeding, regardless of amount, should be considered secondary to cancer until proved otherwise. However, only up to 30% of cases of postmenopausal bleeding are due to a malignant or premalignant condition; the remainder result from various benign causes. Although cancer of the endometrial lining is the most common malignant cause of postmenopausal bleeding, accounting for approximately 15% of cases, other gynecologic malignancies may present with vaginal bleeding and should be considered in the diagnostic work-up. Nongenital sites, such as the urinary and gastrointestinal tracts, also should be examined. Consider the possibility of trauma. Resumption of intercourse may result in lacerations of an atrophic lower genital tract and hemorrhagic bleeding. The emotional nature of this situation should be appreciated.

Causes of Postmenopausal Bleeding

GYNECOLOGIC SOURCES: UPPER GENITAL TRACT	GYNECOLOGIC SOURCES: LOWER GENITAL TRACT	NONGYNECOLOGIC SOURCES
Endometrial polyp	Trauma, vulvar or vaginal	Urethral caruncle
Atrophic endometrial lining	lacerations	Urethral lesions,
Endometrial hyperplasia,	Vaginitis, infection with or	benign or malignant
simple or complex	without atrophy	Hemorrhoids
Endometrial hyperplasia,	Vulvar intraepithelial neoplasia	Rectal polyps or other
with atypia	Vaginal intraepithelial neoplasia	lesions
Endometrial carcinoma	Cervical epithelial neoplasia	
Uterine malignancy of	Vulvar carcinoma	
another nature (sarcoma)	Vaginal carcinoma	
Carcinoma of the fallopian	Cervical carcinoma	
tube		
Ovarian neoplasm		

26. Describe the evaluation of postmenopausal bleeding.

Evaluation includes a thorough history and physical examination to determine the site of origin of the bleeding, a Papanicolaou smear, and an in-office endometrial sampling. Diagnostic hysteroscopy and dilatation and curettage (D&C) are performed if in-office sampling is impossible or insufficient because of cervical stenosis or if results are not conclusive. Ultrasonic evaluation of the endometrial stripe thickness is also used in the work-up of postmenopausal bleeding. A measurement less than 5 mm in a postmenopausal woman not taking HRT is reassuring and may preclude the need for histologic evaluation of the endometrial lining. Additional diagnostic studies, such as pelvic ultrasound and evaluation of the urinary tract or GI tract, may be indicated by the preliminary work-up.

Evaluation of Postmenopausal Bleeding

BASELINE	ADDITIONAL (AS DIRECTED BY ABOVE)
History	Pelvic ultrasound
Physical examination with pelvic and rectal exam	Hysteroscopy and dilatation and curettage
	Urinalysis
Pap smear, Hemoccult stool test	Evaulation of urinary tract
Evaluation of the endometrium	Evaluation of gastrointestinal tract
Endometrial sampling (in office)	
Ultrasonographic evaluation of endometrial stripe	

27. What is the role of selective estrogen receptor modulators (SERMs) in postmenopausal HRT?

SERMs are a class of compounds that act as both estrogen agonists and antagonists, depending on the tissue site of activity. The two SERMs currently available for general use are tamoxifen and raloxifene. Tamoxifen, approved for use in the treatment and prevention of breast cancer, displays an antiestrogen effect in the breast while having an estrogen-like effect on lipid profile, bone metabolism, and the endometrium. Raloxifene, currently approved for use in the prevention of osteoporosis, has a profile similar to tamoxifen except for its anitestrogen effect on the endometrium. Neither tamoxifen nor raloxifene is useful in the management of menopausal symptoms. Both are associated with a mildly elevated risk of thromboembolic events, similar in magnitude to that recently described for HRT.

28. What concerns are unique to the postmenopausal woman who complains of vulvar itching and burning?

Neoplastic conditions of the vulva and vulvar nonneoplastic epithelial disorders, previously known as vulvar dystrophy, occur more often in postmenopausal women and may present with symptoms of pruritus, burning, and painful intercourse. A thorough physical examination with biopsy of visible lesions is indicated in patients presenting with such complaints to ensure appropriate diagnosis and treatment. Because this area does not lend itself well to self-examination, patients often present with significant lesions not previously suspected. A wet mount preparation of any vaginal discharge is examined to identify common causes of vulvovaginitis.

The current classification of vulvar nonneoplastic epithelial disorders accepted by the World Health Organization includes the following categories: lichen sclerosus, squamous cell hyperplasia, and other dermatoses. Diagnosis usually is confirmed with tissue biopsy, which allows proper therapeutic intervention. The current treatment of lichen sclerosus includes the use of high-potency topical corticosteroids (e.g., 0.05% clobetasol cream) for both continuous short-term and intermittent chronic use; good personal hygiene; simple emollients; and avoidance of irritants. Squamous cell hyperplasia usually is managed adequately with short-term administration of medium-potency corticosteroids. Other dermatoses, including conditions such as lichen planus and lichen simplex chronicus, are treated according to the specific tissue diagnosis.

29. How frequently should pelvic exams be done in women over age 65? Why?

There is a noted lack of consensus among national groups about specific recommendations for routine gynecologic screening in women over age 65 for the purpose of health maintenance and disease prevention. No evidence either supports or refutes the recommendations considered to be standard for women in younger age groups. Pelvic exam with Pap smears as part of a problem-focused gynecologic examination is appropriate regardless of age. Since the implementation of the Pap test as a screening tool for cervical cancer, mortality rates for this disease have declined by up to 73%. However, debate continues to surround the issues of frequency and upper age limit of Pap test screening. Approximately 15,000 new cases of cervical cancer and 5,000 related deaths are reported annually. Over 60% of cervical cancer deaths are associated with a Pap smear interval of ≥ 5 years. Forty percent of cervical cancer deaths occur in women over 65 years of age. It is reported that 14% of women aged 65–74 and 39% of women over age 75 have never had a Pap smear, and up to 20% report a lack of regular screening.

Until evidence-based recommendations are available, it is reasonable to continue to screen for cervical cancer in women over 65 whose life expectancy is not limited by other disease states. Screening intervals should be determined by the risk of the individual woman. In women deemed to be at low risk for cervical disease and in whom regular screening has yielded negative results, a screening frequency of 3–5 years represents a consensus of various recommendations. In women thought to be at high risk based on a history of previous disease, high-risk behavior, or lack of regular screening in the previous 10 years, recommended screening intervals are shorter and range from 1–3 years.

The annual gynecologic exam provides a setting to address other health maintenance and screening issues important in women 65 and older, including HRT counseling; osteoporosis prevention and treatment; issues of sexuality, including sexual dysfunction, high-risk behaviors, and prevention of sexually transmitted diseases; and examination of the breast, ovaries, and rectum as part of screening protocols for cancer.

BIBLIOGRAPHY

1. American College of Obstetricians and Gynecologists: Guidelines for Women's Health Care. Washington, DC, American College of Obstetricians and Gynecologists, 1996.
2. American College of Obstetricians and Gynecologists Committee Opinion: Routine Cancer Screening. Number 185. Washington, DC, ACOG, 1997.
3. American College of Obstetricians and Gynecologists Committee Opinion: Recommendations on Frequency of Pap Smear Screening. Number 152. Washington, DC, ACOG, 1995.
4. American College of Obstetricians and Gynecologists Educational Bulletin: Hormone Replacement Therapy. Number 247. Washington, DC, ACOG, 1998.
5. American College of Obstetricians and Gynecologists Educational Bulletin: Vulvar Nonneoplastic Epithelial Disorders. Number 241. Washington, DC, ACOG, 1997.
6. American College of Obstetricians and Gynecologists Technical Bulletin: Pelvic Organ Prolapse. Number 214. Washington, DC, ACOG, 1995.
7. American Medical Women's Association Contemporary Issues in Women's Health: Enhancing Women's Use of Preventive Medicine. Module 1, 1995.
8. American Medical Women's Association Contemporary Issues in Women's Health: Health Maintenance Screening Procedures: Gynecologic Cancers. Module 2, 1995.
9. Baden WF, Walker T (eds): Surgical Repair of Vaginal Defects. Philadelphia, J.B. Lippincott, 1992.
10. Berek JF, Adashi E, Hillard P: Novak's Gynecology. Baltimore, Williams & Wilkins, 1996.
11. Byyny L, Speroff L: A Clinical Guide for the Care of Older Women, 2nd ed. Baltimore, Williams & Wilkins, 1996.
12. Fisher B, Costantino J, for the NSABP investigators: Tamoxifen for prevention of breast cancer: Report of the National Surgical Adjuvant Breast and Bowel Project P-1 Study. J Natl Cancer Inst 90:1371–1388, 1998.
13. Scott JR, DiSaia PJ, Hammond CB, et al (eds): Danforth's Obstetrics and Gynecology, 7th ed. Philadelphia, J.B. Lippincott, 1994.
14. Sobel NB: Primary care of the mature woman. Obstet Gynecol Clin North Am 21:299–314, 1994.
15. Speroff L, Glass RH, Kase NG (eds): Clinical Gynecologic Endocrinology and Infertility, 6th ed. Baltimore, Williams & Wilkins, 1999.
16. U.S. Preventive Task Force: Guide to Clinical Preventive Services. Baltimore, Williams & Wilkins, 1996.

30. DEPRESSION

David S. Miller, M.D.

1. What is the difference between depression and normal sadness?

Depressive illnesses in older people, like those in younger adults, can occur without obvious causes or precipitants. More often, however, late-life depression occurs in the context of medical illness, psychosocial stress, and loss, and so most depressions make sense empathetically and intuitively. Unfortunately, this often leads to the view that depression is a "natural" state of aging rather than a medical symptom requiring evaluation.

Despite these misconceptions, the distinction between depressive illness and normal sadness is straightforward. Depressive illnesses are persistent, lasting for several weeks or longer. Depressive illnesses can be disabling, interfering with social, instrumental, or self-care activities either by themselves or by amplifying the disability associated with medical illness. Although the relationships between depression and disability can be complex and bidirectional, patients who have persistent depression coexisting with functional impairments require medical evaluation.

2. What subtypes of depression are relevant in late life?

Major depressive disorder is characterized by episodes in which the following symptoms persist:

Persistent depressed mood	Hypersomnia
Markedly decreased interest or pleasure in usual activities	Psychomotor agitation or retardation
	Fatigue or loss of energy
Decreased appetite and weight loss	Feelings of worthlessness or excessive guilt
Increased appetite and weight gain (more rarely)	Decreased ability to think or concentrate
	Suicidal thoughts, wishes, plan, or intent
Insomnia	

According to the *Diagnostic and Statistical Manual for Mental Disorders* (DSM-IV), the diagnosis of a **major depressive episode** can be made when patients have depressed mood and/or loss of interests or pleasure and a total of five of the above symptoms to a significant degree for a period of at least 2 weeks.

Major depression can occur as a *single* episode or as part of a *recurring* pattern of episodes. Depressions occurring in the elderly can be of *early onset*, in which the late-life depression occurs as a recurrence of an illness that began in younger adulthood, or *late onset*, in which illness began initially at an older age. Recurrent depression can be *bipolar*, where both depressive and manic or hypomanic episodes occur, or *unipolar*, in which only depressions occur. This distinction between unipolar and bipolar is important because antidepressant treatment of bipolar patients may precipitate manic or hypomanic episodes. Depressions can also be associated with *psychotic* features (hallucinations or delusions). Psychotic depressions do not, as a rule, respond to antidepressants alone and instead require both antidepressants and antipsychotic medications or electroconvulsive therapy.

Although less severe, other types of depressions are also clinically significant. **Dysthymic disorder** is a condition in which lower levels of depressive symptoms exist chronically for a period of 2 years or more. **Minor depressions** include those in which symptoms of depression and anxiety coexist and those in which more severe depressive symptoms occur briefly but recurrently.

3. How is depression related to other medical illness?

The NIH consensus conference on the diagnosis and treatment of late-life depression noted that the hallmark of depression in the elderly was its association with medical illness. Late-onset depressions, in general, emerged in the context of chronic medical or neurologic illness, and a growing body of epidemiologic research demonstrates an increased prevalence of major depression in medical care settings. Major depression occurs in approximately 2–4% of healthy elderly in the community, 10–12% of elderly medical inpatients, and 20–25% of cognitively intact nursing home residents. In addition, as many as 30–50% of patients in medical care settings have clinically significant minor depressions. Clinicians should systematically determine whether comorbid depression is present in all elderly patients with significant medical illness whom they see. Conversely, all elderly individuals who present to mental health care settings for evaluation of depression should be evaluated for significant medical illnesses.

4. How do you treat depression that occurs as part of a medical illness?

When depression complicates significant **acute medical illnesses**, patients require support. Specific treatment is necessary when depression is severe or when it interferes with medical management. For more moderate depressions, continued monitoring of affective symptoms during the course of recovery from the medical illness is necessary. Treatment for depression should be instituted when the depression persists despite improvement in medical status.

When depression occurs in medically stable patients with **chronic illness**, systems should be reviewed to identify possible medical causes of the affective symptoms. Common causes include unrecognized acute illnesses (e.g., heart failure, urinary tract infections), side effects of medications (e.g., beta blockers), electrolyte abnormalities (e.g., hyponatremia, hypercalcemia), thyroid dysfunction, and vitamin B_{12} or folate deficiency. A review of systems is also necessary to identify medical conditions that could complicate treatment; for example, before use of tricyclic antidepressants, patients must be evaluated for disorders of cardiac conduction, prostate hypertrophy, and glaucoma.

5. How can you tell if a particular symptom is due to medical illness or to depression?

Extensive literature in the field of consultation-liaison psychiatry has focused on the possibility that medical symptoms can obscure the diagnosis of major depression. Some symptoms, such as fatigue, can be due to medical illnesses (e.g., heart failure) or to depression. Experienced clinicians can evaluate the etiology of symptoms and "factor" them into their medical and depressive components. Even with truly ambiguous symptoms, utilizing an inclusive approach to diagnosis based on all observed symptoms, regardless of their apparent etiology, can still be helpful. Despite the theoretical difficulties, current approaches to diagnosis have, in fact, been validated in patients suffering from many of the comorbid medical disorders that are common in late life. Controlled clinical trials have demonstrated that depressions diagnosed in patients with medical illnesses as diverse as stroke, parkinsonism, cancer, ischemic heart disease, chronic obstructive pulmonary disease, and arthritis still respond to treatment.

6. What is depressive pseudodementia?

Classically, most textbooks in geriatric psychiatry emphasized the difficulties in identifying patients in whom major depression caused significant cognitive impairment and in distinguishing between these potentially treatable cases of "pseudodementia" and irreversible dementias such as Alzheimer's disease. The use of the term *pseudodementia* has been criticized by some investigators who note that severe depression can cause real cognitive impairment. The name **dementia syndrome of depression** has been proposed to emphasize that although these conditions are treatable, there is nothing "pseudo" about the disability resulting from severe depression.

More significantly, Reifler and colleagues noted that patients with coexisting depression and cognitive impairment could have either one disease or two. Patients could have a pure depressive disorder associated with cognitive impairment (pseudodementia), in which case, treatment of depression could restore normal levels of functioning. Alternatively, they could have an irreversible dementia with a superimposed depressive disorder. In these cases, treatment of depression could reverse only a component of the patient's disability. In either case, recognition, diagnosis, and treatment of depression could be of benefit to the patient.

7. What is the long-term prognosis for patients having dementia syndrome with depression?

Recent research has been reevaluating the long-term prognosis of patients with depression associated with cognitive impairment that is alleviated through treatment. Two generations ago, there were concerns that all depressions with onset in late-life were prodromes of dementia. A generation ago, systematic follow-up studies on patients hospitalized for depression demonstrated that depression and dementia were, in fact, separable disorders and that the long-term outcome of most patients with late-life depression did not include cognitive deterioration. New research in this area, however, suggests that patients with depression associated with reversible cognitive impairment are at increased risk for developing dementia over the subsequent few years. At present, these findings should not be taken to reflect nihilism about outcomes for these patients but rather should underscore the importance of long-term follow-up and treatment.

8. What are the problems associated with untreated depression?

Untreated or undertreated depression is associated with both psychiatric and general medical consequences. Psychiatric morbidity includes chronicity with its associated psychosocial disability, risks of alcohol or substance abuse in attempts at self-treatment, and suicide. The most compelling case for the importance of the recognition of depression by primary care physicians comes from the finding that 75% of older people who kill themselves saw their physicians within 30 days of their deaths.

Suicide can occur not only when depression is missed but at any time during the treatment course of a depressive episode. Closer surveillance is indicated if the patient expresses suicidal thoughts, intent, and/or describes a plan. There is a transient increased suicide risk in the early stages of treatment, as patients gain the energy and capacity to act on their earlier plans.

Medical morbidity associated with depression includes increased disability, protein-calorie undernutrition, increased pain complaints, and greater sensitivity to subjective side effects of medications. There are also increases in utilization of general medical care services (inpatient and outpatient) and in caregiver burden. Finally, there is an increase in mortality, even after controlling for the increased severity of medical illnesses in patients with depression.

9. When should patients receive antidepressant medications?

The efficacy of antidepressant medications has been established for the treatment of patients with major depression. Thus, clinicians should inquire about the presence of the DSM-IV diagnostic symptoms. Significantly (and counterintuitively), evaluating a patient's need for antidepressant medication requires knowledge about symptoms but not about the presence or absence of reasons for the depression.

In addition to their well-established use in the treatment of major depression, antidepressants may be of value in patients with dysthymia or minor depression who either do not respond to psychosocial treatment or are not amenable to it.

10. When should older patients receive psychotherapy?

Structured psychotherapies, such as cognitive-behavioral therapy, interpersonal therapy, or brief dynamic therapies, may be the treatments of choice for dysthymia or minor depression. They may also be a first-line treatment for milder major depression; however, if these patients do not experience a significant amelioration of their symptoms within several weeks, use of antidepressants should be reconsidered.

In general, depression in the elderly frequently has associated functional and social difficulties. Among these are loss of or changed roles, lack of social support, chronic medical illnesses, hopelessness, disability, and bereavement. Therefore, psychotherapy can be extremely useful as an adjuvant to pharmacotherapy in patients with major depression of moderate severity.

11. What are first- and second-line agents used in the pharmacotherapy of depression?

Selective serotonin reuptake inhibitors (SSRIs—e.g., fluoxetine, sertraline, paroxetine, citalopram): Given their tolerable side effect profile and safety in overdose, these agents are appropriate first-line treatments for depression in ambulatory elderly, especially those seen by primary care providers. They have fewer anticholinergic and cardiac side effects but may cause nausea, diarrhea, somnolence, and headache. Their once-daily dosing and tolerability may enhance compliance. However, although SSRIs are somewhat less effective in people over 75-years-old, their efficacy and safety in frail or medically ill elderly patients have not been established. In such patients, SSRIs may cause lethargy, anorexia, and syndrome of inappropriate antidiuretic hormone secretion. In the elderly, who frequently take multiple medications, particular attention must be paid to the effect of SSRIs on hepatic metabolism of other medications via the cytochrome P450 system. Additional problems may include drug interactions, extrapyramidal symptoms, bradycardia, and sexual dysfunction.

Tricyclic antidepressants (TCAs): The secondary amine TCAs nortriptyline and desipramine are preferred for use in the elderly. Their efficacy in the elderly, including patients with significant medical comorbidity, has been well-established. Moreover, these agents are less likely to produce orthostasis (which can lead to falls and fractures), excessive sedation, anticholinergic symptoms, or cardiac toxicity than the tertiary amine TCAs (e.g., amitriptyline or imipramine). The secondary amine TCAs can be used safely in patients who do not have cardiac conduction problems, acute narrow-angle glaucoma, and prostatic hypertrophy with urinary retention. With these agents, plasma level–response correlations have been established, and therapeutic blood levels (80–120 ng/ml for nortriptyline and > 125 ng/ml for desipramine) can be utilized to individualize doses for the individual patient.

	SEDATION	HYPOTENSION	ANTICHOLINERGIC SIDE EFFECTS	CHANGES IN CARDIAC RATE AND RHYTHM
Desipramine	+	+/++	+	+
Nortriptyline	+	+	++	+

Other agents: Among the newer antidepressants, mirtazapine, bupropion, venlafaxine, and nefazodone may be of value in treating older patients. Some of these agents target more than one neurotransmitter system to enhance effectiveness.

12. How do you select an appropriate medication?

Before an antidepressant is chosen one must consider the risks and benefits for that particular patient. Factors to be mindful of are concurrent medical conditions and medications, substance abuse problems (e.g., alcohol abuse), and the likelihood of overdose, either by suicide attempt or secondary to cognitive problems. Several basic principles can be outlined:

- For ambulatory outpatients with major depression that is mild to moderate in severity, the first-line use of SSRIs or other well-tolerated agents is reasonable.
- For patients with more severe depression, early use of the better-established TCAs should be considered.
- In patients who are frail or with specific medical conditions that could complicate use of these agents, hospitalization may be necessary to optimize safety during the institution of treatment. Frequently, an extensive list of medications can and should be pared down (generally in consultation with the geriatric medicine team). This affords the treatment team an opportunity to determine to what degree the patient's presenting symptoms are iatrogenic. Concurrently, as the patient's medical conditions are treated, the depression may lessen or remit. When it does not, antidepressants are indicated.
- Regardless of which medications are used initially, it is necessary to monitor patients to evaluate both therapeutic responses and to identify side effects.
- If patients do not show early signs of response within 4–6 weeks, it is important to consider modifying the treatment plan.

13. Should St. John's wort be used?

The jury is still out. Studies of variable quality and rigor have shown that St. John's wort is better than placebo and as effective as tricyclic antidepressants for mild-to-moderate, but not severe, depression. Studies are currently under way in the United States to determine its effectiveness and to understand more fully the mechanism of its purported antidepressant and antianxiety effects. The Food and Drug Administration has yet to establish clinical guidelines for its use.

14. How long should treatment be continued?

Treatment of depression can be divided into three phases:

Acute phase (goal: to achieve symptom remission)—The median time to recover from the acute phase of an index episode of depression is 12 weeks (longer than for younger patients). Discerning whether a patient is responding can only reliably be done after 4–6 weeks.

Continuation phase (goal: to stabilize patients during a period when they are highly vulnerable to relapse)—All patients recovering from an episode of depression are vulnerable to relapse during the first 6–9 months after symptom remission. All patients should remain in continuation-phase treatment for this period of time.

Maintenance phase (goal: to prevent recurrence)—At the completion of the continuation phase, patients and their physicians must decide whether treatment should be discontinued (by slowly tapering antidepressant doses) or whether the patient should remain on long-term maintenance treatment to decrease the probability of recurrences. If treatment is discontinued, the patient and family should be educated and informed about the need for continued monitoring to facilitate the early identification of recurrences. If the patient has had > 2 episodes of depression, or if the initial episodes were particularly severe or lengthy, long-term (possibly lifetime) maintenance therapy should be considered.

15. When should electroconvulsive therapy (ECT) be considered?

The indications for ECT in both younger and older patients include severe major depression and mania. Older patients with severe depression often present with psychotic symptoms and suicidality (occasionally taking the form of food refusal). They may respond to SSRIs less consistently and may be less able to tolerate the anticholinergic and cardiac side effects of the TCAs. Therefore, the elderly are more likely to require ECT. They actually account for a disproportionate percentage of those who get ECT (receiving > 30% of all ECTs despite representing < 10% of all hospitalized psychiatric patients).

ECT is safe and effective, even when there are physical comorbidities or dementia. It should be considered the treatment of choice when a rapid response is needed for severely depressed patients. It should also be considered in patients who have previously not responded to adequate trials of antidepressant treatment.

16. What can be done when patients don't respond to treatment?

Between 20 and 30% of patients fail to respond satisfactorily to initial treatment with an antidepressant medication. Possible explanations include improper diagnosis, inadequate treatment, and failure to identify and treat concurrent general medical and psychiatric disorders.

Obstacles to administering adequate treatment include:

• Poor compliance by both patient and family (who may fail to understand the illness, its course, and/or the importance of compliance)
• Side effects
• Hidden self-medication (e.g., alcohol)
• Adverse psychosocial factors (which may diminish the desire to comply)
• Medical comorbidities (which can interfere with antidepressant response or attainment of adequate dosages)

Steps the clinician can take to enhance compliance include creating an alliance with and providing education about depression to the patient and family, being mindful of side effects so as to decrease them when they occur, and maintaining a supportive attitude.

Once satisfied on all counts that the initial trial was adequate, one can either augment the present medication or switch to another agent (from another class of antidepressant). Adjuvant treatments include:

- Lithium (a response should be seen within a few days to a few weeks; blood levels indicating therapeutic levels are not clear)
- Thyroid hormone
- Psychostimulants

The anticonvulsants carbamazepine and valproic acid have been used both as primary and adjuvant agents for treatment-resistant depression. Occasionally the clinician will choose an antidepressant that targets more than one neutrotransmitter system. Sometimes, multiple antidepressants are used simultaneously. Combined treatment, however, carries the risk of adverse interactions and may require dose adjustment (e.g., SSRIs can increase TCA blood levels, and thus TCA doses may need to be reduced to avoid toxicity). If a patient fails two separate trials of antidepressant medication, ECT should be considered.

17. Under what circumstances are psychostimulants indicated?

In the elderly, psychostimulants such as methylphenidate (Ritalin) are generally used for two purposes. The first is to treat patients who, although not severely depressed, become apathetic or discouraged, frequently in the context of chronic disease or rehabilitation from illness or surgery. Although not effective in treating major depression, psychostimulants have been found to be helpful in medically ill patients and apathetic nursing home residents. The second use is to augment an ongoing antidepressant trial in which the response has been suboptimal.

Ritalin is well tolerated and works quickly. It should be given in the morning to avoid insomnia. Dosing should begin at 2.5–5.0 mg/day and titrated to a maximum of 20 mg/day (generally divided between 8:00 AM and noon). The most common side effects are tachycardia and mild elevation in blood pressure.

18. What are the most important points about late-life depression for primary care doctors?

1. The diagnosis of late-life depression is as valid as that of other significant medical disorders.
2. Major depression in the elderly is a significant disorder associated with both psychiatric and medical morbidity, increased utilization of general health care services, and increased mortality.
3. Late-life depression is a treatable disorder.

BIBLIOGRAPHY

1. Alexopoulos GS, Meyers GS, Young RC, et al: The course of geriatric depression with "reversible dementia": A controlled study. Am J Psychiatry 150:1693–1699, 1993.
2. Conwell Y: Suicide in elderly patients. In Schneider LS, Reynolds CF, Lebowitz BD, Friedhoff AJ (eds): Diagnosis and Treatment of Depression in Late Life. Washington D.C., American Psychiatric Press, 1994, pp 397–418.
3. Jones BN, Reifler BV: Depression coexisting with dementia: Evaluation and treatment. Med Clin North Am 78:823–840, 1994.
4. Katz IR: Drug treatment of depression in the frail elderly: Discussion of the NIH consensus development conference on the diagnosis and treatment of depression in late life. Psychopharmacol Bull 29(1): 101–108, 1993.
5. Katz IR, Streim J, Parmelee P: Prevention of depression, recurrences, and complications in late life. Prev Med 23:743–750, 1994.
6. Reynolds CF, Alexopoulos G, Katz IR, et al: Treatment of geriatric mood disorders. Curr Rev Mood Disord 1:189–202, 1997.
7. Schneider LS, Reynolds CF, Lebowitz BD, Friedhoff AJ (eds): Diagnosis and Treatment of Depression in Late Life: Results of the NIH Consensus Development Conference. Washington, D.C., American Psychiatric Press, 1994.
8. Wallace AE, Kofoed LL, West AN: Double-blind placebo-controlled trial of methylphenidate in older, depressed medically ill patients. Am J Psychiatry 152:929–931, 1995.

31. PARKINSON'S DISEASE

Howard Hurtig, M.D.

1. Who is Parkinson's disease named after?

James Parkinson is credited with the first detailed description in 1817 of the illness that now bears his name.

2. How is Parkinson's disease different from parkinsonian syndrome?

Parkinsonian syndrome, or parkinsonism, is an umbrella term that applies to a recognizable cluster of neurologic symptoms (fatigue, tremor, slowed mobility, difficulty walking) and signs (bradykinesia, stooped posture, shuffling gait, cogwheel rigidity, rest tremor). Most often symptoms of parkinsonism appear in middle-aged adults and increase in frequency with the advance of old age. Approximately 1% of people in the developed world over age 60 have some form of parkinsonism, although it is prevalent everywhere in the world.

Any combination of signs and symptoms of parkinsonism can occur, most often emerging gradually, or even imperceptibly. Not all components of the symptom complex are present in every patient. Rest tremor is often the only early symptom, but because it is distinctively different from other types of tremor (i.e., action or intention tremor), it is usually recognizable as parkinsonian. Rarely, self-recognition of the signs of parkinsonism is abrupt; for example, in the form of tremor starting in the aftermath of physical or psychological trauma. There is no evidence that either type of trauma actually causes parkinsonism.

Eighty percent to 90% of people who develop the cardinal symptoms and signs of parkinsonism will have *idiopathic* parkinsonism or **Parkinson's disease** (PD). A clinical diagnosis of Parkinson's disease can be made confidently if at least 3 major signs are identified. Parkinson's disease is a *clinical* diagnosis, reached after other causes of parkinsonism have been excluded by a careful history, thorough physical examination, and a few specific laboratory tests. Brain imaging studies, such as magnetic resonance imaging (MRI), are rarely helpful.

Criteria for Diagnosis of Parkinson's Disease*

Unilateral onset and persistent asymmetry	Levodopa-induced dyskinesias
Rest tremor	Levodopa response for $\geq$ 5 yrs
Progressive disability	Clinical course of $\geq$ 10 yrs
Excellent response to levodopa	

* Three or more required for diagnosis of definite Parkinson's disease.
From United Kingdom Parkinson's Disease Society Brain Bank.

3. What are the pathologic findings associated with Parkinson's disease?

The disease is primarily confined to the upper brainstem, where a particular collection of pigmented (melanin) neurons in the substantia nigra undergo progressive degeneration from an unkown cause. The **Lewy body** (LB), an intracytoplasmic inclusion body found at autopsy in the few nigral neurons that survive the process of progressive nigral degeneration, is the histologic signature of PD. LBs are also found at postmortem in the cerebral cortex, especially among people who have significant cognitive dysfunction, the prevalence of which increases with advancing motor disability. Approximately one-third of patients with PD become demented late in the disease course; cortical LBs are found in the great majority.

Nigral neurons, when healthy, are the main source of the brain's supply of catecholamine and the neurotransmitter **dopamine**. Dopamine is transported from the brainstem rostrally via the **nigrostriatal** anatomic pathway, beginning in the substantia nigra and ending at the corpus striatum (caudate and putamen) adjacent to the lateral ventricles. The assemblage of neurons in this brain region is known collectively as the **basal ganglia**. Dopamine plays a major role in the normal physiologic circuitry that connects the basal ganglia to the cerebral cortex and is a major contributor to the complex neurotransmission responsible for programming and executing voluntary movement. Dopamine replacement therapy with the dopamine precursor **levodopa** often alleviates many of PD's most disabling symptoms, but it does not stop the relentless but protracted natural progression of the disease.

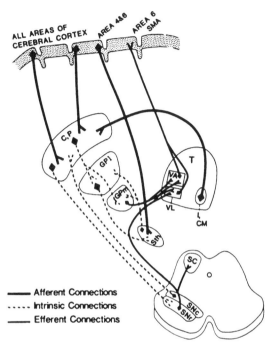

Major afferent, efferent, and internuclear pathways of the basal ganglia. C,P = caudate nucleus and putamen (striatum), GP = globus pallidus (l = lateral, m = medial), SN = substantia nigra (c = compacta, r = reticulata), Sth = subthalamic nucleus, T = thalamus (nuclei: VA = ventral anterior, VL = ventrolateral, CM = centromedian, I = other intralaminar nuclei), SMA = supplementary motor area of cortex, SC = superior colliculus. (From Riley DE, Lang AE: Movement disorders. In Bradley WG, et al (eds): Neurology in Clinical Practice. Boston, Butterworth-Heinemann, 1996, with permission.)

⸻⸻ Afferent Connections
· · · · Intrinsic Connections
⸻⸻ Efferent Connections

4. Name the major and minor signs and symptoms of parkinsonism.

Signs of Parkinsonism

MAJOR	MINOR
Rest tremor (4–6 Hz)	Masked facies
Bradykinesia	Micrographia
Muscular rigidity with cogwheeling	Fatigue
Postural instability	Drooling
	Hypophonia

5. Which other neurologic disorders have parkinsonism as a major clinical feature?
Parkinson-plus syndromes—Approximately 10% of people with parkinsonism have pathology in anatomic sites other than the pigmented neurons of the substantia nigra. Degenerative disorders such as progressive supranuclear palsy (PSP), striatonigral degeneration, and parkinsonism with autonomic failure (Shy-Drager syndrome) often resemble Parkinson's disease early in the course, except that patients with Parkinson-plus syndromes are less likely to have tremor and more likely to have postural instability with significant gait problems at the beginning. The generic term **multisystems atrophy** has become a popular label for a parkinsonian syndrome that is characterized by increasing bradykinesia, rigidity and postural instability, and

findings on neurologic exam that reflect multiple anatomic sites of degeneration (basal ganglia, cerebellum, pyramidal tract). Levodopa usually gives little or no benefit to Parkinson-plus patients, and as a result, the rate of progression is often faster.

Cerebrovascular disease—In the elderly with vascular risk factors, especially hypertension, parkinsonism can evolve as a result of multifocal ischemia and be almost indistinguishable from Parkinson's disease. Early onset of gait instability, presence of frontal release signs, prominent cognitive loss, little or no tremor, and an MRI scan showing multiple infarcts are a few features that help to separate vascular parkinsonism from the other parkinsonian syndromes.

6. Can medications cause parkinsonism?

Any neuroleptic drug used for any length of time can produce signs of parkinsonism and other movement disorders in older patients. It is important to remember that metoclopramide (Reglan) is a neuroleptic with the same potential for causing parkinsonism as the more potent drugs, such as chlorpromazine and haloperidol. Neuroleptics cause Parkinson symptoms by the same mechanism that they relieve the symptoms of psychosis; they block postsynaptic dopamine receptors in the basal ganglia and mesolimbic cerebral cortex. Reserpine, once a standard antihypertensive, is still used occasionally, often in a combination drug. Reserpine causes parkinsonism by depleting the presynaptic stores of catecholamines, including dopamine. It has no effect on dopamine receptors.

7. What disorders of the nervous system are commonly confused with parkinsonism?

1. **Senile gait** is a disorder of locomotion among older people that resembles the shuffle of parkinsonism, but it can be so severe that walking is impossible due to the inability to initiate or sustain the rhythmic sequence of movements basic to normal walking. This condition has been called **lower-body parkinsonism** because the other usual symptoms of parkinsonism found above the waist are missing or relatively mild. Senile gait overlaps with the mincing steps of older persons who have a background of multiple small strokes and with "gait ignition failure," transient freezing that occurs with initiation of walking. The pathophysiology of these nonparkinsonian gait disorders is obscure.

2. **Essential tremor** (ET) is another common idiopathic movement disorder that is usually familial (autosomal dominant) and increases in frequency with aging. It is the mirror image of parkinsonian rest tremor; i.e., it is activated by voluntary movement and subsides at rest. A careful neurologic examination is the key to separating ET from PD. Handwriting is often a clue: micrographic and tight in Parkinson's (usually not shaky), shaky and large in ET.

3. **Stroke** is sometimes diagnosed when problems are actually caused by PD. Since parkinsonism often starts unilaterally, a flexed and rigid arm or leg can look as if it was caused by a stroke (especially if tremor is absent). Yet, examination shows the telltale signs of unilateral parkinsonism (cogwheel rigidity, bradykinesia of fingers and toes) and the absence of findings typically seen in stroke-related neurologic deficits: strength and sensation are normal, reflexes symmetrical, and Babinski signs absent. On the other hand, multiple small strokes can cause a parkinsonian syndrome that highly resembles PD. A markedly abnormal MRI scan (showing strokes in the basal ganglia) and a poor response to levodopa usually delineate the two disorders.

8. What is the relationship between Alzheimer's disease and Parkinson's disease?

Alzheimer's dementia (AD) is by far the most common neurologic disorder of aging in the Western world. Mild parkinsonism occurs in 20–30% of patients with AD, a reflection of the frequent autopsy finding of a moderate decrease in the number of neurons in the substantia nigra of Alzheimer-affected brains. This interesting overlap between AD and PD is also evident in the higher-than-chance occurrence (20–30%) of dementia in a cross-section of elderly patients with PD, a significant number of whom have Alzheimer's pathology and cortical LB at autopsy.

A clinical diagnosis of AD with parkinsonism versus PD with dementia is a common chicken-and-egg dilemma in neurology. It is often unscrambled by identifying the symptom complex that came first as the primary disorder. Under such circumstances, the clinicopathologic correlation is strong. The high rate of coexistence of AD and PD suggests a common but as-yet-unidentified pathogenetic mechanism that gives rise to neurofibrillary degeneration of vulnerable cell groups in particular but different locations in the brain.

9. Describe an appropriate diagnostic work-up for someone with parkinsonism.

In reality, the diagnosis of classic PD is purely clinical and no tests are needed. However, when diagnostic criteria are not met confidently, many doctors choose to do a **brain imaging study**, especially an MRI scan. MRI or computed tomography (CT) scans show no definitive abnormalities in PD and only occasionally are helpful in patients with the atypical forms of parkinsonism. Rarely, **severe hydrocephalus** can cause parkinsonism, and only a CT or MRI can show the large ventricles. A ventriculoperitoneal shunt will improve neurologic function in these cases.

Blood and urine tests for **copper** are mandatory in the work-up of parkinsonism in anyone under 40 to exclude **Wilson's disease**, an inherited disorder of copper metabolism. Parkinsonism in children and young adults also can be part of the phenotype in certain other hereditary conditions, such as the autosomal dominant **Machado-Joseph disease** (MJD).

A strongly positive response to an adequate trial of **levodopa** is usually the best indicator that classic PD is the right diagnosis. As a rule, a weak or absent response suggests one of the atypical parkinsonian states, although a significant response to levodopa may occur early in the course of any patient with any form of parkinsonism.

10. What organ systems does parkinsonism affect?

Gastrointestinal tract
Slowed motility
Constipation
Pseudo-obstruction or megacolon (rarely)
Obstipation and impactions
Urinary tract
Increased frequency
Urgency
Incontinence

Respiratory system
Hypoventilation
Laryngeal stridor
Visual system
Visual blurring
Diplopia
Olfactory system
Anosmia

11. What causes Parkinson's disease?

This is the question that tantalizes everyone. While there is enough circumstantial evidence to permit experts to formulate a unified working causal hypothesis, the mystery of causation for the most part has not been deciphered. The evidence falls into 3 broad categories with many points of convergence and intersection:

1. Although it has been known for most of this century that approximately 10–15% of patients with PD have a positive family history of parkinsonism, autosomal dominant pedigrees with autopsy proof of PD (Lewy bodies) have been rare. Moreover, studies of identical twins have shown a relatively low rate of concordance when one twin has PD. Yet, the occurrence of these autosomal dominant families and the more common, nonspecific familial aggregations of PD gives some weight to the belief that an abnormal gene with variable penetrance and expressivity is fundamentally responsible for *all* cases of PD. This conjecture was given weight in 1997 with the discovery of a gene responsible for familial parkinsonism in several large families with an autosomal dominant pattern of inheritance. The gene lies on chromosome 4 and codes for the presynaptic protein alpha synuclein (a-syn). Subsequent investigations have shown that immunostaining of a-syn in the brain localizes to nigral and cortical LB.

2. Numerous epidemiologic studies have suggested, albeit weakly, that a host of environmental insults, including past head injury, chronic exposure to pesticides (or other toxins), and rural living, might be risk factors for later development of PD.

3. Neurons die slowly as the brain ages, and neural tissue does not regenerate. Consequently, advancing age contributes to the loss of chemical transmitters manufactured by those dying neurons, and the result in susceptible individuals (i.e., those genetically predisposed or environmentally exposed) is age-related neurologic illness, such as PD and AD.

12. What is neuroprotection or neuroprotective therapy?

The basis of neuroprotection is the belief that neural degeneration can be slowed or halted by using agents that stabilize cells and keep them from dying. The fundamental pathogenesis of neurodegeneration is thought to be linked to oxidative stress, which in turn is mediated by the generation of an excess amount of toxic-free radical molecules. Free radicals are highly destructive to cell membranes. The discovery that the drug **deprenyl**, an inhibitor of the B form of monoamine oxidase, could block the formation of MPP+ from MPTP (MPP+ is a highly neurotoxic, oxidized byproduct of the recreational drug MPTP that produces severe parkinsonism) and thereby prevent its toxicity led to the hypothesis that deprenyl could slow progression of the disability of PD by preventing the formation of oxygen free radicals that result from the oxidation of dopamine. In the 1980s, a double-blind, randomized clinical trial of deprenyl in patients with early PD showed that deprenyl delayed the need for levodopa therapy by almost a year when compared with placebo. Unfortunately, solid proof that deprenyl actually does protect neurons has been elusive because it also has a mild but significant potential to reduce parkinsonian symptoms by a separate mechanism. Many neurologists now prescribe deprenyl in early PD for its putative neuroprotective effect, despite the absence of proof.

The recent discovery of a variety of **growth factors** in the human nervous system has created the possibility of an entirely new form of clinically viable neuroprotection. These biologically active substances naturally promote growth and membrane stability of all cells during development.

13. Which drugs are most effective in treating Parkinson's disease?

Drugs for Treatment of Parkinson's Disease

DRUG	MECHANISM OF ACTION	RELATIVE POTENCY	SIDE EFFECTS
Levodopa/carbidopa (Sinemet)	Activates DA receptors	++++	Nausea Dyskinesia Psychosis Hypotension Constipation
Dopamine agonists (bromocriptine pergolide, pramipexole, ropinirole)	Activates DA receptors	++	Nausea Hypotension Leg edema Psychosis
Amantadine (Symmetrel)	Releases DA from vesicles	+	Psychosis Leg edema Livedo reticularis
Anticholinergics (Artane, Cogentin, Kemadrin)	Blocks ACh receptors	+	Memory loss Blurred vision Psychosis Prostatism Dry mouth
Deprenyl (Eldepryl)	MAO inhibitor—blocks reuptake of DA ?Neuroprotection	+	Psychosis Hypotension
Tolcapone	Catechol O methyl transferase inhibition—blocks reuptake of DA	+	Dyskinesia Diarrhea Liver damage

DA = dopamine; ACh = acetylcholine; MAO = monoamine oxidase.

Four important axioms underlie the application of any of these drugs to the treatment of Parkinson's disease:

1. Never start treatment with > 1 drug.
2. Start with the lowest practical dose and increase slowly—there's never a need to rush.
3. Never make > 1 change at a time when raising or lowering doses, unless the patient is in crisis.
4. Multiple drugs at the same time may be necessary. Many neurologists introduce second and third drugs early in the treatment if the primary one (usually levodopa) is not giving adequate benefit.

14. Why is levodopa given with carbidopa?

Levodopa, after almost 30 years since its introduction as a dramatic new treatment for Parkinson's disease, remains the best drug with the best therapeutic margin (fewest side effects in relation to benefit), despite its complicated pharmacology. Levodopa, a precursor of dopamine, is biochemically inert (i.e., not a neurotransmitter), but it easily crosses the blood-brain barrier (BBB) to get into the brain where it is converted to dopamine by the enzyme dopa-decarboxylase (DD). The active transmitter dopamine, on the other hand, is excluded from the brain when used systemically because its molecular structure does not permit it to cross the BBB. The problem is that levodopa is rapidly decarboxylated to dopamine peripherally by DD in the gut and liver before it reaches the brain; thus it is rendered useless for clinical purposes unless given in large amounts to saturate the converting enzyme, in which case intolerable nausea usually occurs. The solution to this therapeutic "catch 22" came in the early 1970s with the development of the DD inhibitor, **carbidopa**. When carbidopa is given in combination with levodopa (Sinemet), it prevents peripheral decarboxylation and reduces by 80% the amount of levodopa required to have a clinical effect. It also eliminates most of the side effects associated with using pure levodopa, and makes levodopa accessible to a much larger population of patients.

15. Do all patients with parkinsonism and all symptoms of parkinsonism respond to treatment?

No, unfortunately. The cardinal symptoms of early disease—rest tremor, rigidity, and bradykinesia—usually respond well but not necessarily at the same time. Tremor tends to lag behind the other two but eventually follows. Only 50% of all responders will grade the response as very good or excellent. A completely negative response to levodopa-carbidopa usually portends an unfavorable prognosis as well as a diagnosis of one of the Parkinson-plus disorders.

The most vexing of all symptoms of parkinsonism is loss of balance or postural instability (PI). Most drugs, including Sinemet, have little or no effect on PI, although occasional significant improvements in balance make the effort of trying the various available dopaminergic medications worthwhile. The relatively poor response of PI to dopamine replacement therapy compared with many of the other symptoms of parkinsonism suggests a nondopaminergic pathophysiology.

16. What are the important adjunctive drugs used in treating secondary problems in Parkinson's disease?

Adjunctive Drugs Used in Parkinson's Disease

DRUG	INDICATION	DRUG	INDICATION
Antidepressants	Depression	Cisapride Lactulase	Constipation
Tricyclics SSRIs		Atypical neuro- leptics	Drug-induced psychosis
Anxiolytics Benzodiazepines	Anxiety, panic	Clozapine Olanzapine	
Carbidopa	Sinemet-induced nausea	Quetiapine Fludrocortisone Midodrine	Orthostatic hypotension
Oxybutinin	Urinary urgency	Hypnotics Benzodiazepines Diphenhydramine	Insomina

SSRI = Selective serotonin reuptake inhibitor.

17. What drugs can interfere with the anti-Parkinson drugs (APDs)?

Drugs That Can Aggravate Parkinsonism

DRUG	HOW USED	ADVERSE PHARM EFFECT
Alpha-methyldopa	Antihypertensive	Depletes presynaptic catecholamines
Amiodarone	Antiarrhythmic	Unknown
Amoxapine	Antidepressant	Blocks reuptake of NE and serotonin, blocks DA receptors
Lithium	Antipsychotic, bipolar disease	Unknown
MAO inhibitors*	Antidepressants	Blocks reuptake of DA and NE
Meperidine	Analgesic	Drug-drug interaction
Metoclopramide	GI promotility	Blocks DA receptors
Neuroleptics (except clozapine) and other atypical neuroleptics	Antipsychotic, schizophrenia	Blocks DA receptors
Papaverine	Vasodilator	?Blocks DA receptors
Reserpine	Antihypertensive	Depletes presynaptic catecholamines

* MAO (monoamine oxidase) inhibitors of subtypes A and B—to be distinguished from deprenyl, which inhibits only type B. But MAO inhibitors can cause severe hypertension when used in combination with Sinemet. DA = dopamine; NE = norepinephrine.

The preceding table lists the drugs that anyone with PD should either avoid or at least be aware of when using APDs. Neuroleptics (major tranquilizers and metoclopramide) head the list because they block dopamine receptors in the striatum and can produce severe "extrapyramidal" (parkinsonian) side effects in patients with or without PD. The introduction of clozapine, an "atypical" neuroleptic which does not produce extrapyramidal side effects, allows control of psychosis in patients with PD, especially when these symptoms are caused by APDs.

Recently a warning was issued against the simultaneous use of deprenyl and the antidepressants that inhibit serotonin uptake (the selective serotonin reuptake inhibitors and the tricyclics) because of the rare occurrence of an acute serotonin crisis (hypertension, sweating, agitation, psychosis).

18. Can nonpharmacologic treatments help?

The most important are physical, occupational, and speech therapy. Each has a place and a time and may be repeated without fear of overdosing. **Physical exercise** is good for conditioning, strengthening, and stretching stiff, underutilized muscles. Working with a good therapist can restore confidence and stability to a deteriorating patient, especially when drug options are limited in the more advanced stages of disease.

Good **nutrition** also keeps the body strong. Most patients are aware that large protein meals may block or truncate the response to a dose of Sinemet taken near mealtime. Transport of the large neutral amino acids in the blood following breakdown of ingested protein uses the same carrier system that delivers absorbed levodopa to the brain. Competition for delivery to the brain via an overloaded transport system in effect reduces access of drugs to the brain and aggravates symptoms.

Acupuncture may relieve pain and even depression associated with parkinsonism. Despite centuries of use, its mechanism of action in the nervous system remains unknown.

19. What surgical procedures are available for the treatment of PD?

Neurosurgical treatment of PD falls into two broad categories:

Ablative procedures destroy small, precisely targeted groups of cells in strategic locations within the basal ganglia. The medial globus pallidus and the ventral-lateral thalamus are specific anatomic targets in the two most common operations, because pathologically hyperactive neurons in these regions contribute to the severity of bradykinesia, rigidity, and rest tremor. **Pallidotomy** was popular in the 1950s but disappeared after the introduction of levodopa in the late 1960s. It began a comeback in the early 1990s when it was shown to relieve some of the more serious motor problems related to chronic levodopa usage (particularly dyskinesias). Sophisticated computerized imaging (not available in the 1950s) has allowed stereotactic localization of anatomic targets to become more precise. **Thalamotomy** has been used specifically to control medically intractable parkinsonian tremor. The other symptoms of PD are alleviated much less by it than by pallidotomy. Preliminary observations suggest that **electrical stimulation** of sites in the basal ganglia that are currently being surgically ablated may become a safer alternative with equivalent or better results.

   Restorative procedures include transplantation with fetal mesencephalon and implantation of various genetically engineered cell lines or devices that deliver dopamine directly into neuron-rich striatal tissue. **Fetal tissue transplantation** is being done in only a few places in the world. Its usefulness is still uncertain after more than a decade of experimental application to humans and primates. Ethical and logistical concerns probably will restrict its application. Other implantation techniques, using genetically altered viral vectors or cultured cells that deliver dopamine and growth factors, are being developed in experimental animals. Human trials are also planned.

20. Can pain and altered sensation be part of the symptom complex of Parkinson's disease?

   Yes, fairly often. It is not uncommon for patients to report stiff, achy joints or numbness and tingling early on before the diagnosis is made. Since Parkinson's disease usually presents as a unilateral or asymmetric clinical disorder, pain and sensory symptoms tend to occur on the side of greater motor involvement. Effective treatment alleviates pain in parallel with the relief of rigidity and improved joint mobility. Physical therapy has the potential for contributing significantly to the patient's well-being.

   Pain also can occur as a side effect from APD therapy. Levodopa sometimes induces painful dystonic contractions of limb muscles, either at peak dose effect or as the drug's effect is wearing off. Painful dystonia of the foot on awakening from sleep in the morning is not uncommon and usually clears after the first dose of Sinemet of the day.

21. How common is depression in Parkinson's disease?

   Very. Depression occurs throughout the course of PD, and although antidepressants or psychotherapy help, depression tends to recur. Serious and unexplained depression, often sudden in onset, may herald or precede the onset of the motor symptoms by months or years.

   Dopamine deficiency in the basal ganglia is the major biochemical abnormality responsible for the motor trouble in PD. Norepinephrine and serotonin also are depleted, but to a lesser extent than dopamine, as a result of a milder loss of neurons in the midbrain. Virtually all of today's antidepressants work in the brain by blocking reuptake of serotonin, norepinephrine, or both at the synapse, so that more of these transmitters are available to stimulate noradrenergic or serotonergic receptors. The major and minor biochemical losses in PD therefore predispose every patient to a combination of motor and mental changes that include depression as a natural expression of the underlying pathology.

22. What cognitive problems occur in PD?

   Most patients with PD, even early in the course of illness, have abnormalities of mental processing. These subtle changes of language and memory are usually clinically insignificant. Many patients, however, complain of mental sluggishness and difficulty with the highest levels of cognition, especially if occupational demands are both physically and intellectually taxing. The term **bradyphrenia** has been applied to this state of slowed thinking. Abnormalities of executive function (decision-making) are well-documented in the intermediate stages of disease progression and may force patients in high-pressure jobs to take early retirement, even when they are still independent in every respect outside the office.

   Mental and motor deteriorations tend to occur in parallel as PD disease progresses. Serious mental disturbances, such as periodic confusion, visual hallucinations, delusions, and agitation with insomnia at night occur much later in the course and are frequently caused or aggravated by the various APDs. Drug-induced delirium is more likely to occur in patients whose cognitive function is already compromised by the underlying illness. Dementia, which affects 20–30% of patients, occurs late in the course in most cases, when motor function is severely impaired, but not always. The dementia of PD has a more complicated effect on social and personal functions than that of Alzheimer's disease because of the additive impact of the motor and mental disabilities. Unlike Alzheimer's dementia, which is classified neuropsychologically as a cortical dementia because of the high frequency of severe language dysfunction in late stages, Parkinson dementia is designated a **subcortical dementia**. Nonlanguage functions, such as memory retrieval, visual-spatial orientation, and frontal lobe executive functions are the most seriously impaired areas of performance.

23. Describe the natural history of PD.

Variability is the single most remarkable feature of the natural history of PD. All patients tend to get worse over many years, but the pace of that progression differs. Few if any features are reliable indicators of prognosis.

Most patients notice a very gradual increase in disability, sometimes over a period of 30 or more years. The timing of the onset of postural instability during the course of illness is also unpredictable, but it usually appears several years after the other symptoms have been treated successfully. When and if it occurs, postural instability signals a major downturn in disability, although steady deterioration does not necessarily follow. Many patients, again unpredictably, remain on the new plateau for variable amounts of time until the next sign of progression occurs.

24. Is chronic levodopa usage harmful?

The possibility that chronic levodopa usage might accelerate progression has been hotly debated without resolution for over 2 decades. Levodopa, with its potential to generate oxygen free radicals and to downregulate dopamine receptors, reaches a point of diminishing returns with prolonged usage, according to the skeptics. Therefore, the doctor should delay starting it for as long as possible and use the other APDs first. Levodopa promoters, on the other hand, point to the normalization of life-span for patients with Parkinsonism, compared to shortened life-spans in the era before levodopa, and to the vastly improved quality of life in most users, irrespective of the complications that often occur. Therefore, why not start it as soon as the patient's disability dictates a need for effective treatment?

Irreconcilable positions notwithstanding, one fact is indisputable: Everyone with PD at some point requires levodopa to achieve maximal functional ability, usually around 4 years into the disease. Postponing the use of the best drug for a year or 2 when the disease often runs a 20- or 25-year course does not buy much time. Besides, there is essentially no hard clinical evidence that witholding levodopa for any length of time makes any difference in the long run.

25. How do people who have PD die?

Patients live a relatively normal life-span now, compared to expectations 30 years ago before levodopa was introduced. Many die in old age or earlier of other causes before they progress to the point of extreme immobility. The general rate of deterioration is usually slow enough that most patients learn to accommodate, although none too happily, as the next level of compromise is reached.

In some instances, deterioration and progression to end-stage disability are unpredictably precipitous after years of stability. The cause of this rare abrupt decline is unknown, but rapid worsening sometimes follows hospitalization (e.g., for surgery, a broken hip, or heart attack) or some other period of forced immobilization associated with an intercurrent illness. Nigral cell loss at postmortem is usually directly proportional to the degree of clinical disability at the time of death. It is likely that an accelerated increase in disability at the end of life reflects the death of the substantia nigra's last few cells. The conversion of levodopa to dopamine in the brain can no longer occur because there are no cells with enough dopa decarboxylase to promote the conversion. The patient's clinical response to Sinemet ceases and voluntary movement becomes impossible. A parallel decline in cognitive function is a common end-stage occurrence. Dementia, especially in very old patients, affects as many as 50% at the very end of life. Pneumonia, urinary tract infections, and pulmonary emboli are often the direct antecedents of death from cardiac arrhythmia or myocardial infarction.

BIBLIOGRAPHY

1. Goetz CG, DeLong MR, Penn RD, Bakay RAE: Neurosurgical horizons in Parkinson's disease. Neurology 43:1–7, 1993.
2. Hoehn MM, Yahr MD: Parkinsonism: Onset, progression and mortality. Neurology 17:427–442, 1967.
3. Jankovic J, Tolosa E (eds): Parkinson's Disease and Movement Disorders, 2nd ed. Baltimore, Williams & Wilkins, 1993.
4. Lang AE, Lozano AM: Parkinson's disease. N Engl J Med 339:1044–1053 (Part I) and 1130–1143 (Part II), 1998.
5. Marsden CD, Fahn S: Akinetic rigid syndromes. In Marsden CD, Fahn S (eds): Movement Disorders, 3rd ed. Oxford, Butterworth-Heinemann, 1994.
6. Quinn N: Drug treatment of Parkinson's disease. BMJ 310:575–579, 1995.

32. DEMENTIA

Jason H. T. Karlawish, M.D., and Christopher M. Clark, M.D.

1. What is dementia?

The term *dementia* describes a clinical syndrome of at least 6 months of chronic and progressive impairments in two or more domains of cognitive function in the absence of delirium or a psychiatric or medical illness that can cause cognitive dysfunction. A key point in this definition is the need for symptoms of dysfunction in two or more domains of cognitive function such as memory and language. A "preclinical" diagnosis of dementia is not logically possible, and memory loss alone is not dementia.

2. Is dementia primarily defined by progressive memory loss?

Dementia is not just memory loss. Alzheimer's disease, the most common cause of dementia, does present with prominent impairments in short-term memory that correspond with the early pathologic changes of neurofibrillary tangles in the hippocampus where short-term memory is processed. But even in its early stages, patients with Alzheimer's disease have deficits in other domains of cognition, especially language and visuospatial skills. The appropriate descriptor for a patient who has a single cognitive deficit, such as memory loss, is *mild cognitive impairment*, not dementia.

3. What is mild cognitive impairment and how is it different from dementia?

The concept of mild cognitive impairment is in transition, but the current consensus is that it is a "diagnosis" reached when a patient has an impairment in only one domain of cognition. In this case, *impairment* is defined as performance that is greater than two standard deviations below the performance of age-matched persons. One significant controversy is whether mild cognitive impairment is a state of "preclinical dementia." Cohort studies suggest that persons with mild cognitive impairment are at high risk to progress to dementia compared to persons without it.

4. Is *any* degree of memory loss "normal"?

Memory loss that may be annoying but not severe enough to interfere with daily function can occur as part of the normal aging process. In addition, intellectual response time slows with aging. It takes nondemented elderly people longer than younger people to complete memory tasks and solve problems. However, accuracy is unaffected. See Chapter 3 for a discussion of cognition and aging.

5. Can a patient who is aware of his or her memory loss have Alzheimer's disease?

Many patients with early-stage Alzheimer's disease are aware of their cognitive deficits, especially the memory loss. However, patients often minimize the deficit's severity and clinical significance. As the disease progresses (sometimes even in the earliest stages), the patient's and caregiver's reports of disease severity begin to diverge. The patient usually rates his or her disease severity far lower than the caregiver does. It is likely similar disparities will occur with quality-of-life ratings.

6. How is dementia clinically different from delirium and affective disorders such as schizophrenia and depression?

A patient's history is the key to sort out the different clinical presentations of these disorders that can affect cognitive function. Of course, a patient can have two diagnoses, especially dementia and depression or dementia and delirium. A patient with delirium may appear to have dementia.

The cognitive impairment seen in delirium starts abruptly (especially during a hospitalization) and is marked by periods of waxing and waning alertness. In contrast, patients with dementia generally retain their level of alertness.

Patients with depression also can seem like a patient with dementia, but again, the patient's history may show that the depressed patient may have an antecedent event, such as the death of a spouse or diagnosis of a significant disease. In addition, the depressed patient characteristically exaggerates the degree of cognitive impairment compared to his performance of cognitive testing.

Patients with schizophrenia have predominant thought disorders, the hallmark of which is beliefs that do not adhere to reality testing (e.g., "I am Napoleon!"). A patient with dementia also can have delusions, but these usually occur in the middle to late stages of the syndrome. Also, the demented patient will have prominent signs of cognitive dysfunction, such as errors in calculation, language, and memory. The schizophrenic will have relatively preserved cognitive function. Finally, schizophrenia typically presents between the ages of 20 and 35. Dementia typically presents after age 60.

7. How common is dementia in America?

In the late 1980s, the United States' Office of Technology Assessment calculated that 4 million persons have dementia. Between 6% and 8% of persons over 65 have dementia. The risk of dementia compounds with age. After age 60, the prevalence doubles every five years: 30% of the population over 85 has dementia. By 2050, an estimated 12 million people will have dementia.

8. Are there risk factors for dementia?

Case-control and cohort studies suggest that the following may place a person at an increased lifetime risk of developing dementia (specifically Alzheimer's disease):

- Lower education (less than 12 years of school)
- Advanced age
- Family history of dementia
- Alcohol abuse
- Previous head injury
- Genes: two copies of the ApoE ε4 allele (not well established in nonwhite races) and mutations on chromosome 1, 14, and 21

9. What diseases can cause dementia?

After a thorough assessment for medical illnesses and medications that can cause or contribute to cognitive impairment, the clinician should consider five common causes of dementia:

DISEASE	PREVALENCE	DESCRIPTION
Alzheimer's disease (AD)	~60–80%	**Onset:** ages 70–80, range 50–90. **History:** initial changes in memory, language, and judgment followed by changes in personality, behavior, and function. Early-stage patients typically preserve social conduct and well-learned roles despite cognitive impairments. **Neurologic exam:** typically normal in early and middle stages.
Frontal dementia	~10%	**Onset:** ages 60–70. **History:** initial changes in personality, behavior, or language *followed* by changes in memory. **Neurologic exam:** signs of frontal reflexes (e.g., palmomental reflex).

(*Table continued on following page.*)

DISEASE	PREVALENCE	DESCRIPTION
Dementia with Lewy bodies	~10%	**Onset:** ages 60–80 **History:** cognitive dysfunction much like AD except for delusions and delirium seen early on. **Neurologic exam:** parkinsonian signs such as a slow gait, masked face, and cogwheeling.
Ischemic vascular dementia	5%	**History:** stroke closely antecedent to onset of cognitive dysfunction and in a neuroanatomic location that may explain cognitive dysfunction. Most cases of small-vessel disease and periventricular white matter changes actually are AD.
Depression	~10–20%	**History:** cognitive dysfunction much like AD, except for complaints of memory loss in excess of cognitive performance and clinical signs of depression; often an antecedent event, such as loss of spouse, is present. Response to antidepressant therapy is a diagnostic clue.

Although it is best to select the fewest diagnoses to explain the most symptoms, a skilled clinician should recognize that a patient may have more than one cause of dementia or that a patient may have a blend of criteria for different diseases. For instance, "Alzheimer's disease—frontotemporal variant" or "Dementia with Lewy bodies and depression" are potential diagnoses.

Other causes of dementia are Huntington's disease, Jakob-Creutzfeldt disease, progressive supranuclear palsy, Parkinson's disease, and corticobasilar degeneration. Key features of these diseases include rapid progression, focal weakness, impaired eye movements, dysarthria and dysphagia, myoclonus, tremor, and movement disorders. With the exception of Parkinson's disease, all are uncommon. The dementia of Parkinson's disease typically occurs later in the course of the illness, a key feature that distinguishes it from dementia with Lewy bodies.

10. What is a caregiver?

Dementia is a disease that impacts the patient's entire family and social network. At the center of this family are at least one caregiver and the patient. The standard of care for the *patient* with dementia must include care for the *caregiver* of that patient. A caregiver occupies at least four roles:

Caregiver Roles

ROLE	FEATURES OF ROLE
Knowledgeable informant about disease progression and response to therapies	Day-to-day experience of the patient provides valuable knowledge of the patient's cognitive and physical function. Physician should teach caregiver how to observe and record these functions.
Decision-maker for the patient	Cognitive impairment can cause a patient to be incapable of making a decision. Caregiver acts as a surrogate decision-maker. Physician should teach caregiver how to serve the patient's best interests.
Caretaker for the patient	Cognitive impairment can cause a patient to be incapable of performing IADLs and BADLs. Caregiver will assume these tasks. Physician should teach caregiver when to expect functional losses and ways to cope with them.
Second patient	Caregivers are likely to experience emotional, social, and financial burden. Physicians should assess caregiver for depression and related illnesses.

IADLs = instrumental activities of daily living (e.g., using the telephone, cooking, cleaning, managing money, using transportation, shopping). BADLs = basic activities of daily living (e.g., feeding, transferring, toileting, dressing, bathing/grooming).

Although one person can fulfill all four of these roles, it is highly likely that multiple persons will share one or more of these roles. Dementia is a disease that requires a biopsychosocial approach that challenges the traditional ethic that autonomous patients self-determine their care. Proper care of the patient requires careful attention to family dynamics. If caregivers are to properly fulfill these roles, they need core knowledge and skills, including information about diagnosis, prognosis, and treatment, and support for emotional and financial burden. Randomized trials demonstrate providing information and support to caregivers may postpone the need for 24-hour nursing care.

The physician should develop skills to respect the balance between the provision of a standard of care and the individuality of each family. This is particularly important for managing issues such as discussing the patient in his or her presence and disclosing the diagnosis to the patient.

11. What is caregiver burden and why should we care about it?

The term *caregiver burden* describes the emotional, social, medical, and financial impacts of caregiving on a person. Manifestations include depression, isolation, stress-related illnesses, and poverty. Caregiver burden is significant for at least three reasons. First, research shows that a caregiver's ability to accurately assess a patient is influenced by the caregiver's mood and burden. Second, research shows that patients and caregivers benefit when caregivers receive interventions to relieve burden. Third, the caregiver is a person, not an instrument, who deserves the dignity and respect accorded to all persons.

12. Discuss the work-up of a patient who has signs and symptoms of cognitive impairment.

A thorough history is the cornerstone of a work-up. The clinician should interview both the patient and the caregiver; and some portion of each person's interview should be separate from the others. A skilled clinician should prompt the caregiver to narrate the patient's history of cognitive dysfunction in as much detail as possible. The clinician should assess for evidence of impairment in several categories:

Categories and Features of Impairment

CATEGORY OF IMPAIRMENT	TYPICAL FEATURES
Memory	Difficulty retaining new information and recalling information acquired in the past
Function:	
Advanced activities of daily living (AADLs): Work, hobbies, and leisure activities, such as going to church, reading, and golf	Inability or partial ability to complete a function that patient was fully capable of doing before. AADLs and IADLs are characteristically lost before BADLs.
Instrumental activities of daily living (IADLs): Using the telephone, cooking, cleaning, managing money, using transportation, shopping	
Basic activities of daily living (BADLs): Feeding, toileting, dressing, grooming, and bathing	BADLs are characteristically lost in the reverse order that they are acquired in infancy*
Language	Substitution of words; agrammatical speech; changes conversation topics without proper cuing; paucity of speech output
Behavior and personality	*Changes commonly seen in frontal lobe dysfunction:* Disinhibited behavior, such as hypersexuality, public nudity, and cursing. Repetition of tasks. *Changes commonly seen other than frontal lobe dysfunction:* Blunting of affect; blunting of social engagement

* A pattern that does not fit these criteria is highly suggestive of an illness other than dementia.

13. Which tests of cognitive function are most useful for evaluating cognitive impairment?

The clinician should be able to administer and interpret a standardized set of cognitive tests that cover the range of cognitive and emotional functions described above. Although the minimental status exam (MMSE) is a common test, it combines tests of multiple cognitive functions to determine whether the patient is cognitively impaired. The following table lists standard tests and their normal values:

Standard Tests and Their Normal Values

FUNCTION	MEASURES	SCORING
Affect	Geriatric depression scale (GDS)—short form; evaluate answers to simple questions "Are you depressed?" and "Are you anxious?"	GDS < 5(+) out of 15
Memory	Five-minute recall of 3 words; recite full date, home address, and telephone number	Recall 2 or 3 out of 3
Language	Naming parts of objects; generating from a category a list of words in one-minute (e.g., "Tell me all the animals you can think of."); following a multi-step command	10 or more words in 60 seconds
Visuospatial	Draw the face of a clock to show that it is 8:20 (the instructions can be repeated if necessary; this is not a test of memory); draw two interlocking pentagons	10 angles and 4 interlocking sides
Judgment	Interpret proverbs (e.g., "What does the statement 'People who live in glass houses shouldn't throw stones' mean?"	Judgment of examiner
Attention and calculation	Spell *world* backwards; count down from 100 to 85 by 3's	No errors for individuals with ≥ 12 years schooling

14. What laboratory and imaging tests are most useful for evaluating dementia?

After medical illnesses have been excluded as the cause of a patient's cognitive impairment, few (if any) clinically useful laboratory tests can diagnose the cause of a dementia. One goal of clinical research is to develop tests that measure biologic markers of disease. At present, candidate biomarkers for Alzheimer's disease are cerebrospinal fluid tau protein (a component of the neurofibrillary tangles) and beta-amyloid (a component of the neuritic plaques). Clinicians should carefully follow the literature that reports the operating characteristics of these diagnostic tests.

Functional and structural neuroimaging tests can be useful to confirm a diagnosis of the cause of dementia. Functional neuroimaging studies such as positron emission tomography (PET) and single photon emission computed tomography (SPECT) scans demonstrate cerebral metabolism (directly with PET, indirectly with SPECT). They can be useful in distinguishing depression (globally decreased metabolism), frontal dementia (uni- or bilateral decreased frontal-temporal lobe metabolism), and Alzheimer's disease (decreased temporal-parietal metabolism). Structural neuroimaging tests such as computed axial tomography (CAT) and MRI scans demonstrate neuroanatomy. MRI is the preferred study for assessing focal or global cortical atrophy, mass lesions, and cerebral infarcts. Two key issues should temper the physician's ordering hand: the administration and interpretation of these tests is operator-dependent (decreasing reliability and validity), and many insurance companies will not reimburse the charges when used for the diagnosis of dementia.

15. What treatments are available for dementia?

There are two classes of treatments for dementia: disease-slowing and symptomatic. At present, few disease-slowing therapies are available. Vitamin E (at doses of 1,000 international units twice a day) has been shown to slow the progression of Alzheimer's disease. Selegiline may do the same. The ability of cholinesterase inhibitors to slow progression is debatable. Clinicians should keep close attention to the literature for developments. The multiple symptomatic treatments may be categorized in categories of behavioral and pharmacologic treatments. They can affect cognition and function, mood, and behavior such as agitation and psychosis.

Multiple Symptomatic Treatments

TREATMENT CATEGORY	COGNITION AND FUNCTION	MOOD	BEHAVIOR
Pharmacological	Cholinesterase inhibitors (e.g., donepezil)	Serotonergic reuptake inhibitors (e.g., sertraline) Tricyclic antidepressants	Antipsychotics (e.g., Risperdal) Benzodiazepines (e.g., ativan)
Behavioral	Remove hazards from environment Emphasize assistance over dependence in early-stage patients	Nonstressful activities during the day (e.g., adult day care) Supportive counseling	Identify and then redirect patient from sources of stress Identify calming activities such as aroma or music therapy

16. How do we know that treatment for a dementia is working?

Patients with dementia lack the insight and judgment to assess their own symptoms. The general goal of all treatment is to maximize the patient's quality of life and function, but how to assess these is unclear. The caregiver is a key person here. The caregiver not only acts as a knowledgeable informant, but also can help to assess the degree of patient response. The physician's role is to help the caregiver assess the areas of function, cognition, mood, and behavior. The goal of the caregiver and clinician is to arrive at a consensus concerning the direction and degree of a patient's global change, whether it is improved, unaltered, or worse.

17. A patient with severe-stage dementia develops aspiration. How can this be managed?

If aspiration occurs in a patient with severe-stage dementia, it is reasonable to approach the problem with exclusive attention to maintaining the patient's dignity and quality of life. The clinician should carefully assess the patient's ability to swallow food and liquid safely and comfortably. A speech therapist may be useful here. In general, careful oral feeding with attention to the pace of feeding and the portion and consistency of foods can significantly decrease complicated episodes of aspiration. The data describing the inability of enteral feeding to reduce aspiration risk and the 6-month and 1-year mortality rates suggest that this intervention should follow only after considerable discussion of its risks and potential benefits in the context of the patient's dignity and quality of life. Time-limited trials of interventions also help to settle uncertainty. Decision-makers must be comfortable with withdrawing an ineffective treatment.

18. How do patients die of dementia?

Most of the research on prognosis comes from patients with Alzheimer's disease. Survival after diagnosis ranges from 2–10 years. Death follows complications of functional impairments in swallowing, movement, and nonstarvation-related loss of lean body mass. Typical causes are pneumonia, urinary tract infection, and infected stage 4 ulcers.

19. How is dementia staged?

Valid instruments that stage the progression of Alzheimer's disease include the Clinical Dementia Rating (CDR) and Dementia Severity Rating Scales (DSRS). The DSRS is administered by the caregiver.

In general, the three broad categories of disease severity are mild, moderate, and severe. The following table describes the typical patient who fits in each category. Note that for a patient with frontal dementia, behavior symptoms may be more prominent in the "mild stage." A patient also may fit in between stages, such as "moderate to severe."

A Clinical Staging System for Dementia

	MILD	MODERATE	SEVERE
Function	• BADL-independent • IADL-independent or assistance needed	• BADL-independent or assistance needed • IADL-dependent	• BADL-dependent • IADL-dependent
Cognition	• Recognizes and communicates with family	• Problems with recognizing and communicating with family	• Cannot consistently recognize family • Communication with family is largely impressionistic
Behavior and personality	• Generally is the "same" person as before the disease except is less engaged	• Behavior problems can be difficult and a source of great stress	• Behavior problems may worsen and patient may seem like "a different person"

20. How do you know if a patient with dementia is competent to make medical decisions?

A diagnosis of dementia *does not* mean that the patient is incompetent, but it does raise clinical suspicion that the patient *may* be incompetent. A physician should be skilled in competency assessment, which relies on assessing the patient's specific abilities to understand, appreciate, and rationally manipulate the information needed to make a decision. A patient's decision-making abilities should be weighed against the balance of the risks and potential benefits of the decision. Because competency is specific to each decision the patient must make, the context of each decision is very important. For instance, a patient with Alzheimer's disease may not be competent to decide to take a nonsteroidal anti-inflammatory drug (which has unproven benefits and real risks such as gastrointestinal bleeding). However, the same patient may be competent to decide whether to take vitamin E to slow the progression of Alzheimer's disease (which has proven benefits and few if any risks).

ACKNOWLEDGMENTS

The authors thank the participants of the Washington University in St. Louis e-mail discussion group on Alzheimer's disease for their thoughtful suggestions (www.biostat.wustl.edu/alzheimer/).

BIBLIOGRAPHY

1. Clark CM, Ewbank D: Performance of the dementia severity rating scale: A caregiver questionnaire for rating severity in Alzheimer's disease. Alzheimer Dis Assoc Disord 10:31–39, 1996.
2. Finucane TE, Bynum JPW: Use of tube feeding to prevent aspiration pneumonia. Lancet 348: 1421–1424, 1996.
3. Geldmacher D, Whitehouse P: Evaluation of dementia. N Engl J Med 335:330–336, 1996.
4. Grisso T, Appelbaum PS: Assessing Competence to Consent to Treatment. A Guide for Physicians and Other Health Care Professionals. New York, Oxford University Press, 1998.
5. Haley WE: The family caregiver's role in Alzheimer's disease. Neurology 48:S25–S29, 1997.
6. Mittelman M, Ferris S, Shulman E, et al: A family intervention to delay nursing home placement of patients with Alzheimer's disease: A randomized controlled trial. JAMA 276:1725–1731, 1996.
7. Neary D, Snowden J, Gustafson L, et al: Frontotemporal lobar degeneration. A consensus on clinical diagnostic criteria. Neurology 51:1546–1554, 1998.
8. Office of Technology Assessment: Losing a Million Minds: Confronting the Tragedy of Alzheimer's Disease and Other Dementias. Washington, D.C., U.S. Government Printing Office, 1987.
9. Rogers S, Farlow M, Doody R, et al: A 24-week, double-blind, placebo-controlled trial of donepezil in patients with Alzheimer's disease. Donepezil study group. Neurology 50:136–145, 1998.
10. Sano M, Ernesto C, Thomas RG, et al: A controlled trial of selegiline, alpha-tocopherol, or both as treatment for Alzheimer's disease. N Engl J Med 336:1216–1222, 1997.
11. Small GW, Rabins PV, Barry PP, et al: Diagnosis and treatment of Alzheimer's disease and related disorders. JAMA 278:1361–1371, 1997.

33. STROKE

Steven E. Arnold, M.D.

1. What is a stroke?
Stroke is an injury to the brain caused by occlusion or rupture of a cerebral artery. It is the third most common cause of death in the United States and, perhaps even more grim, the leading cause of adult disability. The challenges of stroke prevention and care are particularly compelling for geriatricians, given the burgeoning elderly population and the fact that the most significant risk factor for stroke is age.

2. What are the major categories of stroke? Are they important to recognize?
The stroke syndrome is characterized by rapid onset and a pattern of focal neurologic signs and symptoms that reflect injury in a specific vascular territory. The two broad categories of stroke are (1) ischemic stroke, which results from thrombosis or embolism, and (2) hemorrhagic stroke, due to primary intracerebral or subarachnoid hemorrhage. Thrombotic strokes are the most common and account for approximately 65% of all strokes. Embolic strokes account for 20–25%; intracerebral hemorrhage, for 5%, and subarachnoid hemorrhage, for 5%.

Diagnosing the type and location of stroke is critical for appropriate management and prevention of recurrence. For instance, the mortality rate of hemorrhagic stroke is 3–5 times greater than that of ischemic stroke. Hemorrhagic stroke requires more critical and specialized care. Although information about the early temporal profile may be difficult to obtain, the mode of onset may yield clues about whether the lesion is thrombotic, embolic, or hemorrhagic. The symptom profiles for stroke vary according to type and vascular territory.

3. Describe the mode of onset for different types of strokes.
Thrombotic strokes
 Variable onset of neurologic symptoms
 Frequently preceded by transient ischemic attacks (TIAs), which herald permanent deficits
 Neurologic deficits are often rapid in onset but may be fluctuating, stepwise, or stuttering
  (stroke in evolution)
Embolic strokes
 Sudden onset with maximal neurologic deficit present from the start
Intracerebral hemorrhage
 Sudden onset
 Often occurs in setting of elevated blood pressure and during activity
Subarachnoid hemorrhage
 Sudden onset
 Tends to occur during activity and may be associated with elevated blood pressure
 Invariably accompanied by a crushing headache (which is a rare or minor symptom in
  other types of stroke)
 Often proceeds to coma, from which the patient may emerge in a confusional state

4. Describe the major clinical syndromes of stroke.
Middle cerebral artery
 Contralateral hemiplegia
 Contralateral hemisensory loss
 Contralateral homonymous hemianopia
 Ipsilateral gaze preference

Aphasia (dominant hemisphere)
Affective disturbance (especially in nondominant hemisphere)
Neglect (failure to respond to stimuli presented to the side opposite a brain lesion, especially in nondominant hemisphere)

Anterior cerebral artery
Contralateral leg/foot paralysis
Gait disturbance
Abulia (loss or impairment of volition)
Ideomotor apraxia (inability to perform purposeful movements)
Perseveration (inappropriate repetition of word, phrase, or behavior)
Urinary incontinence

Posterior cerebral artery
Contralateral homonymous hemianopia
Dyslexia
Memory impairment
Contralateral hemiparesis (mild)
Contralateral hemisensory loss
Variable brainstem signs (e.g., ipsilateral third nerve palsy, contralateral involuntary movements, hemiplegia, ataxia)

Internal carotid artery
Transient monocular blindness
Watershed signs
    Homonymous hemianopia
    Aphasia (dominant hemisphere)
    Neglect (nondominant hemisphere)
    Variable sensorimotor deficit
Signs of middle, anterior, and posterior cerebral artery infarction (as above)

Vertebral artery
Ipsilateral cerebellar ataxia
Ipsilateral face dysesthesia
Contralateral trunk and limb dysesthesia
Vertigo
Nystagmus
Ipsilateral vocal cord paralysis
Dysphagia
Nausea and vomiting
Ipsilateral Horner syndrome

Basilar artery
Wide spectrum of clinical symptoms
Contralateral hemiplegia or quadriplegia
Contralateral hemisensory loss
Horizontal gaze palsies
Ipsilateral facial paralysis
Internuclear ophthalmoplegia (inability to adduct contralateral eye with voluntary eye movement)
Nystagmus
Nausea, vomiting
Deafness, tinnitus
Coma
"Locked-in" syndrome (intact consciousness but total paralysis except for eyelid and vertical eye movements)

Lacunar syndromes
Pure motor hemiparesis
Pure sensory stroke
Dysarthria/clumsy hand syndrome
Hemichorea/hemiballismus
Homolateral ataxia and crural paresis

5. What causes stroke?

Primary thrombotic occlusion typically occurs in a blood vessel already partially occluded by atherosclerosis. The earliest lesion is a "fatty streak," which evolves into a fibrous plaque. The rate of progression from atheromatous stenosis to virtual occlusion is highly variable but may be as short as weeks. The source of most **cerebral embolisms** is the heart; much less commonly, embolic material may be released from ulcerated atherosclerotic plaques in the aortic arch and origin of the great vessels. The sites of embolic occlusion within the brain are more variable than in atherothrombotic disease, although there is some predilection for right hemisphere lesions, based on tendencies of blood flow. **Lacunar infarcts** are a particular type of ischemic stroke involving the deep perforator arterial and arteriolar branches of the major cerebral blood vessels. Pathologically, they are due to lipohyalinosis or microatheroma.

Intracerebral hemorrhage is usually due either to rupture of the small penetrating arteries of the brain in the setting of hypertension or to amyloid angiopathy. **Subarachnoid hemorrhage** is most commonly due to rupture of a congenital saccular aneurysm, which typically occurs at sites of arterial bifurcation or branching. Most aneurysms are asymptomatic until they rupture. Subarachnoid hemorrhage also may be caused by arteriovenous malformation or tumors.

Thrombotic stroke
1. Atherosclerotic plaque (may be due to stenotic ischemia or local ulcerated plaque embolization)
   - Common carotid bifurcation
   - Proximal vertebral artery
   - Internal carotid siphon
   - Proximal basilar artery
   - Middle cerebral artery stem
2. Rare causes
   - Antiphospholipid antibodies
   - Clotting inhibitory factor deficiencies
   - Arteritides
   - Cerebral vein thrombosis
   - Polycythemia vera

Embolic stroke
1. Cardiac source
   - Mural thrombus
   - Atrial fibrillation
   - Myocardial infarction
   - Valvular disease
   - Patent foramen ovale
   - Bacterial endocarditis
   - Libman-Sacks endocarditis
   - Atrial myxoma
2. Atherosclerotic plaques in aortic arch or origin of great vessels

Lacunar stroke: strongly associated with age, diabetes mellitus, and hypertension

Intracerebral hemorrhage
1. Rupture of small penetrating vessels in setting of hypertension
   - Putamen
   - Thalamus
   - Pons
   - Cerebellum
2. Amyloid angiopathy (tends to be lobar)
3. Hemorrhagic conversion of an ischemic infarct

Subarachnoid hemorrhage
1. Cerebral aneurysm
   - Anterior communicating artery
   - Internal carotid artery at origin of posterior communicating artery
   - Middle cerebral artery bifurcation
2. Arteriovenous malformation
3. Tumor

6. What other conditions may mimic TIAs or stroke?

Various neurologic processes that cause transient as well as nontransient deficits may be misdiagnosed as TIA or stroke. In fact, it has been estimated that 10–15% of initial diagnoses of stroke are incorrect. Seizures (especially simple and complex partial seizures), confusional states, and cardiogenic syncope lead the list of alternative diagnoses confused with stroke. Other conditions that may simulate stroke or TIA include migraine and migraine equivalents, subdural hematoma, brain tumor, hypoglycemia, demyelinating disease, brain abscess, encephalitis, and panic attack. Obviously, management of these various conditions differs greatly.

7. What are the major modifiable risk factors for stroke?

Much of the steady decline in stroke mortality in the past 50 years may be attributed to the identification and treatment of risk factors, particularly hypertension. This decline has been most prominent among the elderly, but it appears to be slowing or even reversing in recent years. Stroke remains the third leading cause of death. Some risk factors, such as age, male gender, African-American heritage, and heredity are nonmodifiable, whereas other medical and lifestyle factors may be modified. To decrease the still high incidence of stroke, there needs to be yet greater emphasis on education and management of modifiable risk factors.

Major Risk Factors for Strokes

MODIFIABLE MEDICAL FACTORS	RELATIVE RISK	LIFESTYLE FACTORS	RELATIVE RISK
Systolic and diastolic hypertension	3–4 times	Cigarette smoking	1.5–2.9 times
Cardiac disease		Excessive alcohol	4 times
Atrial fibrillation	5–17 times	Physical inactivity	Uncertain
Coronary artery disease	2–4 times		
Congestive heart failure	2–4 times		
Left ventricular hypertrophy	2–4 times		
Diabetes mellitus	2–4 times		
Hyperlipidemia	Uncertain		
Hypercoagulable state	Uncertain		
Elevated homocysteine	Uncertain		

Other potential risk factors for stroke include atrial septal aneurysm, patent foramen ovale, aortic arch atheroma, anticardiolipin antibodies, and chronic inflammation. These factors may be especially important in younger populations with cryptogenic stroke. Their significance in the geriatric population is undetermined.

8. What are the options for primary prevention of stroke?

Strategies for stroke prevention target the modifiable risk factors. In general, although the risk factors for stroke are not exactly the same as those for coronary artery disease, the main cause of death in patients with cerebrovascular disease is cardiac disease. Therefore, the same recommendations are made for stroke as for coronary artery disease. Hypertension, diabetes mellitus, hyperlipidemia, tobacco abuse, alcoholism, and obesity should be managed with a combination of dietary and lifestyle changes and medication (when necessary).

9. When should anticoagulation be considered for primary prevention of stroke in patients with cardiac disease?

For primary prevention of stroke in patients with a well-established cardiac source for embolic stroke (chronic atrial fibrillation, dilated cardiomyopathy, valvular heart disease, prosthetic valves), anticoagulation with warfarin is clearly effective and generally has an acceptable risk of bleeding complications. People over the age of 75 share in this decreased risk, although they experience a significantly higher risk of major hemorrhage; thus, the decision to anticoagulate is an individual one. Antiplatelet therapy with aspirin, 325 mg, has fewer bleeding complications and has been shown to reduce the risk of stroke in patients with atrial fibrillation, albeit with significantly less efficacy (about half) than warfarin. Initial results from recent trials combining low-dose warfarin and aspirin have not been encouraging.

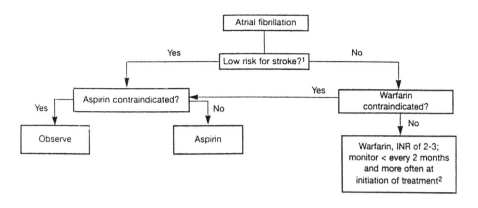

[1] Low stroke risk: age < 60 years with none of the following: previous transient ischemic attack/stroke, hypertension, diabetes mellitus, congestive heart failure, echocardiogram with left atrial enlargement or global left ventricular dysfunction.

[2] INR: International Normalized Ratio is a measure of prothrombin time that adjusts for differences in thromboplastin reagents used by different laboratories. INRs between 2 and 3 are currently considered optimal for atrial fibrillation patients.

Atrial fibrillation.

10. What is the initial management for a patient with an acute stroke?

For all patients with acute stroke, rapid clinical evaluation and initiation of treatment are critical, especially now that thrombolytic therapy for hyperacute stroke is widely available. Treating stroke as anything less than an emergency is substandard care. Patients should be offered tissue-type plasminogen activator if the onset of stroke was less than 3 hours before. Beyond the history and physical examination, the initial emergency evaluation should include an electrocardiogram (EKG), chest radiograph, complete blood count, platelet count, prothrombin and partial thromboplastin times, chemistry profile, erythrocyte sedimentation rate, syphilis serology, and arterial blood gas. It is imperative to distinguish hemorrhage from infarction as soon as possible because further decisions about acute management depend on this distinction. Therefore, a noncontrast computed tomography (CT) scan of the head should be performed and interpreted urgently because it easily differentiates hemorrhage from infarction in almost all cases.

The utility of magnetic resonance imaging (MRI) in the early management of stroke is controversial. Conventional MRI methods (T1-, T2-, and proton density-weighted images) can detect ischemic lesions much sooner after stroke and with much greater anatomic resolution than CT, but the advantages of MRI over CT have not been demonstrated by clinical outcome studies. However, new MRI methods are under development, including diffusion-weighted imaging and perfusion imaging, which can detect within minutes the territory undergoing infarction and the ischemic territory still at risk for infarction. These techniques offer the promise of identifying which patients are most likely to benefit from acute thrombolytic therapy.

In patients with ischemic infarction, high blood pressure should not be lowered rapidly unless it is greater than 220 mmHg systolic or 120 diastolic or unless other indications, such as heart failure or aortic dissection, are present. In contrast, for patients with hemorrhage, elevated blood pressure should be lowered and maintained within the normal range. Other general management strategies include treatment of hypoglycemia or hyperglycemia (> 170 mg/dl), monitoring of cardiac status, oxygen for hypoxemia, and monitoring for cerebral edema and seizures. Accumulating evidence indicates that specialized stroke units can save lives and improve outcome and should be used, if available.

11. What are the guidelines for thrombolytic treatment of hyperacute stroke?

The National Institute of Neurologic Disorders and Stroke has found that tissue-type plasminogen activator is effective for minimizing damage from acute ischemic stroke and preserving functional status in a select group of patients, if initiated within 3 hours of initial symptom onset. Obviously, much depends on the expediency of stroke recognition and triage by the patient, family, emergency medical transport services, and hospital emergency services.

Tissue-type plasminogen activator should be offered if (1) the diagnosis is acute ischemic stroke; (2) the interval between initial onset of symptoms and treatment can be determined to be less than 3 hours; (3) the patient has significant acute focal neurologic deficit; (4) a neurologist has been consulted, concurs with treatment, and will participate in ongoing inpatient treatment; and (5) a head CT scan has been obtained and interpreted by an experienced physician.

Tissue-type plasminogen activator should not be offered if (1) the time of onset is unclear (e.g., the patient awakens from sleep with symptoms); (2) sustained blood pressure is greater than 185/110 mmHg at the time treatment is administered; (3) CT scan shows evidence of hemorrhage; (4) neurologic deficits improve spontaneously and significantly before initiation of treatment (e.g., TIAs); (5) the neurologic deficit is minor; or (6) other contraindications pose a risk for hemorrhage. After treatment, emergent ancillary care must be available in a skilled care facility (intensive care unit or acute stroke care unit) that permits close observation, frequent neurologic assessments, and cardiovascular monitoring.

12. Does a TIA or minor stroke require immediate diagnosis and management?

TIAs and minor strokes should be evaluated and treated according to the same principles as stroke. TIAs are warning signs of stroke, and aggressive management can prevent permanent disability and death. The rate of a completed stroke after TIA may be as high as 57% within 2 years; most occur within the first year. The risk of stroke in the first few days after a TIA is unclear; however, it is considered to be highest during this time. Therefore, all patients with a recent TIA (within 10 days) should be evaluated urgently.

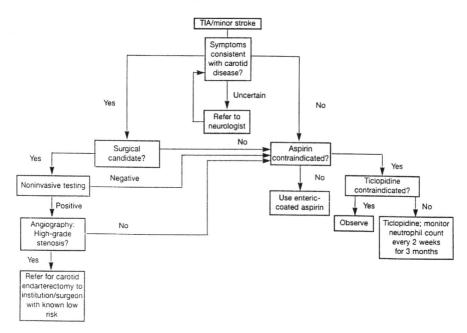

Transient ischemic attack (TIA/minor stroke). (This algorithm is not intended to be a comprehensive management strategy for patients with TIA or minor stroke.)

13. Describe the diagnostic work-up of a new stroke or TIA.

At present, no algorithm for diagnosis of stroke is uniformly accepted. Which tests to perform and how aggressively they should be used are decisions based on individualized factors, such as age, clinical presentation, risk factors, other health considerations, and intent to treat. At a minimum, evaluation should include the above-noted admission tests, head CT, and noninvasive carotid artery evaluation to identify atherosclerotic disease. Duplex scanning is the most revealing noninvasive method because it combines ultrasound real-time imaging with a Doppler probe and is quite accurate in detecting significant disease up to the carotid bifurcation. Ultrasound techniques are of little use for vertebrobasilar disease. Additional diagnostic tests and procedures for selected patients include transthoracic echocardiography (and transesophageal echocardiography in patients in whom a cardioembolic source is highly suspected); transcranial Doppler, MRI, and MR angiography to assess suspected intracranial arterial stenoses; cerebral angiography to identify most sensitively any cerebrovascular disease; and tests for coagulopathies (e.g., proteins C and S, antiphospholipid antibodies, antithrombin III deficiencies, especially in younger patients with no other obvious cause). For cases of suspected subarachnoid hemorrhage, lumbar puncture is indicated if clinical suspicion is high and CT is nondiagnostic. Early angiography also is indicated for subarachnoid hemorrhage, especially in more robust, less impaired patients, for whom early aneurysm repair is the treatment of choice. Positron emission tomography and single-photon emission computed tomography, although not widely available, may be useful in assessing TIAs in patients with no anatomic lesion or early stroke before tissue infarction.

14. What is the role of anticoagulation in acute stroke?

Anticoagulation is clearly effective in preventing recurrent cardioembolic stroke. Patients with cardioembolic stroke due to atrial fibrillation, recent myocardial infarction, valvular disease, or patent foramen ovale should be anticoagulated if no contraindications are present. Heparin should be administered on admission for at least 48 hours before being replaced by warfarin if no systemic contraindications are present, if no hemorrhage is seen on imaging studies, if the infarct is not large (hemorrhagic conversion is a greater risk in large than in smaller strokes), and if no evidence suggests the presence of bacterial endocarditis. For patients with atrial fibrillation who are not candidates for long-term anticoagulation, low-dose heparin may be considered. Aspirin alone also reduces the risk of further embolization in atrial fibrillation, although not nearly as much as warfarin. The role of anticoagulation is more controversial for atherothrombotic ischemic stroke. Many physicians feel compelled to anticoagulate patients with atherothrombotic stroke in evolution, but the value of this strategy has not been demonstrated. Anticoagulation is of no benefit in completed stroke.

15. What is the role of neuroprotective agents in acute stroke?

Various neuroprotective agents are under study for their potential role in interrupting the cascade of molecular events that lead to neuron death after ischemic injury. Examples include calcium entry antagonists, glutamate antagonists, sodium channel antagonists, glycine antagonists, opioid antagonists, and antioxidants/free radical scavengers. Although this strategy offers much promise, as yet little convincing evidence indicates that any neuroprotective drug is effective in either reducing the size of infarction or improving outcome.

16. What are the major complications of acute stroke?

The most common and significant medical complications after stroke include deep vein thrombosis and pulmonary embolism, aspiration pneumonia, urinary tract infections, and decubitus ulcers. Cardiac arrhythmias are also common, and EKG monitoring is indicated in the first few days. Three major neurologic complications, particularly with large strokes, are cerebral edema, seizures, and hemorrhagic transformation of ischemic infarcts. Cerebral edema is especially important in cerebellar infarctions because it may cause brainstem herniation. Hyperventilation, osmotic therapy, or even surgery may be needed for cerebral edema. Corticosteroids have not been shown to be effective in cerebral infarction or hemorrhage with or without edema. Seizures should be treated with anticonvulsants. If anticoagulation is being considered for stroke in evolution or other circumstances, a repeat CT scan should be performed before initiation of heparin to check for hemorrhagic conversion.

17. When should carotid endarterectomy be recommended?

Major controlled studies have demonstrated clearly that carotid endarterectomy (CEA) reduces the risk of subsequent stroke in patients who have had TIAs or minor stroke and who have arteriographically confirmed stenotic lesions > 70%. It appears to be of no benefit in patients with < 50% stenosis. Patients with < 50% stenosis should be evaluated more vigorously for cardioembolic and other causes of stroke. If no other cause emerges, they should be treated medically with risk factor reduction and antiplatelet therapy. For patients with moderate degrees of stenosis (50–69%), CEA may yield a moderate reduction in risk for subsequent stroke, but the decision must take into consideration surgical skill and recognized surgical risk factors. If ulcerated plaque is present in the setting of moderate stenosis, the risk of stroke increases and patients benefit from CEA. Surgical decisions should be made on an individual basis.

Recommendations for Carotid Endarterectomy

GRADE (%) OF STENOSIS	RECOMMENDATION
< 50	No. Search for cardioembolic or other sources
50–69	Individualized decision; yes, if ulcerated plaque is present
≥ 70	Yes
Asymptomatic, ≥ 60, low surgical risk	Yes

18. What are the risks of CEA? Do they differ in the elderly?

Risks of CEA include stroke and death as well as local complications such as hematoma, infection, or false aneurysm formation. Although successful CEA confers a relative risk reduction of 69% in the incidence of stroke over the ensuing 5 years, perioperative and arteriography-related risk for mortality and stroke must be considered. The aggregate risk of stroke or death in the perioperative period with an experienced team, including the risk of stroke associated with arteriography, is approximately 3%.

The results of CEA for the elderly are controversial. Some studies indicate an increased risk of complications with advanced age, whereas one recent study of CEA in octogenarians found the procedure to be as safe and effective as for the general population. Patients with prohibitive surgical risk should be treated with antiplatelet agents and risk factor reduction.

19. What medical therapy can prevent recurrent stroke in patients with established atherothrombotic cerebrovascular disease?

Numerous controlled clinical trials have demonstrated the efficacy of antiplatelet agents for the secondary prevention of stroke in patients who have had TIAs or previous stroke. **Aspirin** has been the most extensively studied, and its use is associated with a 23% decrease in the risk of subsequent stroke or myocardial infarction. Controversy continues over the optimal dose, with recommendations ranging from 30–1300 mg. A recent survey found that most neurologists recommend 325 mg/day in deference to gastrointestinal symptoms; however, recent studies suggest that higher doses may be better for secondary prevention of stroke.

Ticlopidine and clopidogrel are two other platelet antiaggregants with efficacy in secondary prevention of stroke. They work by inhibiting adenosine diphosphate linkage of fibrinogen to platelets and have a greater global inhibitory effect than aspirin. Ticlopidine has been reported to be modestly more effective than aspirin in preventing strokes. However, adverse reactions, including diarrhea, rash, gastrointestinal upset, and neutropenia, have limited its widespread use. CBCs need to be obtained every 2 weeks for the first 3 months to monitor for neutropenia (which occurs in 2.4% of patients and is fully reversible on discontinuation). Clopidogrel is at least as effective as aspirin with a somewhat better safety and side-effect profile.

The role of **warfarin** for prevention of carotid atherothrombotic stroke is unclear and awaits report of a large multicenter trial currently under way (Warfarin Aspirin Recurrent Stroke Study [WARSS]). Dipyridamole and sulfinpyrazone show no efficacy in secondary stroke prevention, either when used alone or in combination with aspirin.

20. How should asymptomatic carotid artery disease be managed?

Stenosis may be identified in asymptomatic patients as a result of bruits heard during physical examination, vascular studies for other reasons, or screening tests for unusual symptoms. Asymptomatic carotid stenosis is an indicator of more extensive atherosclerosis and is associated with an increased risk of stroke. Recently, the Asymptomatic Carotid Atherosclerosis Study (ACAS) reported that, for asymptomatic patients with high-grade stenoses, CEA in combination with aspirin and risk factor reduction lowers the relative risk for stroke compared with medical therapy alone. However, the relative risk reduction is not as great as for patients who have had TIAs or minor strokes. Consequently, consideration of other factors such as age, other medical illnesses, and risks of surgical and arteriographic complications become even more important in reaching a surgical decision. Whether or not surgery is recommended, risk factor modification and antiplatelet therapy should be initiated.

21. Who should be referred for rehabilitation after stroke?

Sensory, motor, cognitive, and language deficits are the presenting symptoms of stroke and, to varying degrees, the permanent residuals. Mortality from stroke has declined with advances in technology and treatment; as a consequence, a greater proportion of patients survive with substantial neurologic impairment. The goal of rehabilitation is not cure but rather adaptation to functional handicap—to maximize function in the service of enhancing quality of life. Numerous factors must be considered in determining the appropriateness of referral for rehabilitation. Consultation with a physiatrist, physical therapist, occupational therapist, and/or speech therapist is recommended to determine the appropriate rehabilitation needs of the patient. Patients with mild deficits probably do not need specialized rehabilitative services, whereas patients who are stuporous, completely immobile, severely cognitively impaired, or severely ill medically derive little benefit. Type and severity of neurologic deficit, presence and degree of cognitive impairment, physical endurance, patient and family goals, available social support, and psychological make-up contribute to the success of rehabilitative efforts and need to be assessed carefully. Age is not a factor; patients of all ages have shown substantial benefit in outcome from rehabilitation.

22. How common are depression and other psychiatric complications after stroke? How should they be managed?

Mood disturbances are common after stroke because of both organic and psychological factors. Depression may play a critical role in the success of a patient's recovery, rehabilitation, and adjustment to disability after stroke and should be assessed and treated aggressively. Depending on the diagnostic criteria, prevalence estimates for depression after stroke range from 23% to 63%. Because of frequent impairments in communication and cognition and the common bias that "anyone would be depressed after a stroke," clinical depression is underdiagnosed and undertreated. Yet its importance is underscored by studies indicating that depression in the postacute phase affects physical recovery and subsequent function in the chronic phase. Treatment with antidepressant medication is as effective in poststroke depression as in generic depressive disorders. The newer selective serotonin reuptake inhibitors (SSRIs), such as sertraline, paroxetine, and fluoxetine, are especially well tolerated and effective.

Other neuropsychiatric complications of stroke include delirium with agitation, paranoid reactions (especially in association with Wernicke's aphasia), impulse dyscontrol, and pseudobulbar affect (emotional incontinence). Such complications can be highly distressing to patients, family, and caregivers alike and are often amenable to psychiatric management.

BIBLIOGRAPHY

1. Adams HP Jr, Brott TG, Crowell RM, et al: Guidelines for the management of patients with acute is-chemic stroke. A statement for health care professionals from a special writing group of the Stroke Council, American Heart Association. Stroke 25:1901–1914, 1994.
2. Anderson DC: Primary and secondary stroke prevention in atrial fibrillation. Semin Neurol 18:451–459, 1998.
3. Barnett HJ, Taylor DW, Eliasziw M, et al: Benefit of carotid endarterectomy in patients with symptomatic moderate or severe stenosis. North American Symptomatic Carotid Endarterectomy Trial Collabo-rators. N Engl J Med 339:1415–1425, 1998.
4. Barnett HJM (ed): Stroke: Pathophysiology, Diagnosis, and Management. New York, Churchill Livingstone, 1998.
5. Biller J, Feinberg WM, Castaldo JE, et al: Guidelines for carotid endarterectomy: A statement for health-care professionals from a special writing group of the Stroke Council, American Heart Association. Stroke 29:554–562, 1998.
6. Dyken ML: Antiplatelet agents and stroke prevention. Semin Neurol 18:441–450, 1998.
7. Gorelick PB, Sacco RL, Smith DB, et al: Prevention of a first stroke: A review of guidelines and a multi-disciplinary consensus statement from the National Stroke Association. JAMA 281:1112–1120, 1998.
8. National Institute of Neurological Disorders and Stroke rt-PA Stroke Study Group: Tissue plasminogen activator for acute ischemic stroke. N Engl J Med 333:1581–1587, 1995.
9. Robinson RG: Treatment issues in poststroke depression. Depression Anxiety 8(Suppl 1):85–90, 1998.

34. FALLS

Elizabeth Capezuti, Ph.D., R.N.

1. How frequently do falls occur in the elderly?

Regardless of living arrangements, accidents are the sixth leading cause of death in the elderly, with falls being the most frequently reported type of accident. Approximately 30–40% of community-residing older adults and 30–60% of nursing home residents fall each year.

2. How do falls affect the morbidity and mortality of older persons?

- > 90% of hip fractures are associated with falls, with the great majority of fractures occurring in persons over age 70.
- Persons with hip fractures have a 12–22% higher mortality rate than those without hip fractures when matched by age and/or gender.
- Survivors of hip fracture are frequently institutionalized for short-term rehab or long-term placement due to permanent disability or coexisting mental or physical problems.
- Of those who return home, many suffer substantial functional deficits requiring assistance by others or mobility aids.
- Treatment and related care due to fall-related injuries account for a disproportionately high use and expenditure of health care resources in the elderly.
- Fractures other than of the hip or pelvis account for about 2–3% of fall-related injuries.
- Serious soft-tissue injuries requiring medical intervention and resulting in impaired functional status occur in approximately 10% of falls.
- Approximately 9500 deaths of older Americans are associated with falls each year.
- 20% of fatal falls occur in nursing home residents.

3. What are the psychological consequences of falling?

A fall may immobilize an older person, who then fears that her or his next fall will result in a hip fracture and eventual institutionalization. For many older persons, fear of falling results in excess disability, with fear leading to dependence and immobility, followed by functional deficits and the greater likelihood of falls.

4. Why should the clinician ask directly about falls? How often?

Because of the fears many elders harbor regarding institutionalization, clinicians should ask specifically about falls and should not expect the older person to provide this information as a chief complaint. Direct questioning regarding falls should occur at least annually.

5. How many falls should signal the clinician to perform a falls work-up?

One fall does not mean that the person is at risk for subsequent falls; it may simply be an isolated event without indicating risk of falling in the future. Recurrent falls (typically defined as ≥ 2 falls in a 6-month period), however, often necessitate a work-up to determine the presence of treatable causes.

6. What are the usual causes of falls?

The frequency of falling in older adults is related to the accumulated effect of multiple disorders superimposed on age-related changes. These multiple disorders, or risk factors, have been studied extensively to predict fall risk. Although risk factors have been categorized in several ways, they can be broadly grouped into intrinsic and extrinsic factors. **Intrinsic factors** are characteristics inherent to the individual and include presence of chronic disease, age-related physical and mental changes, acute health problems or acute exacerbations of disease, and the concomitant effects of medication usage. **Extrinsic factors** include environmental hazards as well as activity-related factors.

7. **Give examples of intrinsic risk factors for falling.**

Demographics	**History** *(cont.)*
Older age	Acute illnesses
Female sex	Infection
White race	Myocardial infarction
History	Dementia
Cane/walker use	Medications
Recurrent falls	Tricyclic antidepressants and selective
Chronic illnesses	serotonin reuptake inhibitors (SSRIs)
Stroke	**Physical findings (deficits)**
Parkinson's disease	Orthostatic hypotension
Other neuromuscular disease	Vision
Arthritis	Walking speed
Diabetes	Lower and upper extremity strength
Heart disease and hypertension	Lower extremity sensory perception

8. **Discuss the chronic and acute illnesses that affect fall risk.**

Multiple chronic illnesses can directly affect mobility status, especially arthritis, cardiovascular insufficiency, and diabetes, as well as most neuromuscular diseases such as Parkinson's disease and stroke. Problems with balance manifested by dizziness or vertigo may indicate seizure disorder, hypothyroidism, or inner ear dysfunction. The associated weakness accompanying some acute illnesses (infection, myocardial infarction) and acute exacerbations of chronic disease (congestive heart failure, diabetes, hypertension) can increase the older individual's tendency to fall. Moreover, the sudden onset of repeated falls is considered a sign of underlying acute pathology. Therefore, when an older person presents with new-onset repeated falls, acute illness must be ruled out.

9. **What points should the clinician focus on in obtaining a history of falls?**

Many patients attribute their falls to "just tripping," but the clinician should attempt to ascertain if the fall is due to an environmental factor and/or if other precipitating causes are present. Ask if the fall occurred after a position change, which may indicate orthostatic hypotension, carotid sinus hypersensitivity, or cervical disc spondylosis. A thorough review of the musculoskeletal and neurologic systems will reveal most intrinsic risk factors as well as identify problems for further inquiry; for example, if there is a history of dizziness or vertigo, you should focus on the cardiovascular, visual, auditory-labyrinthine, and proprioceptive systems. Within these systems, symptoms of orthostatic hypotension (positional dizziness), macular degeneration, acute labyrinthitis (vertigo with nausea and headache), Meniere's disease (vertigo with tinnitus and hearing loss), benign paroxysmal vertigo (positional vertigo with nystagmus), and peripheral neuropathy should be ascertained.

These conditions are often referred to by patients by a wide variety of terms, such as "falling out" and even "fall," which may have a different meaning from the medical definition of fall. The clinician should clarify with the patient what he or she means when describing conditions.

10. **Which drugs may have side effects related to falls?**

Polypharmacy and increased fall risk have been linked in a number of studies. However, examination of specific medications and their individual side effects and potential drug interactions is needed in order to identify a more precise clinical decision. Often it is helpful to ask an older person to bring in all current and past prescribed medications as well as those purchased over-the-counter, which helps to identify medication misuse. Classes of drugs that have been strongly correlated with fall/fracture risk and therefore need to be reviewed include short- and long-acting hypnotics-anxiolytics (including benzodiazepines), tricyclic and SSRI antidepressants, and antipsychotics. Also, overzealous pharmacologic treatment of cardiac and respiratory disease can adversely affect the vestibular system, impair balance, and create side effects such as severe orthostatic hypotension, all of which lead to greater fall risk. A recent meta-analysis of the effects of drugs on fall risk found that, among 14 cardiac and analgesic drugs or drug groups, only diuretics, digoxin, and type IA antiarrhythmic agents significantly increased the risk of falling. It is not clear, however, whether the drug or the underlying illness is the factor most likely to increase fall risk.

Drugs That May Affect Fall Risk

Hypnotics-anxiolytics (including benzodia-zepines)	Tricyclic antidepressants	SSRI antidepressants	Antipsychotics
Chlordiazepoxide (HCl)	Amitriptyline	Fluoxetine	Haloperidol
Chloral hydrate	Amoxapine	Paroxetine	Risperidone
Diazepam	Doxepin	Sertraline	Trifluoperazine
Ethchlorvynol	Imipramine (HCl)		
Flurazepam	Nortriptyline (HCl)		
Quazepam	Protriptyline (HCl)		
Temazepam			

11. What are environmental or extrinsic risk factors for falling?
Most falls occur when older persons are performing their usual activities, such as rising from a chair or walking. Beds and chairs that are too low, soft, on wheels, or on uneven or slippery surfaces can lead to problems. Hazards implicated in patient's homes include inappropriately placed furniture or objects, scatter rugs, carpeted stairs, and lighting that is too dim or causes glare. Some of these problems can be identified by direct interview. Also, observe the patient's footwear. Loose-fitting and/or badly worn shoes, as well as slippers, have been identified to increase fall risk.

Extrinsic Risk Factors or Environmental Home Hazards

Ground surfaces	**Lighting**
Throw rugs or loose carpets	Glare from unshielded windows or lamps
Slippery floors	or highly polished floors
Low-lying objects on the floor,	Absence of night lights
e.g., cords and wires	**Bathroom**
Stairs with rugs or in poor repair	Low toilet seats and/or unsecured grab bars
Furniture	Absence of nonslip surfaces
Clutter	**Other**
Unstable or low-lying furniture	Poorly maintained walking aids and equipment
Low chairs without armrest support or seat back	Improper shoes (not slip-resistant, high-heeled,
Beds/cabinets that are too high or too low	too large)

12. How is an environmental assessment done?
If there are questions regarding the safety of the home environment after interviewing the older person in the office, nurses and physical/occupational therapists in home-care agencies can provide in-home evaluations for potential hazards and offer suggestions such as the installation of grab bars for the tub and toilet.

13. What aspects of the physical exam are important in a falls evaluation?
A thorough head and neck, musculoskeletal, neurologic, and foot examination will help reveal areas of dysfunction and weakness that can contribute to fall risk and may be amenable to

treatment. The sensory exam should include evaluation of vibratory sense of both upper and lower extremities (marker of peripheral neuropathy), vision (acuity and fields), and hearing. Testing of motor functioning should focus on assessment of joint range of motion (flexibility) and muscle strength. If joint range of motion is limited, document the angle of motion, preferably with a goniometer. Particular areas of muscle strength to evaluate include hip abduction, adduction, and extension; knee extension (quadriceps) and flexion (hamstring); and ankle plantar and dorsiflexion.

Observe the person walking, checking for posture and balance. In testing for balance, check for unsteadiness in the following tasks: standing on one leg unsupported (unipedal stance), turning (360°), and after a gentle push or "tap" on the sternum. Specific aspects of an ataxia gait associated with fall risk include increased trunk sway, inability to walk in a straight line (path deviation), and inability to increase walking pace. In evaluating gait, note if the person becomes short of breath or complains of chest pain or palpitations. If so, perform a thorough cardiovascular and chest examination, including changes in vital signs with exercise.

14. Which functional or performance-based tests can be used to assess fall risk?
The physical examination should be supplemented with performance-based tests to improve accuracy in assessing fall risk. Observe the person standing and sitting down, rising from supine to sitting position, lifting a book and reaching to put it on a shelf, picking up a small object from the floor, and climbing stairs. Performance tests of position changes should also include blood pressure and pulse for objective measurement of orthostatic hypotension. (See also Chapter 24.)

15. How can exercise improve function and reduce fall risk?
In a large, multicenter research initiative known as FICSIT (Frailty and Injuries: Cooperative Studies of Intervention Techniques), exercise has been found to improve functional status and reduce the risk of falls and injurious falls. Various modalities have been found to be useful, including resistance training to increase muscle strength and exercises that improve endurance, flexibility, and balance, such as tai chi.

Sedentary lifestyle, especially immobilization, is associated with increased risk of osteoporosis. Although weight-bearing activity (walking, cycling, dancing, swimming) in those with established osteoporosis may only result in minor gains in skeletal mass, it is believed that the effect of exercise on muscle strength, gait, and confidence reduces risk of fracture. This type of exercise improves cardiovascular function, which may be a contributing factor for fall risk and/or sedentary lifestyle.

16. When is a rehabilitation/exercise referral necessary?
Individuals with deficits in gait/balance skills should be evaluated for their potential to improve with a structured exercise program. Evaluation of cardiac risk, including exercise stress testing, depends on significant findings in the history, including cardiac dysrhythmia, severe congestive heart failure, angina, exercise-related chest pain or myocardial infarct, diabetes mellitus, hypertension, elevated cholesterol levels, and current cigarette smoking. Patients with exercise-induced angina, intermittent claudication, chronic obstructive lung disease, degenerative joint disease, orthopedic problems, and neurologic abnormalities require both professional evaluation and supervised exercise programs.

17. What types of supervised rehabilitation/exercise programs are available for referral?
An exercise program should be tailored to the needs of the older person by a knowledgeable exercise professional, such as a physical therapist, occupational therapist, or physiatrist. Many cardiac rehabilitation programs and health clubs with a physical therapy department provide gait and balance evaluations as well as prescribe exercise regimens. Many also provide supervised exercise programs for those with specific health problems. Programs that employ exercise physiologists, physical therapists, occupational therapists,

and/or rehabilitation nurses who work collaboratively with physiatrists, sports medicine specialists, and/or cardiologists are ideal.

18. What is the role of physical restraints in institutionalized elders?

Despite the assumed safety of nursing home environments, falls remain an important clinical problem. Until the late 1980s physical restraints were the primary intervention to prevent falls, although their efficacy in fall prevention has never been demonstrated. Similarly, bilateral, full-length siderails have been viewed as the simple solution to preventing falls from bed. The Omnibus Budget Reconciliation Act was passed in 1987 as a mechanism to reduce, if not eliminate, the use of physical restraint in nursing homes. In 1997, the Health Care Financing Administration issued guidelines to nursing homes directing them to regard siderails as restraints. All restraints, especially vest restraints and "geri-chairs" (chairs with fixed tray tables), have been correlated with the negative sequelae of immobility as well as reports of restraint-related injury and death. Interventions including regular ambulation and other exercises that increase strength, balance, and coordination have been shown to be the most effective measures in preventing falls.

19. Are physical restraints useful in preventing falls in the hospitalized elder?

No. Fall prevention is essential if injuries leading to increased morbidity, length of hospital stay, institutionalization, and even death are to be prevented. Recent Joint Commission for Accreditation of Health Care Facilities (JCAHO) guidelines restrict physical restraint use to limited situations. New interventions individualized to specific patient needs are beginning to be used to prevent falls in the hospital. Interventions such as beds equipped with transfer "enablers" ($\frac{1}{4}$ or $\frac{1}{2}$ length siderails with narrow bars to prevent head entrapment), motion-activated lights, open monitors with the nursing station, bedside commodes, bed alarms, and video monitoring are useful for those who require assistance with transferring but who choose not to or are not cognitively or physically able to seek assistance. Encouraging families to stay overnight with hospitalized older adults or use of companions also can be helpful.

20. How can the risk of legal liability be reduced?

American physicians and nurses continue to believe that failure to restrain elder persons places clinicians and facilities at risk for legal liability. In the past, many cases favored plaintiffs against hospitals when fall-related injuries occurred in the absence of physical restraints. However, the current standard of care (as demonstrated in clinical and research literature and government regulations) reflects elimination or at least minimal usage of restraint; settlement and court decisions in fall-related injury cases have begun to shift. Although a number of reported cases assert the so-called failure to restrain, a careful reading of these cases demonstrates that the real basis of liability is a lack of care addressing fall risk. Only falls that are the proximate result of a deviation from the current standard of care are a liability risk. In fact, suits are being won against nursing homes and hospitals for physical restraint use leading to adverse consequences of enforced immobility or to restraint-related deaths.

21. What can be recommended for a nonambulatory older person at risk of falling?

Falls in nonambulatory persons usually occur as a result of sliding or slipping out of chairs or transferring unassisted from a chair or bed. If the person falls because he or she is attempting to get out of an uncomfortable chair, individualized seating "alternatives" are currently available. Recliner chairs and wedge or other support cushions may prevent such unassisted ambulation while assuring comfort. Replacing siderails with a low-height bed coupled with floor mats may prevent fall-related injuries from bed. For elders who wish to be mobile despite their inability to ambulate, interventions that improve wheelchair skills along with more user-friendly wheelchairs have been found to increase mobility. Physical and occupational therapists can provide guidance in prescribing these interventions.

BIBLIOGRAPHY

1. Capezuti E, Strumpf N, Evans L, et al: The relationship between physical restraint removal and falls and injuries among nursing home residents. J Gerontol A Biol Sci Med Sci 53A:M47–M53, 1998.
2. Capezuti E, Talerico KA, Strumpf N, Evans L: Individualized assessment and intervention in bilateral siderail use. Geriatr Nurs 19:322–330, 1998.
3. Northridge ME, Nevitt MC, Kelsey JL, et al: Home hazards and falls in the elderly: The role of health and functional status. Am J Public Health 85:509–515, 1995.
4. Province MA, Hadley EC, Hornbrook MC, et al: The effects of exercise on falls in elderly patients: A pre-planned meta-analysis of the FICSIT trials. JAMA 273:1341–1347, 1995.
5. Ray WA, Taylor JA, Meador KG, et al: A randomized trial of a consultation service to reduce falls in nursing homes. JAMA 278:557–562, 1997.
6. Thapa PF, Gideon P, Cost TW, et al: Antidepressants and the risk of falls among nursing home residents. N Engl J Med 339:875–882, 1998.
7. Tinetti M, Baker D, McAvay G, et al: A multifactorial intervention to reduce the risk of falling among elderly people living in the community. N Engl J Med 331:821–827, 1994.
8. Tinetti ME, Williams SC: Falls, injuries due to falls, and the risk of admission to a nursing home. N Engl J Med 337:1279–1284, 1997.

35. ANEMIA

Janet Abrahm, M.D,

1. Are all patients with a low hemoglobin and hematocrit anemic?
No. Patients with a normal red cell mass may appear to be anemic if they have an increased plasma volume. Patients with congestive heart failure, hypothyroidism, or hyperviscosity syndrome may therefore appear to be anemic when they are not. All three of these conditions are seen more commonly in older adults than in middle-aged and young individuals.

2. What are the common types of anemia in the elderly?
Common microcytic anemias include iron deficiency, lead poisoning, and congenital disorders not previously diagnosed (hemoglobinopathies or hereditary spherocytosis). The anemia of chronic disease and infiltrative marrow processes are usually normocytic. Macrocytic anemias are usually due to B_{12} or folate deficiency, but a significant portion reflect myelodysplasia. Patients can also have congenital or acquired hemolytic anemias.

3. How are iron deficiency and lead poisoning diagnosed?
In otherwise healthy patients, an iron saturation (Fe/total iron-binding capacity [TIBC]) of < 15% indicates **iron deficiency**. However, in patients with inflammatory, infectious, or hepatocellular disease, the iron saturation may appear to be >15% despite an iron-deficient status. In these patients, a ferritin level ≤ 100 μg/dl indicates iron deficiency.

The anemia of **lead poisoning** can mimic that caused by iron deficiency. Lead poisoning may arise from an untreated occupational exposure (welders, metal workers) or from ingestion of lead leached into fluids from earthenware or lead-glazed pottery. In both iron deficiency and lead poisoning, the cells are microcytic, but in lead poisoning, the red cells have a characteristic basophilic stippling. Abdominal complaints, neuropathy, and hypertension may also be present. Chelation therapy is required.

4. How should patients with iron deficiency be treated?
Iron is poorly absorbed in the elderly. Patients should ingest foods that contain heme iron, such as red meats or liver, or foods containing non-heme iron along with foods rich in vitamin C, such as citrus fruits or dark-green leafy vegetables. (Vitamin C enhances the absorption of non-heme iron.) Iron supplements are usually poorly tolerated in elderly patients because they exacerbate constipation and cause gastric irritation. Enteric-coated iron supplements, however, should not be used; their iron is released distal to its site of intestinal absorption. Parenteral iron replacement with Infed should be considered for patients with ongoing iron losses (e.g., from inflammatory bowel disease or vascular malformations).

5. What are the common microcytic congenital disorders? How are they diagnosed?
The alpha- and beta-thalassemias and hemoglobin E disease. Alpha-thalassemias occur in people of African origin, beta-thalassemia in persons of Iranian or Mediterranean origin, and hemoglobin E disease in those of Southeast Asian descent.

In the thalassemias, cells are microcytic, but the red cell count is elevated. Patients with beta-thalassemia also have target cells, fragments, and basophilic stippling. Hemoglobin electrophoresis will be diagnostic in both iron-replete patients with beta-thalassemia and in hemoglobin E disease. The alternate hemoglobins (E, F, and rarer variants) and increased levels of A_2 appear. Electrophoresis is normal in alpha-thalassemia, and genetic studies are required for its diagnosis.

6. What is the "anemia of chronic disease"?

This is a normocytic, normochromic anemia that occurs in most patients with an inflammatory chronic disease, such as rheumatoid arthritis or active infection, that has persisted for 1–2 months. While the exact mechanism is unknown, contributing factors likely include the many cytokines released, including interleukin-1, tumor necrosis factor, and interferons alpha and gamma. Re-utilization of iron is impaired, and serum iron and TIBC levels are decreased despite normal or increased amounts of marrow iron.

7. How can the anemia of chronic disease be distinguished from that of other causes?

The figure illustrates one way to diagnose an anemic patient whose red cell indices are reported to be normal. The first step is to review the peripheral blood smear, as that can often make the diagnosis.

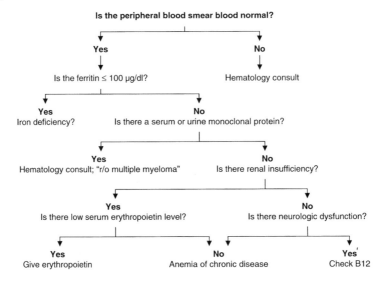

Evaluation of patients with normocytic, normochromic anemia.

1. If the marrow is infiltrated by cancer, many of the red cells will have abnormal shapes (e.g., teardrops), platelets often are large, and both red and white cell precursors are seen. This blood smear is termed *myelophthistic* or *leuko-erythroblastic*. A bone marrow aspirate and biopsy are necessary to confirm this diagnosis.

2. If there is a primary marrow process, such as acute or chronic leukemia or the myelodysplastic syndromes, abnormalities of the white cells and platelets will also be present. Review of the peripheral smear is often diagnostic. In most cases, however, bone marrow aspirate or biopsy is required to make this diagnosis, as well. If the laboratory reports or you see these types of abnormalities, then a hematology consultation is required.

3. If, however, the smear is normal, a serum ferritin level will distinguish iron deficiency from the anemia of chronic disease. For example, a patient with rheumatoid arthritis who takes nonsteroidal agents and whose ferritin is ≤ 100 µg/dl is iron-deficient, whereas a patient with a level > 100 µg/dl has the anemia of chronic disease.

4. In patients who are not iron-deficient, multiple myeloma must be excluded by serum and urine protein electrophoreses. Myeloma occurs most commonly in the fifth and sixth decades but can occur in older patients as well. If a monoclonal protein is present, it can be caused by one of a number of plasma cell disorders, including multiple myeloma. A hematology consultation is therefore required here, as well.

5. In patients without iron deficiency or myeloma who have renal insufficiency, low serum erythropoietin levels confirm that the anemia is due to renal failure. Treatment with erythropoietin reverses this anemia.

6. In those without renal insufficiency, it is important to exclude B_{12} deficiency. While this disorder usually produces a macrocytic anemia (see question 10), about 15% of patients with neurologic dysfunction from B_{12} deficiency (loss of position sense, loss of sensation, or dementia) have normal red cell size. Therefore, in the elderly population with any of these neurologic findings, evidence for B_{12} deficiency must be sought.

8. Do all patients with macrocytic anemias have megaloblastic anemias?

No. Macrocytic anemia in the elderly may be due to a megaloblastic process, myelodysplasia, or, rarely, hypothyroidism or severe liver dysfunction.

9. How should an elderly patient with macrocytic anemia be evaluated initially?

Thyroid function tests should be obtained, and the peripheral blood smear should be reviewed to distinguish macrocytosis from megaloblastosis and from myelodysplastic syndromes (MDS). Patients with hypothyroidism will have macrocytosis alone; those with liver failure will have target cells and acanthocytes. The white cells will appear normal and the platelets will be normal (in hypothyroidism) or reduced (in liver failure).

In megaloblastic disorders, macro-ovalocytes appear and granulocytes are hypersegmented. In patients with MDS, the neutrophils may be hypogranulated or hyposegmented. Pseudo-Pelger-Huët cells (with nuclei resembling a pair of glasses) are seen in about 20–30%.

10. What are the common causes of megaloblastic anemias in the elderly? How should they be treated?

Megaloblastic anemias arise from tissue deficiencies of B_{12} or folic acid due to inadequate intake or impaired utilization. As many as one-third of elderly patients with a history of gastric surgery may be B_{12}-deficient. Even in those without gastric surgery, atrophic gastritis or agents that inhibit acid production (e.g., cimetidine or omeprazole) can cause B_{12} deficiency. While intrinsic factor production is usually normal in these patients, the lack of acid and pepsin renders them unable to liberate B_{12} from the food protein that binds it. Diet is otherwise not implicated in B_{12} deficiency, as B_{12} is found in all animal products. However, vegans can become deficient in 5–6 years. B_{12}-deficient patients need 5 days of parenteral B_{12} (1000 µg/day) followed by weekly shots for 1 month and then monthly shots for life. Oral replacement using 2 mg B_{12} is also effective. Those with neurologic manifestations require more intensive replacement.

Folate deficiency usually occurs from lack of dietary intake, increased excretion (in alcoholics), or impaired absorption due to achlorhydria. Rarely, folate deficiency occurs in patients with a marked increase in folate requirement from a severe exfoliative skin disease (such as psoriasis) or aggressive hemolytic anemia. Dark-green leafy vegetables, the best source of folate, are not usually a major part of the diet of the elderly. Oral folic acid (1 mg/day) is adequate replacement.

A number of medications cause folate deficiency. The folate deficiency induced by methotrexate (used in dermatologic and rheumatologic diseases), phenytoin, or trimethoprim-sulfamethoxazole can be reversed by concomitant administration of folic acid, without interfering with the therapeutic effect of the drugs. That induced in AIDS patients receiving trimethoprim-sulfamethoxazole, however, cannot be reversed, even by folinic acid. Patients receiving zidovudine or antineoplastic chemotherapy will also have megaloblastic anemias that do not respond to supplemental B_{12} or folate.

11. When is a bone marrow aspiration/biopsy indicated in an elderly patient with a macrocytic anemia?

If macrocytic and megaloblastic processes are eliminated, a bone marrow should be considered to diagnose MDS and obtain prognostic information. MDS includes a number of related stem cell disorders: refractory anemia, refractory anemia with ringed sideroblasts, refractory anemia with excess blasts, refractory anemia with excess blasts in transformation, and chronic myelomonocytic leukemia. Patients with MDS have deficiencies in one or more cell lines (red or white cells, or platelets) and may develop a form of acute leukemia that is unresponsive to conventional anti-leukemic chemotherapy. The cause of MDS is often unknown, but in many patients it is caused by chemotherapy-induced marrow injury. Patients who receive adjuvant chemotherapy for ovarian or breast cancer or chemotherapy for myeloma or lymphoma are at increased risk of developing MDS.

The most important prognostic information is obtained from the karyotype abnormalities of the malignant clone. Patients with multiple chromosomal abnormalities or who have deletion of the long arm of chromosome 7 (7q–) have a median survival of only 1 year. Those with no detectable abnormalities or deletion of the long arm of chromosome 5 (5q–), on the other hand, have an excellent prognosis. Marrows are usually obtained, therefore, both to make the diagnosis and to obtain this prognostic information.

12. How is MDS treated in elderly patients?

Unfortunately, patients over age 60 are not candidates for the only curative therapy, bone marrow transplantation. They experience much more toxicity than younger patients from this procedure, and the consequent risks outweigh the benefits. Besides supportive care, there are few tolerable, effective treatments for the associated cytopenias or leukemias. Some advocate a trial of pyridoxine, though this is rarely effective. Combinations of growth factors can sometimes reverse the cytopenias, though transfusion support is often needed. Occasionally, removal of a massively enlarged spleen that is sequestering red cells is effective. Patients die either from complications resulting from the cytopenias or from leukemic transformation.

13. When should hemolysis be considered as the cause of anemia in an elderly patient?

Acute hemolysis in the elderly presents in the same way as it does in younger patients, with jaundice, dark urine, and weakness, though cardiovascular complaints may also occur. Chronic hemolysis, however, may be asymptomatic except for gallstones, early satiety from splenomegaly, or shoulder pain from splenic infarct. Patients may not even appear jaundiced, though most have splenomegaly. They will, however, have a low haptoglobin level and an elevated reticulocyte count, bilirubin, and lactate dehydrogenase.

14. What are the common causes of congenital hemolytic anemias?

Hereditary hemolytic anemias are usually due to hereditary spherocytosis, enzymopathies, or hemoglobinopathies. Hereditary spherocytosis may first present in the seventh decade. Gallstones may become clinically apparent, or splenomegaly may be noted for the first time during a physical exam for a life insurance policy. Glucose-6-phosphate dehydrogenase (G6PD) deficiency may manifest when the patient is first exposed to a medication causing an oxidant stress. Phenazopyridine, primaquine, and the sulfa drugs sulfamethoxazole (found in Septra and Bactrim), sulfacetamide, sulfanilamide, and sulfapyridine all must be avoided in patients with G6PD deficiency.

Mild hemoglobinopathies (e.g., sickle trait, alpha-thalassemia, or mild variants of beta-thalassemia) similarly may have gone undiagnosed. Hematuria in an elderly patient might be the first presentation of sickle cell trait. However, sickle trait and the other hemoglobinopathies mentioned do not affect the patient's life-span, except in unusual circumstances. A parvovirus infection, for example, may cause a severe, symptomatic anemia. In these patients the red cell survival is shorter than normal. A parvovirus infection will transiently stop red cell production, causing the anemia to worsen significantly and become symptomatic, possibly for the first time. In addition, some thalassemic patients may have incorrectly been thought to suffer from iron deficiency, as their cells are also small. If they received iron for prolonged periods, they may develop iron overload, which can present as heart or liver failure or as arthritis.

15. How are the hereditary hemolytic anemias diagnosed?

In hereditary spherocytosis, spherocytes appear on the smear, and the direct and indirect Coombs' tests (see question 19) are negative. The diagnosis can be confirmed by performing an osmotic fragility test, along with a 48-hour autohemolysis test.

G6PD levels are assayed in the red cells after the reticulocytosis following the hemolysis resolves. Testing the red cells for G6PD during the period of reticulocytosis can give a falsely normal value because reticulocytes have higher levels of G6PD than older cells. Except for alpha-thalassemia, hemoglobinopathies are detected by hemoglobin electrophoresis, as noted earlier.

16. What are the common types of acquired hemolytic anemias in the elderly?

Acquired hemolytic anemias are caused by microangiopathic or immune processes. The antibodies causing the immune hemolytic anemias may be autoantibodies (idiopathic, disease-related, or drug-induced) or alloantibodies (from a transfusion).

17. How are microangiopathic hemolytic anemias diagnosed and treated?

Elderly patients develop microangiopathic hemolytic anemia from uncontrolled hypertension, aortic dissections, leaking artificial valves (especially aortic), widespread metastatic cancer, or certain chemotherapeutic agents. Very rarely, they develop idiopathic thrombotic thrombocytopenic purpura (TTP).

Red cell fragments and early red cell precursors are present on the blood smear; in TTP, there will also be very few platelets. Medication for blood pressure, surgery to correct the vascular or valvular disease, or plasmapheresis for those with idiopathic TTP is usually effective. There is usually no effective therapy for patients with TTP caused by widespread cancer or chemotherapy.

18. What are the causes of immune hemolysis in the elderly?

The usual causes are autoimmune hemolytic disorders. These are either idiopathic or associated with underlying lymphoproliferative disorders (e.g., chronic lymphocytic leukemia, lymphoma). The antibodies are of the IgG or IgM class. The former are active at usual body temperatures and so are considered "warm" antibodies; the latter are most active in the cold and so are called "cold" antibodies. The cold antibodies cause **cold agglutinin disease**, a very difficult form of hemolytic anemia to treat.

Drugs can also produce antibody-mediated hemolytic anemia. Ten percent of patients on methyldopa or L-dopa develop antibodies, but rarely (in 10% of those with antibodies) does the patient develop hemolysis. Penicillin-induced hemolysis is mediated through a hapten mechanism, while sulfa drugs and quinidine induce an immune complex-mediated hemolysis.

A less common antibody-mediated process is the **delayed hemolytic transfusion reaction**. These reactions are caused by alloantibodies raised in response to a non-ABO red cell antigen that was absent on the patient's red cells but present on red cells in the transfusion. Seven to 10 days after the transfusion, the newly formed antibodies cause lysis of transfused red cells that have the foreign antigen. The patient suddenly develops dark-colored urine, jaundice, and, if a large number of units were transfused, symptoms of anemia.

19. How are the autoimmune hemolytic anemias diagnosed and treated?

Immune hemolytic anemias are diagnosed by performing a direct and an indirect Coombs' test, which detects the presence of IgG, IgM, or complement on the patient's red cells (direct Coombs) or IgG or IgM in the patient's serum (indirect Coombs). In the direct Coombs' test, the patient's red cells are incubated with reagents that cause red cells coated with antibodies to agglutinate. The test is positive in patients with immune hemolytic anemias, as the cause of the anemia is the coating of the patient's cells with antibody. The indirect Coombs' test detects antibodies in the serum. The patient's serum is reacted with red cells from a variety of donors, and the cells are examined for agglutination. Usually, this test is also positive, because patients with immune hemolytic anemias usually make more antibody than can bind to the red cells. The excess antibody appears in the serum.

Steroids are the initial therapy for idiopathic **warm antibody-mediated hemolysis**, but splenectomy is also often required to remove the major site of antibody recognition and red cell destruction. However, in addition, specific chemotherapy for the underlying cancer is required to reverse the immune hemolysis associated with lymphoma or chronic lymphocytic leukemia.

For patients with **cold agglutinin disease** associated with mycoplasma or Epstein-Barr virus infection, no therapy is usually required. For the idiopathic forms, the patient is usually advised to stay in a warm climate. Steroids are not routinely effective and immunosuppresive chemotherapeutic agents have mixed success.

20. How are the drug-induced immune anemias diagnosed and treated?

Drug-induced antibodies are also detected by the Coombs' tests. They are positive for IgG in the case of penicillin and methyldopa/L-dopa-induced hemolysis, but the direct Coombs will be positive only for complement in hemolysis induced by quinidine and sulfa drugs. If patients on methyldopa or L-dopa have antibodies but no evidence of hemolysis, the drugs can be continued. If hemolysis has occurred, however, the drugs must be stopped.

21. And the delayed hemolytic transfusion reaction?

A delayed hemolytic transfusion reaction is confirmed by an indirect Coombs' test, which, in this case, detects the specific serum antibody responsible for the hemolysis. The direct Coombs' test will usually be negative, because the red cells that had bound the antibody (and would have made the direct Coombs positive) have been hemolyzed.

As the process is self-limited, no specific therapy is usually required. Patients subsequently receive transfusions only with red cells lacking the antigen to which the antibody was directed.

22. Which patients benefit from erythropoietin?

Erythropoietin can be beneficial to elderly patients in a variety of clinical circumstances. To achieve optimal effect, concomitant iron replacement (oral or intravenous) is required when the serum ferritin falls to ≤ 100 ng/ml. Anemic patients on dialysis and patients with lesser degrees of renal insufficiency who do not produce adequate levels of erythropoietin benefit significantly from erythropoietin replacement. Doses for dialysis patients average 100 U/kg/wk subcutaneously; the average wholesale price is about $450/month. The target hemoglobin is ~ 11–12 gm/dl (hematocrit > 33 and ≤ 36), even for patients with coronary artery disease. Patients no longer require blood transfusions and report significantly improved energy levels and quality of life. The anemia of chronic disease associated with active rheumatoid arthritis also has responded to erythropoietin.

Erythropoietin also is indicated in patients scheduled for elective surgery, including total joint replacement and cardiac procedures. Preoperative erythropoietin is usually effective in enabling adequate autologous blood donation, reducing the need for transfusion with allogeneic blood, and raising the postoperative hemoglobin level in both nonanemic and anemic patients, even those with rheumatoid arthritis. The average wholesale price for erythropoietin in these preoperative regimens ranges from $1000 for low doses to $2500 for higher doses.

The anemia of patients with HIV infection or nonmyeloid malignancies also usually responds to erythropoietin plus iron. The target hemoglobin is 12–13 gm/dl. Cancer patients whose hemoglobin rises ≥ 2 gm/dl in response to erythropoietin need fewer transfusions. They consistently report less fatigue, improved ability to perform daily activities, and improvement in overall quality of life even while they are receiving chemotherapy, regardless of whether the cancer is in complete or partial remission or is stable. The standard erythropoietin dose is 40,000 U/week subcutaneously; the dose is raised to 60,000 U/week subcutaneously for patients who have no response after 4 weeks at the lower dose. If during the subsequent 4 weeks there is no response at the higher level, the erythropoietin is discontinued. For 40,000 U/week, the average wholesale price per month is about $2000.

BIBLIOGRAPHY

1. Atony AC: Megaloblastic anemias. In Benz EJ, et al (eds): Hematology: Basic Principles and Practice, 2nd ed. New York, Churchill Livingstone, 1994, pp 4552–4586.
2. Brittenham GM: Disorders of iron metabolism: Iron deficiency and overload. In Benz EJ, et al (eds): Hematology: Basic Principles and Practice, 2nd ed. New York, Churchill Livingstone, 1994, pp 492–523.
3. Demetri GD, Kris M, Wade J, et al: Quality of life benefit in chemotherapy patients treated with erythropoietin alpha is independent of disease response or tumor type: Results from a prospective community oncology study. J Clin Oncol 16:3412–3425, 1998.
4. Greenberg PL: Myelodysplastic syndrome. In Benz EJ, et al (eds): Hematology: Basic Principles and Practice, 2nd ed. New York, Churchill Livingstone, 1994, pp 1098–1121.
5. Guyatt GH, Oxman AD, Ali M, et al: Laboratory diagnosis of iron deficiency anemia: An overview. J Gen Intern Med 7:145–153, 1992.
6. NKF-DOQI clinical practice guideline for the treatment of anemia of chronic renal failure. Am J Kidney Dis 30(Suppl 3):S192–S240, 1997.
7. Peeters HR, Jongen-Lavrencic M, Vreugdenhil G, Swaak AJ: Effects of recombinant human erythropoietin on anaemia and disease activity in patients with rheumatoid arthritis and anaemia of chronic disease: A randomised, placebo-controlled, double-blind 52-week clinical trial. Ann Rheum Dis 55:739–744, 1996.
8. Red Book. Montvale, NJ, Medical Economics Company, 1999.
9. Schilling RF: Anemia of chronic disease: A misnomer. Ann Intern Med 115:572–573, 1991.
10. Schwartz E, Benz EJ Jr, Forget BG: Thalassemia syndromes. In Benz EJ, et al (eds): Hematology: Basic Principles and Practice, 2nd ed. New York, Churchill Livingstone, 1994, pp 586–610.
11. Schwartz RS, Silberstein LE, Berkman EM: Autoimmune hemolytic anemias. In Benz EJ, et al (eds): Hematology: Basic Principles and Practice, 2nd ed. New York, Churchill Livingstone, 1994, pp 710–729.
12. Spivak JL: The biology and clinical application of recombinant erythropoietin. Semin Oncol 25(Suppl 7):7–11, 1998.

36. ORAL ANTICOAGULATION IN THE ELDERLY

Diane Hershock, M.D., Ph.D., and Stephen I. Chavin, M.D.

1. What are the major indications for use of antithrombotic agents in the elderly?

Thromboembolic events are quite common in the elderly, usually in the setting of atherosclerosis. Among the most common are stroke and myocardial infarction, which generally result from occlusive thrombi forming within arteries already compromised by stenosed or ulcerated atherosclerotic plaques. Because blood flow through these vessels becomes sluggish as a result of luminal narrowing, a highly thrombogenic milieu results. Other common maladies associated with arterial thrombosis or embolism in the elderly include atrial fibrillation and valvular heart disease. Venous thrombosis and pulmonary embolism are frequently encountered as well. Thus, the use of anticoagulation or antiplatelet agents in the elderly encompasses a variety of clinical settings.

2. What are the major classes of agents used for anticoagulation?

1. **Anticoagulants**, which affect the fluid phase of coagulant proteins and include warfarin, heparin, and hirudin.

2. **Antiplatelet drugs**, which inhibit platelet function.

3. **Thrombolytic agents**, which activate the fibrinolytic system and include plasminogen and plasminogen activators. In contrast to anticoagulants and antiplatelet agents, which act primarily before thrombi are formed, fibrinolytic agents can attack both soluble fibrinogen and preformed thrombi.

3. Which agents are most commonly used for oral anticoagulation?

Warfarin, a member of the coumarin family, alters vitamin K metabolism and thereby inhibits a vitamin K–dependent posttranslational addition of carboxyl groups to the amino terminal end of coagulation proteins II, VII, IX, and X, the inhibitory proteins C and S, and the bone matrix protein, osteocalcin. The reduction in number of these glutamic acid residues causes a reduction in the activity of the vitamin K–dependent proteins.

Antiplatelet agents:

Drugs with Platelet-inhibitory Activity

Aspirin and other NSAIDs	Inhibitors of GPIIb/IIIa
Ticlopidine and clopidogrel	Fish oils/n-3 fatty acids
Dextran	Heparin
Sulfinpyrazone	Nitrates
Vitamin E	Calcium channel blockers
β-adrenergic blocking agents	

Aspirin: This is the most common nonsteroidal anti-inflammatory drug (NSAID) and is used specifically as an antiplatelet agent. Aspirin irreversibly acetylates, and thereby inhibits, platelet cyclo-oxygenase. This reaction blocks the production of thromboxane A_2, a potent vasoconstrictor and platelet aggregating agent. As little as 81 mg/day is effective, but optimal dosing has yet to be determined. The effect of a single dose may last for more than one week due to the half-life of platelets in the circulation. Other nonsteroidal agents, such as ibuprofen and indomethacin, have a similar but reversible effect on platelet cyclo-oxygenase. Aspirin pharmacology has not been well evaluated in the elderly. As is common to patients of any age, aspirin can cause gastric bleeding, urticaria, or renal dysfunction, especially in patients with lupus nephritis.

Ticlopidine and clopidogrel are known to prolong bleeding times and inhibit platelet aggregation by adenosine diphosphate (ADP) even at high agonist concentrations. It apparently decreases the ability of ADP to initiate changes in the GPIIb/IIIa receptor needed for fibrinogen binding. Neutropenia is a major side effect of ticlopidine (incidence 0.8%) but occurs much less frequently with clopidogrel.

4. Have pharmacokinetic studies of warfarin been done in the elderly?

Pharmacokinetics includes absorption, half-life, distribution, and excretion. Warfarin is absorbed rapidly and completely with peak plasma concentrations reached one hour after ingestion. Absorption is delayed but not reduced by food. Warfarin in plasma is 98–99% bound to albumin. Ultimately, warfarin is metabolized in the liver by conversion to biologically inactive alcohols, which are then excreted in urine and stool.

No difference in the half-life was determined in a study comparing young individuals (average age 31 years) to elderly people (average age 83 years). The half life was 37 versus 44 hours in the elderly. No differences were seen regarding volume of distribution (193 ml/kg versus 200 ml/kg), clearance (3.8 ml/kg/hr versus 3.26 ml/kg/hr) or protein binding (98.6% versus 98.5%).

The rate of synthesis of functionally active vitamin K–dependent factors was significantly less in the elderly for any given concentration of warfarin, suggesting that the clinical effect of warfarin may be greater in the elderly population and that lower initial and maintenance doses may be prudent.

5. Are the pharmacodynamic effects of warfarin different in the elderly?

Pharmacodynamics are the biological and clinical effects of a drug. A retrospective study has suggested that increasing age may be associated with an increased response to warfarin and other oral anticoagulant agents, even after controlling for other medications, body weight, gender, and comorbidities. The mechanism for this effect is unknown but may be due to a change in the activity of vitamin K epoxide reductase or its affinity for warfarin in elderly subjects.

6. How much warfarin is required for anticoagulation of an elderly person?

Because elderly people appear to be more sensitive to oral anticoagulants, their response to loading doses may be exaggerated and their ultimate steady-state dosage may be lower than that required for a younger person. For this reason, it has been recommended that loading doses of warfarin not be used in the elderly and that a reasonable starting dose would be 2.5 mg/day. The following table is based on the above information and adjusted for age.

Daily Dose of Warfarin (mg) by Age of Patients

AGE	GURWITZ ET AL.	JAMES ET AL.
< 50	6.4	6.1
50–59	5.1	5.3
60–69	4.2	4.3
70–79	3.6	3.9
≥ 80	NA	3.5

7. What are the current recommendations for anticoagulation for atrial fibrillation in the elderly?

Atrial fibrillation occurs in approximately 2% of the population and its prevalence increases with age; 5% of patients over the age of 60 reportedly have atrial fibrillation. Atrial fibrillation is associated with a twofold increase in mortality; 6–24% of patients who have ischemic strokes are noted to have atrial fibrillation, and up to 50% of patients with atrial fibrillation have cardioembolic strokes.

Recently, published studies have stratified the need for anticoagulation in nonrheumatic atrial fibrillation. The results are as follows:

• Patients < age 60 with atrial fibrillation alone do not need to be anticoagulated, because the risk of stroke is not significantly different from those without fibrillation.
.• Patients aged 60–75 with only atrial fibrillation can be treated with 325 mg/day of aspirin. However, some believe that anticoagulation decreases the 2% incidence/year of stroke in patients with atrial fibrillation alone.
• Patients < 75 with one risk factor for stroke have been shown to benefit from anticoagulation with an INR normalized to 2.0–3.0. (For further details, see chapter entitled "Stroke.")
• Patients > 75 even without other risk factors benefit from oral anticoagulation because of the high risk of stroke with advanced age.

8. What are the risks of anticoagulation in atrial fibrillation using warfarin in the elderly?

With the exception of hypersensitivity reactions and warfarin-induced skin necrosis, bleeding is the single largest complication of anticoagulant therapy. The risk of a patient developing an anticoagulant-induced hemorrhage is generally affected by two factors: the intensity of anticoagulation and the duration of therapy. The risk of hemorrhage is generally increased 5–10 fold during the first few months of warfarin therapy. Generally, after 3–6 months the rate stabilizes and remains fairly constant. It has been suggested that the high initial rate of bleeding is due to intensive, excessive warfarin, the concurrent administration of heparin, or undiagnosed gastrointestinal or genitourinary tract pathology. However, how does this apply to the elderly population?

The extent of age on the risk of bleeding is very controversial. Recent studies using either longitudinal-cohort or randomized prospective designs revealed no association between age and bleeding risk. However, other reports contraindicate this, showing an increased rate of hemorrhage in patients older than age 65–75 with major bleeding rates 1.8–3.2 times higher than rates in those younger than 65 years.

The risk of bleeding from anticoagulation therapy has declined over the last several decades. Bleeding rates cited in studies from 1960–1979 compared to those from 1980–1991 have decreased almost 50%. There are several explanations for this phenomenon: recommended therapeutic ranges for prothrombin time (PT) are lower; the INR measure is now an acceptable standard for reporting PTs; and refinements in outpatient monitoring and the use of shorter-acting warfarin (Coumadin) derivatives also have contributed to the decreased risk of bleeding.

9. What are the risks associated with anticoagulation for secondary prevention of stroke in the elderly?

A recent study looked at the complication rates for aspirin, warfarin, and intravenous heparin given as secondary stroke prevention after an initial episode of either ischemic stroke, transient ischemic attack, or amaurosis fugax in a population in which the mean age was 76 years.[8] The results showed that warfarin administration was associated with higher risks of complication compared to aspirin and that the degree of risk was higher in older persons. However, fatal risks were not different in either group. This study did not suggest that patients with ischemic cardiovascular disease were at any greater risk for hemorrhage than those who received warfarin for other indications. The results for each agent are shown below.

Aspirin: It was ascertained that aspirin therapy is not without risk. A fatality rate of 0.2/100 person years of treatment was documented. Standardized morbidity ratio estimates for gastrointestinal hemorrhage and intracerebral hemorrhage were 1.5 and 1.7, respectively. These findings are consistent with the fourfold risk for intracerebral hemorrhage among elderly aspirin users found in an earlier study.

Warfarin (Coumadin): The complication rates were lower than previously reported. Of 145 patients, the major complication rate, which included cerebral vascular bleed or gastrointestinal bleed, was 7.9 (95% CI, 3.4–15.6).

Heparin: The rates of complications with intravenous heparin in this study were lower than rates derived from previous clinical trials when using heparin for cerebrovascular disease, but the risk is still higher with heparin than for aspirin or warfarin. The standardized morbidity ratio estimate of gastrointestinal hemorrhage for heparin was greater than the estimates for warfarin or aspirin. However, the risk for the development of an intracerebral hemorrhage during heparin therapy was low.

10. What are the risk factors for over-anticoagulation in elderly patients?

A recent study of 131 patients ranging in age from 64–71 diagnosed with atrial fibrillation, deep venous thrombosis (DVT), prosthetic heart valves, and antiphospholipid syndrome were evaluated for risk factors. The highest relative risk of 7.3 was associated with a target INR of 3.5 compared to a lower target of 2.5. Five of the 31 patients with high INRs suffered major hemorrhages with a relative risk of bleeding of 5.4. Thus, patients with an INR of 3.5 are more likely to become over-anticoagulated and more likely to bleed than patients with a target of 2.5. A change in medication, particularly antibiotics, also was associated with an increased risk of bleed. This was especially true if the antibiotics included co-trimoxazole, erythromycin, fluconazole, isoniazid, metronidazole, or miconazole. Infection also was a risk factor for an elevated INR. Those treated with decentralized care were not more likely to be over-anticoagulated than patients in a hospital-based setting.

11. Should certain patients be targeted for a higher INR in spite of the increased risks of bleeding?

Patients requiring a higher INR include those with mechanical heart valves, patients with thrombosis associated with antiphospholipid syndrome, and those with recurrent venous thromboembolism despite therapy with warfarin and an INR of 2.0–3.0. Careful consideration should be given to anticoagulating patients in whom clear benefit has not been demonstrated, such as those with arterial thrombotic disease not of antiphospholipid origin, thrombotic stroke in the absence of atrial fibrillation, peripheral vascular disease, arterial grafts, and coronary thrombosis. These patients may benefit more from aspirin.

12. How frequently should the INR be measured in the elderly?

There is an increased risk of intracranial hemorrhage in patients > 70 taking warfarin, especially as the INR approaches 3.0. This population of patients also may have an increased incidence of mild bleeding and excessive bleeding. It has therefore been recommended that an INR be assessed every 3–4 weeks. Furthermore, any time a patient's medications are changed or a significant intercurrent illness is present, the anticoagulation status should be re-evaluated and the INR checked as indicated.

13. Which drugs have major impacts on warfarin metabolism as reflected by the INR?

Common Drug Interactions with Warfarin

DRUGS THAT INCREASE LEVEL ANTICOAGULATION	DRUGS THAT DECREASE LEVEL ANTICOAGULATION	MINOR INTER- ACTIONS INCREASED ANTI- COAGULATION EFFECT	DECREASED ANTI- COAGULATION EFFECT
Amiodarone	Barbiturates	Allopurinol	Thiazide diuretics
Cimetidine	Carbamazepine	Omeprazole	Aminoglutethimide
Androgens (17-alkyl)	Antithyroid drugs	Ranitidine	Spironolactone
Clofibrate	Rifampin	Chloral hydrate	Ethchlorvynol
Erythromycin	Cholestyramine	Dextropropoxyphene	Griseofulvin
Clarithromycin	Glutethimide	Acetaminophen	Cyclophosphamide
Disulfiram		Ciprofloxacin	Sucralfate
Metronidazole		Fluconazole	Ascorbic acid
High-dose salicylates		Tricyclics	
Tamoxifen			
Thyroid hormone			
TMP-sulfamethoxazole			
Sulfinpyrazone			
Glucagon			

14. Does diet affect warfarin kinetics in the elderly?

Foods high in vitamin K, such as coriander, parsley, mint, chard, kale, brussel sprouts, broccoli, watercress, turnip greens, green beans, asparagus, avocado, beef liver, and green tea, can inhibit the anticoagulant response to warfarin in any population. Diets deficient in vitamin K may result in an increased anticoagulant response, especially in those with hepatic dysfunction, which may be common among the older population. Hypoproteinemia, often a problem in the elderly, can affect volume distribution and half-life of warfarin. However, even in the elderly, it is unlikely that differences in serum albumin are responsible for varied anticoagulation responses.

15. Are there other factors that may influence the clinical effects of warfarin?

Biliary obstruction, small bowel dysfunction, and any disorders that affect the biosynthetic functions of the liver such as alcohol- or drug-induced hepatic disease, cirrhosis, and congestive heart failure may result in increased anticoagulation.

16. Is osteoporosis a long-term risk factor of warfarin therapy in the elderly?

A recent study suggests that neither warfarin nor heparin was associated with an increase in risk of osteoporosis. Six thousand two hundred one postmenopausal elderly women were evaluated. Compared to warfarin nonusers (6,052), warfarin users (149) had poor health, involuntary weight loss, and frailty but had similar bone mineral density at the hip. Users and nonusers had similar rates of bone loss and fractures, suggesting that warfarin did not decrease bone mineral density or increase fracture rates.

17. What is the role of antiplatelet agents in elderly patients?

Aspirin has been the mainstay of long-term prevention of stroke and myocardial infarction. More recently, agents such as ticlopidine and clopidogrel have been used for prevention of initial or recurrent stroke. In the Ticlopidine Aspirin Stroke Study (TASS) evaluation, ticlopidine reduced the overall risk of nonfatal stroke by 21% compared with aspirin alone.

18. What are the risks of concurrent antiplatelet agents and warfarin?

Concurrent use of aspirin and oral anticoagulants has not been recommended in recent years due to significant drug interactions leading to unacceptably high rates of bleeding. Whether aspirin has direct anticoagulant effects potentiating that of warfarin is unclear. The frequency of minor bleeds was higher in patients treated with warfarin and acetylsalicylic acid. With this combination of drugs, the mean ages of patients who developed minor bleeds, major bleeds, and fatal bleeds were, respectively, 64.6, 64.4, and 70.1 years. However, an overall comparison of combination therapy with aspirin and warfarin to warfarin alone showed no increase in major bleeds or fatal hemorrhages.

Another study analyzing the effects of ticlopidine co-administration with warfarin in nine elderly men (age range 65–76) receiving anticoagulation for chronic atrial fibrillation, heart valve, and stroke was performed. Ticlopidine did not adversely affect warfarin levels as exemplified by no change in the overall anticoagulation response. In the above TASS evaluation, neutropenia was a major side effect in those who received ticlopidine. Gastrointestinal hemorrhage was noted in only one patient who received ticlopidine but not aspirin.

19. Is there an increased risk for bleeding with concurrent use of acetaminophen and warfarin in the elderly?

A recent study suggests that in patients using more than 9100 mg/week of acetaminophen in addition to warfarin, the odds of having an INR greater than 6.0 were increased tenfold. The population studied was an older cohort (mean age 70). The data suggest that acetaminophen is an underrecognized cause of over-anticoagulation in approximately 30% of patients evaluated. Thus, physicians should take a more detailed drug history, especially with unexplained increases in an INR.

BIBLIOGRAPHY

1. Gurwitz JH, Avorn J, Ross-Degnan D, et al: Aging and the anticoagulant response to warfarin therapy. Ann Intern Med 116:901–904, 1992.
2. Hass WK, Easton JD, Adams HP, et al; The Ticlopidine Aspirin Stroke Study Group: A randomized trial comparing ticlopidine hydrochloride with aspirin for the prevention of stroke in high-risk patients. N Engl J Med 321:501–507, 1989.
3. He J, Whelton PK, Vu B, Kiag MJ: Aspirin and risk of hemorrhagic stroke: A meta-analysis of randomized controlled trials. JAMA 280:1930–1935, 1998.
4. Hurjen M, Erikssen J, Smith P, et al: Comparison of bleeding complications of warfarin and warfarin plus acetylsalicylic acid: A study of 3166 outpatients. J Int Med Res 236:299–304, 1994.
5. Jamal SA, Browner WS, Bauer DC, Cummings SR: Warfarin use and risk for osteoporosis in elderly women. Study of Osteoporotic Fractures Research Group. Ann Intern Med 128:829–832, 1998.
6. James AH, Britt RP, Rankino CL, Thompson SG: Factors affecting the maintenance dose of warfarin. J Clin Pathol 45:704–706, 1992.
7. Landefeld CS, Beyth RJ: Anticoagulant-related bleeding: Clinical epidemiology, prediction, and prevention. Am J Med 95:315–328, 1993.
8. Petty GW, Brown RD, Whisnant JP, et al: Frequency of major complications of aspirin, warfarin, and intravenous heparin for secondary stroke prevention: A population-based study. Ann Intern Med 130:14–22, 1999.
9. Sherman DG, Dyken ML, Harrison JG, et al: Antithrombotic therapy for cerebrovascular disorders. An update. Chest 108(Suppl 4):444S–456S, 1995.
10. Stroke Prevention in Atrial Fibrillation Investigators: Bleeding during antithrombotic therapy in patients with atrial fibrillation. Arch Intern Med 156:409–416, 1996.
11. Stroke Prevention in Atrial Fibrillation Investigators: Warfarin versus aspirin for prevention of thromboembolism in atrial fibrillation: Stroke prevention in atrial fibrillation II study. Lancet 343:87–91, 1994.

37. CORONARY ARTERY DISEASE

Susan E. Wiegers, M.D., and Joseph R. McClellan, M.D.

1. Is coronary atherosclerosis a universal consequence of aging?

The incidence of significant coronary atherosclerosis progressively increases with age, but the disease is not a universal accompaniment of the aging process. All coronary events, including angina, unstable angina, and acute myocardial infarction (MI), increase in frequency with aging. Epidemiologic studies demonstrate that approximately 30% of patients over the age of 75 have evidence of symptomatic coronary artery disease. At necropsy, approximately 60% of octogenarians and more than 90% of nonagenarians have one or more coronary arteries with a 75% or greater reduction in luminal cross-sectional area caused by an atherosclerotic plaque. In addition, in older patients coronary disease is often extensive and diffuse, with generalized coronary calcification and a higher proportion of multivessel and left main disease.

2. Are the symptoms of coronary artery disease different in the elderly?

Acute and chronic coronary syndromes are less frequently recognized in the elderly. Reduced sensitivity to pain results in a high incidence of silent myocardial ischemia and unrecognized acute MI. The Framingham study found that in patients aged 75–84, 42% of MIs in men and 36% of MIs in women were clinically unrecognized. Studies have shown that elderly patients present to the hospital later than younger patients when having an MI. This delay is clinically important, because early delivery of thrombolytic therapy is essential for myocardial preservation. Although decreased pain perception may account for some of the delay in seeking treatment for acute ischemic syndromes, various other factors may prevent elderly patients from prompt presentation for evaluation, including social isolation, cognitive dysfunction, and socioeconomic status. Concerns about the cost of emergency department services have prevented patients from seeking evaluation for symptoms. In addition, women make up a higher portion of the elderly population and are known to present later than men for acute MI at all ages. Finally, the role of the physician's assessment of elderly patients should not be ignored. Discounting the patient's symptoms because of a presumption of cognitive dysfunction may cause the physician to miss the diagnosis. Some physicians also may believe erroneously that excessive somatization is a common feature of aging. This belief may lead to inappropriate diagnoses.

The presenting features of acute MI are also different in the elderly:

- In patients over 85 years of age, dyspnea is the most common symptom. Chest pain is the second most common symptom.
- Most patients under 75 years of age have chest pain.
- Other common symptoms include syncope, confusion and mental status changes, and other neurologic symptoms.

The development of angina in elderly patients strongly correlates with the presence of coronary artery disease. In addition, patients older than 75 years with chronic angina have a high likelihood of severe, multivessel coronary disease.

3. Should the diagnostic approach to coronary artery disease be altered in elderly patients?

Noninvasive strategies are preferable for the initial diagnosis of patients in all age groups except those with unstable symptoms. The electrocardiogram (EKG) tracing may be abnormal in up to 96% of patients over the age of 85, even in patients with no evidence of atherosclerotic disease. T-wave inversions and ST changes are present in the majority. The EKG abnormalities limit the usefulness of routine exercise testing, because a baseline normal EKG is required for diagnostic accuracy. Many elderly patients are unable to reach 85% of their maximally predicted heart rate via treadmill exercise. The standard Bruce protocol has a high VO_2 demand in the initial minutes of the test and may not be the optimal protocol in ambulatory elderly patients. The modified Balke protocol is often performed in this age group. Unfamiliarity with treadmill apparatus and fear of falling also may limit the usefulness of treadmill exercise in the elderly population. In such situations, pharmacologic stress testing is recommended. Dipyridamole and dobutamine stress testing with either thallium or Cc-99m SestaMIBI provides accurate diagnostic and prognostic information equal to maximal exercise testing. Similarly, dobutamine stress echocardiography and adenosine echocardiography are highly sensitive and specific for the diagnosis of coronary artery disease. Because left ventricular ejection fractions and coexisting valvular disease are important determinants of clinical outcome in older patients, echocardiographic assessment of cardiac function should be considered.

Cardiac catheterization remains the gold standard for the diagnosis of coronary artery disease but carries a higher complication rate in elderly patients. In all patients, the decision to undertake cardiac catheterization should be preceded by a therapeutic plan based on the potential results. If revascularization is precluded by the patient's other medical conditions, it is wise to forego cardiac catheterization. Similarly, in elderly patients with normal left ventricular function, chronic stable angina, and no evidence of extensive ischemia in the left anterior descending territory, catheterization may not be indicated.

4. Is modification of coronary risk factors less important in the elderly?
The importance of the well-known coronary risk factors persists in the elderly, and attempts at modification should remain vigorous.

- Hypertension, including isolated elevation of systolic pressure, is a major risk factor in older patients for the development of coronary artery events as well as stroke (see chapters 20 and 36). Treatment of isolated systolic hypertension in the elderly results in a substantial reduction in stroke, cardiac death, nonfatal MI, and all cardiovascular events.
- Cigarette smoking in patients over the age of 65 is associated with a 50% increase in coronary mortality compared with nonsmokers. Cessation of smoking probably lowers this risk substantially.
- Hypercholesterolemia is also a significant independent predictor of increased coronary events in the elderly. However, less information is available about the value of treatment in older patients. Recent secondary and primary prevention trials from Scandinavia and West Scotland demonstrated a striking reduction in cardiac mortality and nonfatal MI, respectively, in patients with elevated cholesterol who were treated with 3-hydroxy-3-methylglutaryl coenzyme A (HMG CoA) reductase inhibitors. Of importance, significant risk reduction was seen in the first 6 months of treatment. Although these results may not be totally reproducible in the elderly, the early benefit of therapy suggests that improvement of hypercholesterolemia with these agents also will be valuable in older patients.
- Physical activity, even at moderate levels, has been associated with an improvement in risk factor profile in the elderly. Sedentary patients had higher levels of low-density lipoprotein and lower levels of high-density lipoprotein that persisted after correcting for differences in obesity, age, and cigarette smoking
- Other well-recognized risk factors, including elevated blood sugar, homocysteine, and left ventricular hypertrophy, also are associated with increased coronary risk in older populations.
- Family history is also a risk factor for coronary artery disease in elderly patients. ApoE genotype conferred increased risk in several longitudinal studies of elderly men after accounting for other common clinical risk factors.

5. Is age an important risk factor in patients with an acute MI?
Age is a significant independent risk factor for mortality and serious morbidity in patients with an acute MI. Various clinical trials have documented the important effect of age on in-hospital mortality. In the first cooperative Italian streptokinase trial (GISSI), the mortality in the

control group was 7.7% in patients under 65 and 33.1% in patients over 75. Similarly, the Worcester Heart Attack Study reported that mortality progressively increased with advancing age. Other major complications, including stroke, heart block, cardiogenic shock, congestive heart failure, pulmonary edema, cardiac rupture, and other mechanical complications, also increase in frequency with advanced age. This significant increase in mortality and complication rates makes the administration of prompt, effective therapy most important in elderly patients with an acute MI.

6. Are elderly patients candidates for thrombolytic therapy?
Yes. Elderly patients definitely should receive thrombolytic therapy for MI if they do not meet the standard exclusion criteria. Many trials of thrombolytic therapy for acute MI excluded patients over the age of 70. However, data from GISSI, the second International Study of Infarct Survival (ISIS-II), and the recent International Trial Comparing Four Thrombolytic Strategies for Acute Myocardial Infarction (GUSTO trial) have demonstrated or suggested significant benefit of thrombolytic therapy in patients older than 65 years.

Results of Recent Trials of Thrombolytic Therapy

TRIAL	TREATMENT	MORTALITY (%)
GISSI	Streptokinase	28.9
	Placebo	33.1
ISIS-II (patients over 69)	Streptokinase	18.2
	Placebo	21.6
GUSTO (patients over 75)	Tissue plasminogen activator	20
	Streptokinase	20

Because of the high mortality rate in the elderly compared with other age groups, the greatest absolute benefit of thrombolysis was obtained in the older population. The GUSTO trial indicated a decreased combined mortality rate in older patients compared with historical controls treated with placebo. This finding suggests a significant benefit of treatment in elderly patients.

Thrombolytic therapy should be used in elderly patients with anterior MIs in the absence of absolute or strong relative contraindications. Some controversy surrounds the use of thrombolytics in stable patients with uncomplicated inferior MIs. The contraindications include:
• Presentation later than 6 hours after the onset of pain if there is no clinical evidence of ongoing ischemia
• Major surgery within the past 3 weeks
• Major trauma in the past 2–4 weeks
• Active internal bleeding
• Ischemic stroke within the past year or hemorrhagic stroke at any time
• Bleeding diathesis
• Severe diabetic retinopathy, which is a strong relative contraindication because of the risk of retinal hemorrhage and subsequent blindness
The incidence of stroke after thrombolytic therapy is increased in elderly patients. However, the reluctance to precipitate stroke should not deter the physician from definitive treatment with thrombolytic therapy in elderly patients because they benefit substantially. In patients who have an absolute contraindication to thrombolytic therapy, strong consideration should be given to the use of emergent direct coronary angioplasty for the treatment of acute MI.

7. Should other medical therapies be altered in elderly patients with coronary artery disease?
In general, effective treatment strategies and beneficial therapies have a similar impact on morbidity and mortality in elderly and younger patients. Aspirin and beta blockers maintain a

central role in treatment of coronary artery disease and prevention of recurrent cardiac events. In elderly patients, however, various alterations in drug absorption, distribution, and metabolism may affect both physiologic responses and toxicity. Both hepatic metabolism and renal excretion diminish with age. Extracellular volume diminishes, and the volume of distribution of hydrophilic drugs also decreases. In addition, end-organ responsiveness may be altered. For example, the decrease in responsiveness to adrenergic stimulation with aging may affect the cardiovascular response to beta blockade. The incidence of significant bradycardia and congestive heart failure after beta-blocker therapy increases with advancing age. Therefore, beta-blocker therapy should be monitored carefully but not withheld. Elderly patients may be more prone to digitalis toxicity because of reduced volume of distribution and renal clearance.

Another important physiologic alteration in older patients is a reduction in the sensitivity of the carotid baroreceptors, which blunts the cardiovascular responses to vasodilation and positional changes. Altered baroreceptor function and decreased extracellular volume increase the likelihood of orthostatic hypotension and adverse reactions to vasodilating drugs such as nitrates. In addition, significant volume reduction with diuretics may have magnified effects on posture-related changes in blood pressure. Concomitant valvular disease, especially senile calcific aortic stenosis, may change drastically an individual's response to cardiac medications. An elderly patient with a fixed cardiac output due to critical aortic stenosis may have fatal hypotension precipitated by nitroglycerin therapy.

Polypharmacy in elderly patients is a well-documented problem. Patients with multiple medical problems and many physicians are more likely to be prescribed medications with negative interactions. Cardiac effects of noncardiac medications, such as bradycardia from eyedrops used to treat glaucoma, should not be overlooked. The cost of medications also should be a consideration when prescribing for any patient population. Overall, careful individualization of drug therapy is especially important in elderly patients.

8. How useful is coronary artery bypass surgery in older patients?

A randomized prospective trial comparing the impact on survival of coronary artery bypass surgery and medical therapy in elderly patients has not been performed. Older patients were excluded from the major randomized trials, including the Veterans' Administration Cooperative Trial, the Coronary Artery Surgical Studies, and the European Cooperative Trial. Nevertheless, coronary artery bypass grafting alone or combined with valvular surgery is carried out in an increasing number of elderly patients. In fact, elderly patients now make up a large proportion of patients undergoing coronary revascularization in the United States. In general, elderly patients have similar benefits, with symptomatic improvement after revascularization, as younger groups. However, operative mortality rates are higher and have been reported at 9–30% in octogenarians. Most studies have shown an improvement in functional status and satisfaction with the quality of life in elderly survivors of bypass surgery.

Elderly patients, in general, have a higher preoperative risk factor profile. Many more patients have class III or IV symptoms and decreased left ventricular ejection fraction. Surgical morbidity occurs in approximately 30% of elderly patients undergoing bypass surgery. Atrial fibrillation is more common than in younger patients and leads to a longer length of stay. Deep sternal wound infections are more common. Other significant concerns are postoperative delirium, mental confusion, and stroke. Studies have shown small changes in neuropsychologial parameters in some patients after bypass surgery. One study failed to show any long-term association between coronary artery bypass surgery and cognitive dysfunction in elderly patients. In general, however, while the percentage of surgery done on older patients has increased, operative mortality has decreased. Evidence suggests that older women have similar results from coronary artery bypass grafting as older men. However, women may have a higher incidence of recurrent angina.

In the highest-risk groups—patients with severely decreased ejection fraction, previous coronary artery bypass grafting surgery, or severe chronic obstructive pulmonary disease—medical therapy may be the only reasonable option.

9. Are catheter-based interventions such as percutaneous transluminal coronary angioplasty (PTCA) useful alternatives to surgery in older patients?

Coronary angioplasty has been used successfully in elderly patients for relief of symptoms and improvement in functional status. However, PTCA in elderly patients has a lower initial success rate and higher rates of morbidity, mortality, and clinical restenosis compared with younger patients. Older data from the 1980s demonstrated a higher mortality rate in patients over 65 after PTCA. More recent studies with coronary artery stenting continue to demonstrate significantly higher rates of procedural complications. The rates of MI (2%), emergency coronary artery bypass grafting (3.7%), and death (2.2%) are significantly higher than in the younger age group. Restenosis is also more common in older patients.

However, elderly patients have more advanced disease and more angiographically complex lesions than their younger counterparts, which increase the difficulty of angioplasty and stent procedures. Angioplasty directed against the culprit lesion (i.e., the active lesion responsible for an acute presentation) may obviate the need for surgery in patients with multivessel coronary disease. Enhanced interventional technique, coronary artery stents, intracoronary ultrasound, and new anticoagulation agents and strategies are likely to improve the results of interventional procedures in the future for all age groups.

BIBLIOGRAPHY

 1. Bayer AJ, Chadha JS, Farag RR, Pahy MS: Changing presentations of myocardial infarction with increasing old age. J Am Geriatr Soc 34:263–266, 1986.
 2. Cane ME: CABG in octogenarians: Early and late events and actuarial survival in comparison with a matched population. Ann Thorac Surg 60:1033–1037, 1995.
 3. Craver JM, Puskas JD, Weintraub WW, et al: 601 octogenarians undergoing cardiac surgery: Outcome and comparison with younger age groups. Ann Thorac Surg 67:1104–1110, 1999.
 4. De Gregorio J, Kobayashi Y, Albiero R, et al: Coronary artery stenting in the elderly: Short-term outcome and long-term angiographic and clinical follow-up. J Am Coll Cardiol 32:577–583, 1998.
 5. Goldberg RJ, Gore JM, Gurwitz JH, et al: The impact of age on the incidence and prognosis of initial acute myocardial infarction: The Worcester Heart Attack Study. Am Heart J 117:543–548, 1989.
 6. Herd JA, Wood AJ, Blumenthal J, et al: Medical therapy in the elderly. J Am Coll Cardiol 10:29A–34A, 1987.
 7. Ivanov J, Weisel RD, David TE, et al: Fifteen-year trends in risk severity and operative mortality in elderly patients undergoing coronary artery bypass graft surgery. Circulation 97:673–680, 1998.
 8. Jeffrey DL, Vijayanagar RR, Bognolo DA, Eckstein PF: Results of coronary bypass surgery in elderly women. Ann Thorac Surg 42:550–553, 1986.
 9. Lloyd-Jones DM, Larson MG, Beiser A, Levy D: Lifetime risk of developing coronary heart disease. Lancet 353:89–92, 1999.
10. Petrovitch H, White L, Masaki KH, et al: Influence of myocardial infarction, coronary artery bypass surgery, and stroke on cognitive impairment in late life. Am J Cardiol 81:1017–1021, 1998.
11. Shirani J, Yousefi J, Roberts WC: Major cardiac findings at necropsy in 366 American octogenarians. Am J Cardiol 75:151–156, 1995.

38. HEART FAILURE

Iris Reyes, M.D., and Jerry Johnson, M.D.

1. Why is heart failure considered an especially relevant medical condition in the elderly?
More than 2 million Americans have heart failure, with approximately 400,000 new cases developing each year. The total treatment costs for heart failure, including drugs, physician costs, and nursing home stays, are estimated to consume > $17 billion in health care expenditures yearly. Heart failure shortens life expectancy, resulting in 5-year mortality rates of 50%. The incidence of heart failure rises markedly above age 65, and its prevalence approaches 10% in people over age 80. As the elderly population encompasses a higher percentage of the general population, the importance of proper management with reductions in morbidity and mortality increases.

2. What causes heart failure?
- Coronary artery disease is the most common cause of heart failure, accounting for 50–75% of patients with heart failure.
- Hypertension is the second most frequent cause of heart failure. In women and elderly African-Americans, it holds particular significance because of relative undertreatment.
- Cardiomyopathy is the third most common cause of heart failure. The various causes of cardiomyopathy include high alcohol intake, viruses, asymmetric hypertrophic cardiomyopathy, and idiopathic disease.
- Valvular heart disease causes heart failure less commonly. The two most common forms of valvular heart disease in the elderly are mitral regurgitation (usually secondary to left ventricular dilatation but may be due to degenerative or rheumatic disease) and aortic stenosis (most commonly due to degenerative disease).

3. What are the major pathophysiologic abnormalities leading to heart failure?
Although multiple diseases can lead to heart failure, the pathophysiologic abnormalities fall in two categories: (1) left-ventricular (LV) systolic dysfunction with an ejection fraction < 35–40%, in which cardiac contractility is reduced, and (2) LV diastolic dysfunction, in which LV filling is impaired because of stiffness or abnormal relaxation. The prevalence in the community of heart failure due to diastolic dysfunction is unknown, but data from clinical studies suggest 20–40%. In elderly patients, this figure may be higher because of increased LV stiffness due to age and the increased prevalence of hypertension. Of interest, the most common causes of heart failure—ischemia and hypertension—may result in systolic or diastolic dysfunction. Knowledge of the pathophysiologic mechanism is necessary to plan an effective and safe management strategy.

4. What symptoms suggest heart failure?
Symptoms do not reliably distinguish heart failure due to systolic function from heart failure due to diastolic dysfunction. Patients who complain of dyspnea at rest or on exertion, paroxysmal nocturnal dyspnea, or orthopnea should be evaluated for heart failure unless the history and physical examination point to a noncardiac cause. Dyspnea on exertion is probably the most sensitive symptom among patients with heart failure. Decreased exercise tolerance, due to dyspnea or generalized weakness, may be a nonspecific symptom of heart failure. The interpretation of leg edema may be complicated. If found with symptoms such as dyspnea, leg edema may indicate heart failure, but in isolation it is caused more often by venous insufficiency. In demented elderly patients, nonspecific symptoms such as worsening cognitive function, fatigue, and decreased food intake may be due to heart failure.

5. Can physical findings suggest the diagnosis of heart failure?
In patients with suspicious symptoms, an elevated jugular venous pressure, hepatojugular reflux, laterally displaced apical pulse, and a third heart sound may indicate heart failure. The presence of rales with this complex of signs and symptoms indicates heart failure. Some patients with mild-to-moderate LV systolic or diastolic dysfunction, however, have none of these signs. In such patients, the physician must rely on diagnostic studies. The finding of wheezing, especially in a patient with no prior history of lung disease, should alert the physician to the possible presence of heart failure.

6. What diagnostic studies should be performed once heart failure is suspected?
The diagnostic studies chosen should provide information about the possible precipitating, complicating, or primary causes of heart failure. However, no test should be ordered unless the result will influence a management decision. Even a seemingly benign test can tax a frail elder.
Chest radiograph. In symptomatic patients, cardiomegaly is highly suggestive of heart failure, especially when accompanied by evidence of pulmonary vascular congestion. Although a normal chest radiograph makes the diagnosis of heart failure unlikely, it does not rule it out.
Electrocardiogram (EKG). Although there is no specific EKG finding for heart failure, the tracing may reveal possible precipitating factors, such as acute ischemia, prior myocardial infarction, arrhythmias, LV hypertrophy, and conduction abnormalities.
Oxygen saturation. Measurement of oxygen saturation by a pulse oximeter or arterial blood gas helps to determine the severity of heart failure.
Complete blood count (CBC). Anemia may aggravate underlying heart failure by decreasing oxygen-carrying capacity. Anemia may trigger signs and symptoms of heart failure, even in patients with no underlying cardiac abnormalities.
Serum electrolytes may be helpful in drug selection.
Creatinine. An elevated serum creatinine may indicate renal insufficiency, requiring adjustments of drug selection or dosage.
Albumin. Hypoalbuminemia may lead to increased extravascular fluid.
Urinalysis. The finding of proteinuria or hematuria may indicate renal causes as precipitants of heart failure.
Thyroxine/thyroid-stimulating hormone. Thyroid studies should be obtained in all elderly patients with heart failure with or without atrial fibrillation. Hyper- or hypothyroidism may present with heart failure as its initial manifestation in patients over age 65.

7. List the general criteria for admitting a geriatric patient with heart failure.
Patients in whom heart failure is present or suspected should be admitted if any of the following is present:
• Evidence of acute myocardial ischemia
• Pulmonary edema or severe respiratory distress
• Oxygen saturation < 90%
• Other severe complicating medical illness, such as syncope, hypotension, or anasarca
• Heart failure unresponsive to outpatient therapy
• Inadequate outpatient social support to manage the condition safely
Some patients with these findings may be managed as outpatients if adequate monitoring and follow-up care can be arranged. Home visits by physicians, nurse practitioners, or registered nurses have demonstrated effectiveness in outpatient management of heart failure.

8. Do echocardiography and radionuclide imaging have roles in the evaluation of patients with heart failure?
Because clinical symptoms and signs do not reliably distinguish heart failure due to systolic versus diastolic dysfunction, it is essential to measure LV function in patients with suspected

heart failure. Noninvasive studies, such as radionuclide scanning or echocardiography, can distinguish reliably between systolic and diastolic dysfunction—a necessary step in planning therapy. Echocardiography also has the ability to determine the presence of vascular and pericardial disease. The distinction between diastolic and systolic dysfunction is particularly relevant in the elderly population. All cardiovascular medications may carry significant risks and should be used only in patients with objective evidence of heart failure.

9. **When should diuretics be started in older patients with heart failure?**
   Diuretics are useful in patients with heart failure and evidence of volume overload, whether due to systolic or diastolic dysfunction. Patients with heart failure and signs and symptoms of volume overload, such as peripheral edema and pulmonary congestion, should be started on diuretics immediately. Patients with evidence of mild heart failure can be managed with thiazide diuretics. Patients with findings indicating moderate or severe heart failure require loop diuretics. Thiazides are ineffective when the creatinine clearance is less than 30 cc/min (serum creatinine: 1.8–2.0). The dosage is severity- and patient-dependent. It is important, however, to consider starting elderly patients on low dosages (e.g., 25 mg of hydrochlorothiazide or 20–40 mg of furosemide) and titrating upward as needed. The timing of diuretic administration is also relevant, especially in patients with urinary urgency or incontinence. Patients managed with diuretics need to be monitored for possible volume depletion, hypokalemia, hyponatremia, hypomagnesemia, and azotemia.

10. **What is the role of the angiotensin-converting enzyme (ACE) inhibitors in the management of heart failure?**
    ACE inhibitors should be started in all patients with heart failure due to LV systolic dysfunction unless a specific contraindication exists. Several studies provide strong evidence that ACE inhibitors reduce mortality in patients with LV ejection fraction below 35–40% and symptoms of mild-to-advanced heart failure. Prolonged survival also has been documented in asymptomatic patients with low ejection fractions due to coronary artery disease. ACE inhibitors have been shown to improve cardiac hemodynamics and functional status. Contraindications include:
    • Serum potassium > 5.5 mEq/L
    • History of adverse drug reaction
    • Symptomatic hypotension
    ACE inhibitors should be used with caution in patients with serum creatinine > 3.0 mg/dl or creatinine clearance < 30 ml/min.
    Although the largest randomized clinical trials have used captopril or enalapril, the reduction in mortality in patients with heart failure due to systolic dysfunction is probably a class effect. In using any of these drugs in the elderly, the physician should start with a low dose equivalent to 2.5–5 mg of enalapril or 12.5 mg of captopril while monitoring the patient's blood pressure and electrolytes. If the initial dose is tolerated, titrate upward to the equivalent of 20 mg of enalapril per day.

11. **What are the side effects of ACE inhibitors?**
    Hypotension is a possible side effect of ACE inhibitors, especially when starting or titrating the dose upward. Therefore, patients should be euvolemic, not hypovolemic, when therapy with an ACE inhibitor is initiated. Increases in serum creatinine and potassium also have been noted in some patients. ACE inhibitors should be used with caution in patients with renal insufficiency. However, chronic renal insufficiency is not an absolute contraindication. Potassium supplements and potassium-sparing diuretics should be discontinued before starting ACE inhibitors. Cough is a common complaint. Because cough is also a symptom of heart failure, such patients should be evaluated for possible pulmonary vascular congestion. Angioedema has been reported in some patients; involvement of the oropharynx is an absolute contraindication to continuing ACE inhibitors.

12. When are direct vasodilators indicated in the management of heart failure?

Vasodilators such as isosorbide dinitrate and hydralazine are appropriate alternatives for afterload reduction in patients who are intolerant of ACE inhibitors. In one trial this combination was shown to decrease mortality from 19% to 12% at 1 year and from 47% to 36% at 3 years compared with placebo. Side effects, including palpitations, headache, and nasal congestion, are somewhat more likely with these agents. Anti-ischemic agents also are indicated when transient episodes of ischemia are suspected.

13. What is the role of digoxin in the management of heart failure?

Although digoxin is used routinely in patients with heart failure, atrial fibrillation, and a rapid ventricular response, its use remains controversial in patients with sinus rhythm. Evidence suggests that digoxin improves functional status and can prevent clinical deterioration in some patients with LV systolic dysfunction, but it does not prolong survival. These findings indicate that it is beneficial to start digoxin in patients with severe heart failure due to LV systolic dysfunction who remain symptomatic despite treatment with ACE inhibitors and diuretics.

In initiating treatment with digoxin, lower dosages should be used in elderly patients, patients with renal insufficiency, and patients with baseline conduction abnormalities. Patients should be aware of signs of toxicity, including confusion, nausea, visual disturbances, and anorexia. The clinician should be aware that digoxin levels may be raised by medications such as quinidine, verapamil, amiodarone, antibiotics, and anticholinergic agents. Therefore, digoxin levels should be checked approximately 1 week after starting any of these medications. Digoxin's narrow therapeutic window means that it must be used with care in older patients. More frequent monitoring than in younger patients is warranted.

14. How should diastolic dysfunction be treated?

The survival of older patients with heart failure due to diastolic dysfunction, although not as poor as with systolic dysfunction, is still reduced with an annual mortality rate of 8–22%. However, randomized clinical trials to determine the efficacy of alternative pharmacologic approaches in treating patients with diastolic dysfunction have not been conducted. Beta blockers and calcium channel blockers are recommended to treat diastolic heart failure. Pharmacologic therapy should have the following goals:

- Decreasing central blood volume with diuretics
- Controlling heart rate with calcium channel blockers or beta blockers, because tachycardia further decreases ventricular filling
- Enhancing the rate of relaxation with calcium channel blockers
- Decreasing left ventricular wall thickness with antihypertensive agents such as calcium channel blockers

ACE inhibitors theoretically should benefit patients with diastolic dysfunction.

15. What is the role of angiotensin receptor blockers, beta blockers, calcium channel blockers, and anticoagulants in treating heart failure in older adults?

An angiotensin type II inhibitor should be prescribed for patients with heart failure due to systolic dysfunction who are unable to tolerate ACE inhibitors because of cough, rash, or altered taste sensation. At 48-week follow-up in the Evaluation of Losartan in the Elderly (ELITE) Study, the angiotensin receptor antagonist losartan, in doses of 50 mg/day, was found to be superior to captopril in doses of 50 mg 3 times/day in reducing total mortality. Hospitalization rates for congestive heart failure were similar for both drugs. Longer comparisons with losartan and studies using other angiotensin receptor blockers are necessary to determine whether the preliminary findings of the ELITE study are justified and whether the benefits of losartan can be considered a class effect.

Growing evidence indicates that modulation of the sympathetic nervous system by beta receptor blockade can favorably affect patients with heart failure. Therefore, stable patients with systolic heart failure should be started on a beta blocker. Theoretical evidence suggests that counteracting cardiac beta-receptor stimulation may be beneficial in advanced heart failure. Indeed, the Metoprolol in Dilated Cardiomyopathy (MDC) trial found that the administration of metoprolol to symptomatic patients with a low LV ejection fraction slowed clinical deterioration and improved symptoms and cardiac function. Similar benefits plus an improvement in survival have been found with carvedilol, a new beta blocker that also has alpha blocker activity and antioxidant effects. Carvedilol is recommended in patients with class II and III heart failure who are taking ACE inhibitors, diuretics, and digoxin. Because of side effects (hypotension, dizziness, and worsening heart failure) carvedilol must be used by practitioners experienced in its use and limitations. Beta blockers should not be initiated during acute heart failure in the absence of an arrhythmia or unstable angina.

The negative inotropic effects of calcium channel blockers and their undesirable activation of the renin-angiotensin and sympathetic nervous systems remain a major concern in patients with heart failure. In several studies, the degree of clinical deterioration was greater in patients treated with nifedipine or diltiazem than in patients receiving placebo or isosorbide dinitrate. However, a deleterious effect has not been observed in other reports of diltiazem or in reports of amlodipine in the elderly.

In the absence of atrial fibrillation anticoagulant use in heart failure is controversial. Most experts recommend anticoagulants for patients with a left ventricular aneurysm or cardiac thrombus.

16. What are the important nonpharmacologic issues in management?
Diet and lifestyle are crucial aspects of the management of heart failure. In addition to avoidance of smoking and limitation of salt intake to about 2 gm/day of sodium, exercise is beneficial. Exercise training does not improve cardiac function, but it may increase peak cardiac output, leading to a reduction is symptoms such as dyspnea and fatigue. As part of the overall management, home-based interventions involving nurses and other health professionals have decreased the rate of unplanned readmissions and improved mortality rates. In nursing homes one should not adopt a nihilistic nontreatment approach to heart failure. Even if the goal is not prolongation of survival, the treatment of the elderly nursing home resident can improve quality of life by reducing hospitalizations and improving functional status.

17. How should patients be monitored and educated to prevent hospitalizations?
Readmission to the hospital for heart failure is common. It has been reported that patients with heart failure over age 70 have a readmission rate as high as 57% within 90 days of discharge. Factors associated with readmission include inadequate follow-up, poor social situations, noncompliance with a low-salt diet, and noncompliance with medication. These issues must be addressed as soon as heart failure is diagnosed, whether on an inpatient or outpatient basis. Patients should be taught the symptoms of worsening heart failure, particularly dyspnea on exertion and weight gain, and advised to notify the physician if these symptoms arise.

The physician should arrange for follow-up contact by phone or in person within 1 week of instituting new medications or after discharge from the hospital. During this contact, the proper use of medication and compliance with diet should be addressed. Because weight gain is a crucial objective sign of fluid overload, patients should be instructed to weigh themselves almost daily and to report a weight gain of 3–5 lb. Laboratory studies, including electrolytes, blood urea nitrogen, and creatinine, should be checked during this visit, and medications should be adjusted as needed. Repeat imaging studies of the heart offer little value in monitoring the progress of heart failure once its pathophysiology has been characterized.

BIBLIOGRAPHY

1. American College of Cardiology/American Heart Association Task Force Report: Guidelines for the evaluation and management of heart failure. J Am Coll Cardiol 26:1376, 1995.
2. Aronow W: The ELITE Study: What are its implications for the drug treatment of heart failure? Drugs Aging 12:423–428, 1998.
3. Digitalis Investigation Group: The effect of digoxin on mortality and morbidity in patients with heart failure. N Engl J Med 336:525–533, 1997.
4. Frishman W: Carvedilol. N Engl J Med 339:1759–1765, 1998.
5. O'Neill CJ, Bowes SG, Sullens CM, et al: Evaluation of the safety of enalapril in the treatment of heart failure in the very old. Eur J Clin Pharmacol 35:143–150, 1988.
6. SOLVD Investigators: Effect of enalapril on survival in patients with reduced left ventricular ejection fractions and congestive heart failure. N Engl J Med 325:293–302, 1991.
7. Stewart S, Vandenbroek AJ, Pearsons S, Horowitz J: Prolonged beneficial effects of a home-based intervention on unplanned readmissions and mortality among patients with congestive heart failure. Arch Intern Med 159:257–261, 1999.
8. Tresch DD, McGough MF: Heart failure with normal systolic function: A common disorder in older people. J Am Geriatr Soc 43:1035–1042, 1995.
9. Wang R, Mouliswar M, Denman S, Kleban M: Mortality of the institutionalized old and old hospitalized with congestive heart failure. Arch Intern Med 158:2464–2468, 1998.
10. Wong WF, Gold S, Fukuyama O, et al: Diastolic dysfunction in elderly patients with congestive heart failure. Am J Cardiol 63:1526–1528, 1989.

39. THYROID DISORDERS IN THE ELDERLY

Mary Ann Forciea, M.D.

1. Why is the thyroid gland important to aging?

The spectrum of thyroid dysfunction in the elderly is broad. Illnesses due to thyroid dysfunction are common enough to be seen regularly in any primary care practice with significant numbers of elderly patients. Alterations in thyroid hormone have even been proposed as the cause of aging itself.

2. What does the thyroid gland do?

The thyroid gland secretes thyroid hormone and parathyroid hormone. Parathyroid hormone is important in calcium regulation. The primary role of thyroid hormone is the regulation of metabolism. In humans, the thyroid gland incorporates dietary iodide molecules into the storage compound, thyroglobulin. When affected by the pituitary hormone thyroid-stimulating hormone (TSH), glandular epithelium releases L-thyroxine (T4), which contains four iodide molecules, and modest amounts of triiodothyronine (T3), which contains three iodides. T4 usually circulates bound to serum proteins and is converted in peripheral tissues to T3. T3 is the active form of the hormone at the cellular level in most tissues. Pituitary TSH production and release are triggered by hypothalamic thyrotropin-releasing hormone (TRH).

3. Is thyroid function different in older patients?

Healthy aging produces very little change in thyroid hormone homeostasis. No clinically significant alterations in circulating levels of T4, T3, or TSH are seen. Circulating levels of T4 are preserved despite alterations in both thyroidal production and peripheral degradation of T4. Pituitary response to exogenous TRH administration is also preserved. Age-related alterations in the ability of the thyroid to concentrate dietary iodine (as measured by the radioactive iodine uptake) does decrease with age; one study has shown that the absolute iodine uptake in 80–90-year-olds is 60% of that seen in subjects aged 20–39 years. End-organ responsiveness to T4 also varies in reports: in humans, the basal metabolic rate (BMR) is unchanged, but in animals, liver enzyme induction decreases.

4. How is thyroid function evaluated in older patients?

The evaluation of thyroid function is safe, reliable, and relatively inexpensive. Serum levels of circulating T4 and TSH are widely available. T4 is usually measured as **total T4**, i.e., T4 bound to serum proteins and the small amount of T4 circulating free. Because T4-binding proteins can fluctuate in various situations (e.g., exogenous estrogen use), most laboratories also report a measurement of binding protein availability, the **T3 resin uptake** (T3RU). This measurement has nothing to do with the patient's T3; the T3 in the name refers to *exogenous* radioactive T3 (*T3) added in the laboratory to the patient's serum. A known amount of resin that will adsorb the "leftover" *T3 is also added. If large numbers of binding protein sites are unoccupied in the patient sample (as in hypothyroidism), most of the *T3 will stick to the protein and little will be available on the resin—thus, the T3RU will be low. In hyperthyroidism, binding sites will be full of the patient's T4, little *T3 will stick to the patient's proteins, and large amounts of *T3 will adhere to the resin—thus, the T3RU will be high. In patients on estrogen, total T4 will be high because of increased binding proteins; many sites will be available so that the resin contains little *T3, and the T3RU is low. The T3RU is reported as the percentage of added *T that appears in the resin, usually 35–45%. In many laboratories, the T3RU result is normalized to the value seen in control serum in that assay. The T3RU is then reported as a number (0.85–1.15, with the control sera as 1).

Correcting the total T4 by the T3RU generates an estimate of active hormone. This product is often called the **free thyroxine** index (FTI). Actual measurements of **free T4** and **total T3** can be obtained and are useful in special situations. **Thyroid autoantibodies** can be measured in most clinical laboratories. **Iodine uptake** is measured in the nuclear medicine laboratory; images generated are used as the thyroid scan.

5. What types of hypothyroidism are usually seen in the elderly?

Hypothyroidism is seen frequently in older patients. The prevalence of overt hypothyroidism is approximately 5%, with more women affected than men. Subclinical hypothyroidism (also called the "failing gland" syndrome) may precede overt hypothyroidism and can be seen in up to 15% of patients in some series. These patients are clinically euthyroid and serum T4 levels are normal, but TSH levels are elevated.

A group of patients at special risk for late hypothyroidism are those with laryngeal cancer who undergo extensive neck surgery and radiation or those who have undergone prior thyroid surgery and neglected follow-up. Myxedema coma is a severe form of hypothyroidism with altered consciousness and is an emergency.

Autoimmune thyroiditis is the most common cause of hypothyroidism in the elderly, with prior thyroid surgery or ablation the next most common cause. Pituitary insufficiency can produce thyroid hypofunction, a state referred to as secondary hypothyroidism.

6. How is hypothyroidism recognized?

Patients with hypothyroidism are often unaware that anything is wrong. The onset of symptoms, such as lethargy, depression, confusion, dry skin, constipation, myalgia, and cold intolerance, are often mistaken by the patient and family as part of "old age." On physical exam, hypothyroid patients often appear pale and sallow (due to carotenoid pigments that can accumulate in the skin). The voice may sound low and hoarse. Classically, the outer third of the eyebrows is thinned or absent, but this finding is not specific for hypothyroidism in the elderly. The skin feels dry; the hair also is dry and brittle. The thyroid gland itself may be small. The examiner may occasionally find a surgical scar across the lower neck in a patient who underwent thyroid surgery and subsequently neglected follow-up or thyroid medication. Carpal tunnel syndrome may develop due to myxoid infiltration of the tendon sheath. The hallmark physical finding in hypothyroidism is a change in the patient's reflexes, with a relatively normal upstroke but a delay in the relaxation phase. This change is sometimes best appreciated by palpating the muscle belly while percussing the tendon.

Because of the occult nature of many of the signs and symptoms in older patients, hypothyroidism is often diagnosed with laboratory screening tests. All older patients should have a TSH determination as part of their health evaluation. Experts disagree as to the periodic need for repeat testing in a healthy older patient with a normal TSH, but most suggest a minimum of testing every 3 years. Patients with pituitary disease or in special situations should be screened with T4 and T3RU.

Hypothyroidism is associated with abnormalities in serum lipids. In a study of community-dwelling elderly women with elevated TSH levels, low-density lipoprotein (LDL-C) was 13% higher and high-density lipoprotein (HDL) was 12% lower. These lipoprotein levels may help to explain the increase in atherosclerotic cardiovascular disease seen in older hypothyroid patients.

7. Is the treatment of hypothyroidism different in the elderly?

Thyroid hormone replacement is simple and relatively inexpensive. Patients should understand that they are almost certain to require thyroid replacement for life. Older patients may require lower doses of exogenous T4 to achieve full replacement. Replacement therapy is done with T4 (L-thyroxine), which can be given once daily. Therapy should be begun gradually because of the cardiac stimulation that can be associated with T4.

In the elderly, therapy is often begun with L-thyroxine, 0.0125 mg daily. In 2 weeks, if no cardiac problems have developed, the dose can be increased to 0.025 mg daily. Thereafter, the dose can be increased by 0.025 mg every 3–4 weeks, to a total dose of 0.075 mg. Each patient's final replacement dose must be individually assessed. After 3 months at 0.075 mg of L-thyroxine, a TSH level is checked. If the TSH remains higher than normal, the dose can be increased by 0.025 mg, and the process repeated until the TSH level remains in the normal range. If the TSH is suppressed (below normal), the dose of L-thyroxine can be reduced by 0.025 mg and the process repeated.

Patients with pituitary insufficiency present special difficulties in treatment because the correction of thyroid homeostasis may precipitate adrenal insufficiency and adrenal crisis. An endocrinologist should guide treatment in such patients.

8. What is the failing gland syndrome?

Early in the development of hypothyroidism, patients will develop elevations in TSH levels as their production of T4 begins to fall. The laboratory pattern will be that of a modest elevation in TSH with still normal T4. In former years, these patients were followed with repeat blood tests at 4–6 month intervals, and when a progressive pattern of TSH elevation was seen, L-thyroxine replacement was begun. Recent studies have shown that the presence of antithyroid antibodies in serum assays closely predicts which patients will progress to hypothyroidism. These antibody-positive patients can begin replacement therapy immediately.

9. When do you suspect hyperthyroidism in an older patient?

In most adults and many elderly patients, hyperthyroidism causes symptoms and signs related to "adrenergic" excess: agitation, tremor, sweating, palpitations, prominent stare, and weight loss. Patients may report heat intolerance, hyperdefecation (multiple formed stools each day), and hair and skin changes, but these are rarely the presenting complaint.

Apathetic hyperthyroidism is an unusual presentation of thyroid overactivity seen almost exclusively in older patients. Such patients appear depressed instead of agitated and display few of the adrenergic symptoms of hyperthyroidism. They are most often discovered through diagnostic evaluations of weight loss, depression, or atrial fibrillation. Diagnostic strategy and therapy of the apathetic variant are identical to classical hyperthyroidism. Research into the physiologic basis of the apathetic variant has focused on possible alterations in the adrenergic receptor family during aging.

10. Describe the physical findings in a hyperthyroid patient.

Physical examination in patients with classic hyperthyroidism reveals a nervous, agitated patient. He or she is likely to be dressed in lightweight clothing and may display a fine tremor with a rapid frequency. The skin is soft and smooth and may be slightly sweaty. Examination of the eyes reveals a bulging appearance of the globes (proptosis), a low rate of blinking, and sometimes a rim of white sclera circling the iris (exophthalmos). Extraocular movement may be impaired, especially on lateral gaze, due to myxoid infiltration of the rectus muscles. While asking the patient to track an object from upward gaze to downward, the examiner may note a delay in the lid following the iris (lid lag).

The thyroid gland is usually enlarged; auscultation may reveal a bruit over the thyroid due to increased blood flow. Older patients may have developed fibrosis in the thyroid gland, which restricts enlargement; older patients may be hyperthyroid even with a small thyroid gland. The cardiac rhythm may be rapid but sinusal (sinus tachycardia) or may be rapid and irregular (atrial fibrillation). The fingertips may be red and painful (thyroid acropaxia); the nailbeds may separate from the fingers, leaving dystrophic finger and toenails. Examination of the shins may disclose large thickened areas due to myxoid infiltration of the muscles, lesions which are called pretibial myxedema. Bone mineral density is reduced.

The ocular involvement in hyperthyroidism due to Graves' disease may precede other organ involvement or may occur alone (euthyroid Graves' ophthalmopathy). Computed tomography (CT) scans of the orbit reveal the characteristic muscle infiltration.

11. Are the causes of hyperthyroidism different in older patients?

Graves' disease, which is produced by autoimmune stimulation of the thyroid gland by antibodies resembling TSH, is the most common cause of hyperthyroidism in the elderly.

Overproduction of thyroid hormones by isolated areas of thyroid glandular epithelium that has escaped control and has become autonomous is the next most common cause; it is seen much more commonly in the elderly than in young patients. This autonomous area may be confined to a **solitary nodule** or, more often, to one nodule in a **multinodular goiter**. When the overproduction reaches levels that produce hyperthyroidism, the state is called **toxic multinodular goiter**, or Plummer's disease.

12. What diagnostic tests are indicated in hyperthyroidism?

The clinical suspicion of hyperthyroidism is confirmed initially with serum assays of T4, T3RU, and TSH. The TSH level is low due to suppression of the pituitary by elevated levels of circulating T4. Rarely, elderly or iodine-deficient hyperthyroid patients may secrete more T3 than T4, revealing an elevated T3 with a normal T4 (T3 toxicosis). A total T3 level should be requested in these patients. In early hyperthyroidism, the only abnormality may be a reduced response of pituitary TSH secretion in response to exogenous TRH. The etiology of the hyperthyroidism can be sought with nuclear medicine studies of thyroidal uptake of I-123. In Graves' disease, which is caused by autoimmune stimulation of the thyroid gland by an antibody similar to TSH, uptake is high and diffuse. In thyroiditis, the gland itself is undergoing inflammatory destruction; uptake is low. In toxic multinodular goiter, uptake is high in the autonomous nodule but suppressed in the rest of the gland. A characteristic image will be seen on a thyroid scan. Factitious hyperthyroidism, due to intentional or accidental overdose of exogenous thyroid hormone, can be suspected when I-123 uptake is low and screens for thyroid autoantibodies are negative.

Laboratory Results in Commonly Encountered Clinical Thyroid Syndromes

	TOTAL T4	T3RU	TSH	SPECIAL STUDIES
Hypothyroidism	Low	Low	High	—
Hypopituitarism	Low	Low	Low	—
Hyperthyroidism	High	High	Low	I-123 uptake scan for etiology TRH suppression for diagnosis in borderline cases
T3 toxicosis	Normal	High-normal	Low	T3 level should be measured in old or iodine-deficient patients
Factitious hyperthyroidism	High	High	Low	I-123 uptake is low Thyroid autoantibodies negative
Exogenous estrogen	High	Low	Normal	—
Malnutrition	Low	High	Normal	—
Failing gland	Low-normal	Low-normal	Slightly high	—
Euthyroid sick	Low	Low	Normal	—

13. What are the options in the treatment of older hyperthyroid patients?

Therapy for hyperthyroidism is aimed at relief of symptoms and cure. Historically, thyroidal overactivity was treated with surgical removal of most of the thyroid gland (subtotal thyroidectomy), but suppressive therapy with medications and organ-specific radioisotopes has largely replaced surgery. Beta-blockers, such as propranolol (Inderal), are very effective in curtailing the adrenergic symptoms such as agitation and tremor and may reduce heart rate. Thyroidal production of T4 and T3 can be reduced by antithyroid medications such as propylthiouracil (PTU) and methimazole. These drugs must be taken daily and have a high rate of serious side effects, such as granulocytopenia.

Thyroid tissue can be ablated by oral doses of I-131, which has a longer half-life than I-123. After treatment with I-131, overall production of thyroid hormones is reduced. In the elderly,

I-131 is generally the safest treatment regimen: no long-term medications are required, the fall of T4 is gradual, and theoretical risks of late malignancies are less concerning. Some endocrinologists recommend 2–4 weeks of pretreatment with antithyroid drugs before I-131 to reduce the amount of preformed T4 released during thyroid destruction.

After any form of treatment, patients must be monitored at regular intervals for late hypothyroidism due to either the primary disease process or therapy.

14. Define thyroid storm.

Patients with hyperthyroidism who undergo physiologic stress, such as infection, illness, or surgery, may develop a complication known as thyroid storm. They exhibit high fever (even to 106°F) and severe cardic dysfunction. Treatment is an emergency and should be directed by an endocrinologist.

15. What is factitious hyperthyroidism?

Factitious hyperthyroidism is caused by overdoses of thyroid replacement medication, either intentional or accidental. Patients may misunderstand instructions or may intentionally overdose in the hopes of losing weight. Errors in prescription may occur by physicians or pharmacists. The risk of error is greatest with L-thyroxine at the low dose of 0.025 mg being mistaken for the suppressive dose of 0.250 mg. The doses of L-thyroxine are universally color-coded, and patients should be instructed to report any unexpected change in the color of their tablets. Thyroidal uptake of I-123 will be low in these patients.

16. What causes a goiter?

Goiters are enlarged thyroid glands caused by long-term overproduction of colloid within the gland. This overproduction is caused in most elderly patients by congenital partial defects in the enzymes involved in incorporation of iodide into colloid. T4 production is slightly reduced, TSH is slightly elevated, and the gland slowly enlarges. The enlargement can be stopped by providing exogenous T4 (L-thyroxine) in replacement doses large enough to suppress TSH production. Very large goiters can compress the trachea and may need partial surgical resection. In areas of the world where dietary iodide is unavailable (generally areas far from the sea), iodide deficiency is the most common cause of goiter. In the United States, dietary goiter is now mainly seen in recent immigrants.

17. What is toxic multinodular goiter?

Also known as Plummer's disease, toxic multinodular goiter is a hyperthyroid state produced when one nodule in a goiter becomes autonomous and is no longer subject to pituitary regulation. This condition is seen almost exclusively in the elderly. Patients appear hyperthyroid and have the classic thyroid I-123 scan. Therapy with I-131 is ideal: the active nodular tissue is destroyed, and the normal tissue that was suppressed escapes damage and returns to normal function. Patients with small amounts of autonomous tissue may rapidly develop hyperthyroidism when exposed to large amounts of exogenous iodide, as in radiographic contrast dye or iodinated drugs such as amiodarone.

18. How are "cold" thyroid nodules detected?

In palpating the thyroid gland, the examiner may note an asymmetry that on further exam is felt to be a nodule. In the elderly, this nodule often represents the most superfical nodule of a goiter, it may be an isolated colloid cyst, or it may represent a focus of thyroid cancer. In former years, the next diagnostic step would be a thyroid I-123 scan; nodules that concentrated the I-123 ("hot" nodules) were believed to be composed of functioning tissue and were likely benign. Nodules that failed to concentrate I-123 ("cold" nodules) could not be assessed. Surgery to remove cold nodules was usually recommended, but many specimens revealed normal tissue. In the last 15 years, the initial diagnostic step has become a fine-needle aspiration of the nodule. The cytopathologist can help differentiate benign nodules from malignant ones. Patients with benign nodules are often begun on thyroid replacement therapy to inhibit TSH-directed enlargement, and the nodules are monitored by sequential measurement in the office. An increase in size on replacement therapy is usually an indication for repeated aspiration.

19. Is thyroid cancer seen in older patients?

Primary cancer of the thyroid is uncommon but not rare. Cancers present most often as thyroid nodules. Unfortunately, since thyroid cancers cause so few symptoms, many cancers are not found until metastases have developed. The most common cancer diagnosed in nodules is well-differentiated and likely to be completely resected. Follicular carcinoma is less common but more aggressive. Anaplastic thyroid carcinoma is a very aggressive malignancy often diagnosed because of metastatic lesions before a primary nodule is appreciated.

20. What is the euthyroid sick syndrome?

Patients who are ill are often catabolic: they must breakdown their own protein stores to supply their metabolic needs. The body responds to this stress by suppressing TSH production and allowing T4 levels to fall slightly to spare further protein degradation. This physiologic state can be confirmed by documenting elevated levels of reverse T3, produced by an alternative pathway of T4 degradation. Studies have shown that replacement with exogenous T4 makes these patients sicker. Ill patients with low-normal T4 and T3RU levels and low TSH levels should not be started on L-thyroxine. Their thyroid function should be monitored as they recover.

BIBLIOGRAPHY

1. Bauer DC, Ettinger B, Browner WS: Thyroid function and serum lipids in older women: A population-based study. Am J Med 140:546–551, 1998.
2. Francis T, Wartofsky L: Common thyroid disorders in the elderly. Postgrad Med 92(3):225–233, 1992.
3. Griffin JE: Hypothyroidism in the elderly. Am J Med Sci 299:334–345, 1990.
4. Hansen JM, Skousted L, Siersboek-Nielson K: Age dependent changes in iodine metabolism and thyroid function. Acta Endocrinol 79:60–65, 1975.
5. Hershman JM, Pekary AE, Berg L, et al: Serum thyrotropin and thyroid hormone levels in elderly and middle aged euthyroid persons. J Am Geriatr Soc 41:823–828, 1993.
6. Isley WL: Thyroid dysfunction in the severely ill and elderly. Postgrad Med 94(3):111–128, 1993.
7. Mokshagundaom S, Barzel US: Thyroid disease in the elderly. J Am Geriatr Soc 41:1361–1369, 1993.
8. Rae P, Farrar J, Beckett G, Toft A: Assessment of thyroid status in elderly people. BMJ 307:177–180, 1993.

40. DIABETES MELLITUS

Paula McCrae-Patton, M.D., Cheng-An Mao, M.D., M.P.H., and Mary Ann Forciea, M.D.

1. What is diabetes mellitus?

Diabetes mellitus is a metabolic disorder in which energy obtained from food or carbohydrate stores in the body cannot be utilized by target organs and cells. The hallmark of diabetes is an elevated blood glucose level. If blood glucose levels are high enough, glucose also appears in the urine.

2. What are the criteria for diagnosing diabetes mellitus in older patients?

The National Diabetes Data Group's criteria for diagnosing diabetes are based on fasting plasma glucose levels, which are relatively unchanged by age. Studies have shown that fasting plasma glucose level increases by 1–2 mg/dl for each decade after the age of 50 years. Useful criteria for diagnosis (in the absence of infection or other physiologic stress) are as follows:

1. Fasting plasma glucose level > 126 mg/dl on > 1 occasion

                            or

2. Random plasma glucose levels > 200 mg/dl, accompanied by symptoms

In patients without symptoms, random plasma glucose levels > 200 mg/dl should be followed by determination of fasting plasma glucose levels. Interpretation of glycosylated hemoglobin (HbA1c) levels in the elderly may result in a high false-positive rate of diagnosis. HbA1c levels are elevated with aging and medical conditions such as chronic renal failure and hypoxia.

Impaired fasting glucose (fasting glucose level ≥ 110 mg/dl and < 126 mg/dl) and impaired glucose tolerance (blood glucose ≥ 140 mg/dl and < 200 mg/dl 2 hours after eating) have been associated with an increased risk of cardiovascular disease and subsequent development of diabetes mellitus. Patients who are obese, who have a family history of diabetes, or who have a personal history of gestational diabetes are also at risk of developing diabetes mellitus; random plasma glucose measurements should be part of periodic health examinations.

3. How prevalent is diabetes mellitus in the elderly?

The prevalence of diabetes mellitus is 7–10% in people over age 65 years and increases with age. The rate may be as high as 15% in nursing home populations. Possible factors contributing to the increased prevalence are (1) weight gain, (2) reduced physical activity, (3) postreceptor defects, and (4) impairment of insulin-mediated glucose uptake. In elderly African-American and Hispanic populations the prevalence exceeds 20%. This increased relative risk of diabetes remains throughout the life span of the patient.

4. How is diabetes mellitus classified?

Type 1 diabetes mellitus (also called insulin-dependent diabetes mellitus [IDDM] and juvenile-onset diabetes) is characterized by autoimmune destruction of pancreatic beta cells, which results in absolute insulin deficiency. The incidence of new-onset type 1 diabetes is very low in the elderly. Patients with type 1 diabetes often present with ketoacidosis.

Type 2 diabetes mellitus (also called non–insulin-dependent diabetes mellitus [NIDDM] or adult-onset diabetes mellitus) is characterized by impaired insulin secretion without autoimmune destruction of pancreatic beta cells. Peripheral tissue sensitivity to insulin is often impaired. Type 2 diabetes is not associated with absolute insulin deficiency, at least until the late stages.

5. How are the symptoms of diabetes different in elderly patients?

Elderly patients present with a continuum ranging from no symptoms to weight loss, weakness, confusion, and even coma. Elderly diabetics may present with urinary incontinence instead of polyuria. Weight loss may be a sign of osmotic diuresis, anorexia, and poor oral intake. Because elderly people have decreased thirst perception, they are less likely to present with polydipsia. They may present with orthostasis and unsteadiness or confusion secondary to volume depletion.

Various factors can affect glycemic control in patients with type 2 diabetes. Excessive calories at meals or snacks, infection, trauma, surgery, and emotional stress can promote hyperglycemia. Conversely, factors such as reduced dietary intake, malnutrition, malabsorption, alcohol, renal insufficiency, and hepatic failure can promote hypoglycemia.

6. What syndromes are associated with diabetes in the elderly?

1. Painful shoulder periathrosis: characterized by a moderate-to-severe decrease in range of motion with pain in the glenohumeral joint.

2. Diabetic amyotrophy: characterized by asymmetric weakness, pain, and wasting of the pelvic girdle and thigh muscles with minimal sensory changes. This neuropathic syndrome usually occurs in older men and resolves within 1 year.

3. Diabetic neuropathic cachexia: characterized by painful peripheral neuropathy, severe weight loss, and depression. Patients usually have a good recovery.

4. Diabetic dermopathy with intraepidermal bullae of the feet: usually seen in diabetics over the age of 70 years and usually resolves spontaneously.

7. What tests should be ordered in the initial evaluation of the elderly diabetic patient? What maintenance regimen is recommended for prevention and detection of diabetic complications?

Initial evaluation	Maintenance
Plasma glucose	Office visits at least quarterly
HbA1c	History and physical exam
Serum creatinine	HbA1c every 3 months
Urinalysis for proteinuria and microalbuminuria	Eye exam annually
Electrocardiogram	Podiatry exam annually
Lipid profile	Urine microalbumin analysis
Creatinine clearance	
Ophthalmology consultation	

8. What are the office treatment goals for patients with type 2 diabetes?

The American Diabetes Association recommends a fasting glucose level < 120 mg/dl, a 2-hour postprandial glucose level < 180 mg/dl, a bedtime glucose level of 100–140 mg/dl, and a glycosylated hemoglobin level < 7%. Therapy should be modified if hypoglycemia (glucose < 80 mg/dl) is seen or if HbA1c is > 8%. These recommendations are not age-specific and need to be modified for individual patients. Multiple comorbidities may limit therapy. Hypoglycemia is a serious condition in the elderly and must be avoided.

9. How are the treatment goals for diabetics in nursing homes different from those for diabetics in the community?

Nursing home residents tend to have special problems that complicate their care: confusion, poor appetite, recurrent infections, pressure ulcers, and dementia. These conditions may affect communication of personal needs to alert staff to signs of hypoglycemia. Levels of glycemic control may have to be adjusted modestly upward to avoid recurrent hypoglycemia. Regular determinations of blood glucose with finger-stick monitors are essential.

10. What are the treatment goals for hospitalized elderly diabetics?

Diabetes tends to be poorly controlled in hospitalized patients. Intensive therapy with subcutaneous insulin has significantly improved the short- and long-term survival rates in diabetic patients. If blood glucose exceeds 200 mg/dl, poor wound healing, leukocyte dysfunction, and osmotic diuresis may result. Thus, 120–200 mg/dl is an acceptable target range for glycemic control in hospitalized patients.

11. How is dietary control used in managing diabetes mellitus?

Dietary therapy has few side effects, but dietary habits are not easily changed, especially in older persons. A good diet for diabetics should be a balanced diet, with restricted saturated fat. The requirement of daily calories varies but should be around 30–35 kcal/kg of ideal body weight, depending on the patient's situation. Acutely ill patients may need higher daily calories. Obese patients can have caloric restrictions for weight reduction, but minerals and vitamin supplements may be required if daily caloric intake is restricted too low. The diet can contain 50–60% of the calories from carbohydrates. Because many older diabetic patients are not obese when they are diagnosed, caloric restriction may not be indicated. Malnutrition is a potential risk for older patients and should be carefully evaluated when prescribing a restricted calorie diet.

Clinicians often suggest that patients avoid simple sugars, though there is no evidence to demonstrate that sugar can cause more adverse effects than other carbohydrates. Fructose elevates plasma glucose only slightly, and thus patients should not avoid fruits or vegetables. Alternative sweeteners, such as saccharin and aspartame, can be used safely to increase flavor, if the daily consumed doses of alternative sweeteners are below the acceptable dose recommended by the FDA. Alcohol is relatively contraindicated in diabetic patients because alcohol can induce hypoglycemia, especially in patients treated with hypoglycemic agents.

Poor dietary compliance is the main reason for treatment failure. Allowing diverse options of food can encourage patients to adhere to the dietary program. Educating both patients and family members is important because some patients rely on families to prepare food for them.

12. Can older patients benefit from exercise?

Many studies demonstrate the benefits of exercise for older patients. Exercise improves obesity, glucose tolerance, lipid profiles, and physical abilities and may also reduce cardiovascular risk. Noncompetitive, low-impact, aerobic exercise is favored. Walking is a simple and inexpensive exercise. Swimming is non–weight-bearing and good for patients with arthritic disorders. Tai chi and stretching exercises are other good examples. Wearing appropriate shoes and socks, monitoring orthostatic hypotension, and warming-up before exercise can prevent unnecessary injuries (see also Chapter 16).

Diabetic patients should have a complete physical examination before starting exercise. For those beginning energetic exercise programs, an exercise stress test should disclose coronary artery disease. Patients should attempt to reach their targeted heart rate slowly because sudden cardiac death may occur during vigorous exercise. Patients with proliferative retinopathy need to avoid isometric exercise, such as lifting, that increases intraocular pressure and can cause further damage.

13. What treatment adjustments are warranted for exercising patients?

Exercise expends more glucose than ordinary activities and therefore can be associated with hypoglycemia if treatment adjustments are not made. In normal persons, hypoglycemia is avoided by production of glucose through hepatic glycogenolysis and gluconeogenesis. In patients treated with insulin, the high insulin concentration suppresses hepatic glucose production and causes hypoglycemia. Oral hypoglycemic agents may also increase the chance of hypoglycemia during exercise. Several strategies can be used to prevent this hypoglycemia:

• Eat 15–30 gm carbohydrates before exercise.
• Reduce the regular dosage of hypoglycemic agents before exercise.
• Avoid drinking alcohol.

• Keep insulin injection sites away from exercising muscles.
• Never skip meals.
• Take medications after morning exercise.

14. How are drugs used in the treatment of diabetes mellitus?

If diet and exercise fail to control hyperglycemia, **oral hypoglycemic agents** are often the next therapy because they are painless and easy to use. **Sulfonylureas** have been the most commonly prescribed oral hypoglycemic agents. Their mechanism of action is related to enhanced insulin secretion and tissue sensitivity. **Glyburide** and **glipizide** often are chosen as initial agents. Starting doses should be low; patients must be monitored for the development of hypoglycemia. **Repaglinide** is a short-acting agent given before each meal.

Metformin, a biguanide, is believed to act through inhibition of hepatic glucose production; it also may interfere with intestinal glucose absorption. Metformin is associated with less hypoglycemia and less weight gain. A crucial side effect, however, is that biguanides are associated with lactic acidosis. Lactic acidosis following x-ray studies with iodinated contrast dye has been reported in patients taking metformin. Metformin must be discontinued 48 hours before contrast x-ray studies. Metformin almost always should be discontinued in acutely ill, hospitalized diabetics.

Acarbose is an alpha-glucosidase inhibitor that acts in the small intestine to inhibit enzymes involved in carbohydrate metabolism and thus delays carbohydrate absorption. This action may result in a decrease in postprandial hyperglycemia. Almost 80% of patients taking acarbose experience flatulence, bloating, and diarrhea due to bacterial metabolism of undigested carbohydrate. The flatulence often subsides with time.

Troglitazone is a thiazolidine agent that decreases insulin resistance in target tissues. Serious sequelae of troglitazone use are reported with increasing frequency, including hepatic dysfunction with liver failure. Liver functions tests must be checked at baseline, monthly for the first 8 months, then every 2 months for the first year. If liver function remains normal, testing may be done every 3 months during chronic use.

15. How is insulin therapy initiated if the patient no longer has adequate glycemic control with oral diabetic agents?

A moderately long-acting insulin such as neutral protamine Hagedorn (NPH) is often used to initiate therapy; 0.1 or 0.2 U/kg ideal body weight can be given once or twice daily. After insulin requirements have been established, some patients prefer a premixed form of insulins (70% long-acting, 30% short-acting), which can be given as a once-daily dose. Patients using insulin must be able to test blood glucose at home to facilitate management. They also must eat on a predictable schedule. In patients receiving tube feeding at home or in the nursing home, dosing intervals should be adjusted to tube feeding schedules.

16. Discuss the vascular complications of diabetes mellitus.

Diabetic patients have a 2–3-fold higher risk of myocardial infarction and stroke than nondiabetic persons. In type 2 diabetes, 60% of mortality is from vascular diseases. Hyperglycemia, hyperinsulinemia, and hyperlipidemia are all associated with vascular disease and are commonly seen in older diabetics. In addition, diabetic patients are prone to hypertension, which is also a risk factor for coronary artery diseases.

When choosing medications for hypertension control in diabetic patients, angiotensin-converting enzyme (ACE) inhibitors are preferred because they decrease the rate of proteinuria and preserve renal function. Hydrochlorothiazide and furosemide may induce hyperglycemia and may worsen glycemic control. Beta-blockers should be used carefully, as they may mask tachycardia induced by hypoglycemia.

Peripheral vascular disease can be caused by both macro- and microvascular angiopathy. When peripheral vascular disease combines with neuropathy, there is a high rate of diabetic foot ulcers.

17. Which ophthalmologic complications occur in diabetes?

Vision impairment is a common problem in patients with type 2 diabetes. One-third of the blindness in these patients is due to diabetic retinopathy. Diabetic patients are also prone to cataract formation and macular edema.

The prevalence of retinopathy tends to increase with the duration of disease. Studies have demonstrated that intensive glycemic control can reduce the incidence of retinopathy in patients with type 1 diabetes; the same correlation has been shown in patients with type 2 diabetes.

Intensive treatment always brings the worry of possible hypoglycemia in older patients. Early detection and laser photocoagulation therapy seem to be the best strategies to manage diabetic retinopathy. Annual eye examinations by ophthalmologists are recommended.

18. Describe the diabetic complications affecting the nervous system.

Nerve damage in diabetes mellitus may be due to either ischemic changes or exposure of the neurons to high glucose concentration or abnormal glucose metabolites (e.g., sorbitol and fructose). The prevalence of **polyneuropathy** in patients with type 2 diabetes increases with the disease duration. Studies have shown that intensive glycemic control decreases the incidence of neuropathy in patients with type 1 diabetes, but no well-controlled trials prove this decrease in patients with type 2 diabetes. Peripheral polyneuropathy usually presents with numbness and paresthesia. Tricyclic antidepressant drugs, phenytoin, carbamazepine, and topical capsaicin have been used to treat painful peripheral neuropathy.

Autonomic neuropathy has multiple presentations and is difficult to treat. Postural hypotension can result in falls; nausea and vomiting can be from gastroparesis; urinary tract infections may be secondary to urinary retention caused by dysfunction of bladder contractions. Other complaints, such as constipation, diarrhea, and impotence, are not uncommon. Treatment is mainly for symptom relief. Gastroparesis is treated with optimal glycemic control and medications such as cisapride or metoclopramide. Tetracycline may be helpful in diabetic diarrhea. Increased salt intake, elastic stockings, position modification, and mineralocorticoids have been used in treating postural hypotension.

Diabetic **amyotrophy** is an unusual syndrome of atrophy and weakness of pelvic girdle and upper leg muscles accompanied by anorexia and depression. The muscular problem is asymmetric and associated with severe pain. The syndrome usually resolves spontaneously within 1 year.

Cognitive impairment is noted more frequently in diabetic patients than nondiabetic patients. This impairment can be due to ischemic strokes, recurrent hypoglycemic episodes, and osmolarity changes. Mental status evaluation and follow-up are necessary.

19. What are the renal complications of diabetes mellitus?

About 10–20% of patients with type 2 diabetes develop end-stage renal failure. The classic form of diabetic renal disease is characterized by basement membrane thickening and abundant glomerular mesangial material, although end-stage diabetic renal disease may have other contributing pathology (such as hypertensive renal damage). The appearance of microalbuminuria (urinary albumin of 30–300 mg/24 hr) is a strong predictor of nephropathy and may be present in many elderly diabetics at the time of presentation. All diabetic patients should have yearly screens for microalbuminuria.

Both optimal glucose control and administration of ACE inhibitors have been shown to slow the progression of diabetic nephropathy. Because they slow the decline in glomerular filtration rate by decreasing intraglomerular pressure, ACE inhibitors are recommended for all diabetic patients, even those with normal blood pressure. Any other conditions that affect renal function (such as hypertension and hyperlipidemia) should be treated aggressively.

End-stage renal failure in elderly diabetics usually is treated with dialysis (hemodialysis or chronic peritoneal dialysis), although diabetic patients on dialysis do not survive as long as nondiabetic patients. Renal transplantation in elderly diabetics is offered rarely.

BIBLIOGRAPHY

1. Bailey CJ: Biguanides and NIDDM. Diabetes Care 15:755–772, 1992.
2. Betts EF, Betts JJ, Betts CJ: Pharmacologic management of hyperglycemia in diabetes mellitus: Implications for physical therapy. Phys Ther 75:415–425, 1995.
3. Clark M, Lee DA: Prevention and treatment of the complications of diabetes mellitus. N Engl J Med 332:1210–1227, 1995.
4. Diabetes mellitus in elderly people. Diabetes Care 13(Suppl 2):1990.
5. Franz MJ, Horton ES Sr, Bantle JP, et al: Nutrition principles for the management of diabetes and related complications. Diabetes Care 17:490–518, 1994.
6. Hazzard WR, Blass JP, Ettinger WH, et al (eds): Principles of Geriatric Medicine and Gerontology, 4th ed. New York, McGraw-Hill, 1999.
7. Holbrook JH (ed): Endocrinology and metabolism. Med Self Knowl Assess Progr 11:881–882, 1998.
8. Lilley SH, Levine GI: Management of hospitalized patients with type 2 diaetes mellitus. Am Fam Physician 57:1079–1088, 1998.
9. Morley JE: An overview of diabetes mellitus in older persons. Clin Geriatr Med 15:211–224, 1999.
10. Reikel W: Care of the Elderly: Clinical Aspects of Aging, 4th ed, Baltimore, Williams & Wilkins, 1995.
11. Samos LF, Roos BA: Diabetes mellitus in older persons. Med Clin North Am 82:791–803, 1998.
12. Turner R: UK Prospective Diabetes Study. A review. Diabetes Care Suppl 3:C35–C38, 1998.
13. Turner R, Cull C, Frighi V, Holman R: Glycemic control with diet, sulfonylurea, metformin, or insulin in patients with type 2 diabetes mellitus. JAMA 281:2005–2012, 1999.
14. UK Prospective Diabetes Study Group (UKPDS): Intensive blood-glucose control with sulphonylureas or insulin compared with conventional treatment and risk of complications in patients with type 2 diabetes (UK PDS 33). Lancet 352:837–853, 1998.
15. UK Prospective Diabetes Study Group (UKPDS): Tight blood pressure control and risk of macrovascular and microvascular complications in type 2 diabetes: UKPDS 38. BMJ 317:703–713, 1998.

41. RHEUMATOLOGIC CONDITIONS IN THE ELDERLY

Edna P. Schwab, M.D.

1. What are the characteristic features of polymyalgia rheumatica?

Polymyalgia rheumatica is a common cause of musculoskeletal pain in older individuals. The etiology is unknown. In a survey of Olmsted County, Minnesota, conducted by the Mayo Clinic, its prevalence was found to be 700/100,000 persons over age 50. Most patients are at least 50 years old. Female sex predominates by a ratio of 2.5:1.

Bilateral aching and stiffness of the shoulder girdle and upper arms, neck and torso, hip girdle, and thigh muscles in association with constitutional symptoms and an elevated Westergren erythrocyte sedimentation rate (ESR) characterize polymyalgia rheumatica. These symptoms are most common in the morning and frequently are associated with malaise, weight loss, and low-grade fever. Physical examination is remarkable for tenderness and limitation of motion of the shoulders and hips. Weakness, however, is not evident. Synovitis has been demonstrated by arthroscopy and biopsy of shoulder joints. The diagnosis of polymyalgia rheumatica is made when symptoms of pain and morning stiffness are present for at least one month and other diagnostic possibilities have been excluded.

The onset of polymyalgia rheumatica may be gradual but more often is sudden. This condition rarely responds to nonsteroidal anti-inflammatory drugs and often requires the initiation of corticosteroids. Low doses of prednisone (10 mg/day) usually result in an excellent therapeutic response. Polymyalgia rheumatica is a self-limited disease but also may have a more prolonged course. In patients whose ESR is normal, the diagnosis is made if characteristic symptoms are present and the response to prednisone is rapid and complete. Sometimes, it may be difficult to distinguish between the diagnosis of polymyalgia rheumatica and rheumatoid arthritis because of the similarities in presentation and lack of positive serologies in older patients. A high index of suspicion should be maintained for a closely associated disease, temporal arteritis, which occurs in 15–20% of patients with polymyalgia rheumatica.

2. Which laboratory findings are characteristic of polymyalgia rheumatica?

The ESR is often elevated to > 40 mm/hr and commonly to > 100 mm/hr. Evidence of an anemia due to chronic disease along with mildly elevated liver function abnormalities is usually present. Radiographs of the joints may demonstrate soft-tissue inflammation without evidence of erosions.

3. Define giant cell arteritis and describe its features.

Giant cell arteritis is a large-vessel vasculitis that often affects the vessels of the aortic arch. It has a reported prevalence of 200/100,000 people over age 50, as surveyed by the Mayo Clinic in Olmsted County, Minnesota. Superficial vessels, such as the occipital and external carotid and its branches, including the temporal, lingual, and facial arteries, may be involved. Deeper vessels also may be affected, including the vertebral artery and internal carotid along with its branches. Vessels lacking elastic tissue, such as the intracranial arteries, are spared. Most often, however, the branches of the aorta, occipital, or temporal artery become inflamed, with patients developing symptoms associated with the involved vessels.

Common symptoms consist of occipital or temporal headaches in 90% of patients, along with jaw claudication and tenderness over the temporal artery. Diplopia may occur as a result of ischemia to the extraocular muscles. The most dreaded complication is irreversible visual loss, which occurs in 15% of patients, most commonly due to ischemic optic neuritis with involvement of the ciliary branches of the internal carotid. Stroke is a rare complication of giant cell arteritis. As in polymyalgia rheumatica, these symptoms are often accompanied by constitutional symptoms of fever, malaise, anorexia, and weight loss. These nonspecific symptoms often prompt an evaluation for an occult malignancy. Polymyalgia rheumatica may be present in up to 50% of cases of giant cell arteritis.

4. Which laboratory and histologic features are diagnostic for giant cell arteritis?

In a patient who has characteristic findings of giant cell arteritis, laboratory evaluation usually demonstrates an elevated ESR usually > 100 mm/hr. Anemia and mildly elevated liver function tests also may be present.

The diagnosis is made by a temporal artery biopsy demonstrating destruction of the internal elastic lamina associated with granulomatous inflammation. Histologic examination reveals areas of inflammation of the media and fragmentation of the elastic lamina of the artery. This pattern of involvement follows those vessels that contain internal elastic lamina. Granulomas contain lymphocytes, histiocytes, and giant cells. Inflammatory edema or thrombus may occlude the vessel, leading to ischemic symptoms typically seen in this disorder. It is important to remember that the entire vessel is generally not involved. Skip lesions, areas of inflammation interspersed with normal-appearing vessel, may be found on a temporal artery biopsy. Biopsies should include at least 1 inch of vessel.

5. How is giant cell arteritis treated?

When the diagnosis of giant cell arteritis is considered, temporal artery biopsy should be obtained. Treatment should be started promptly with high-dose corticosteroids, at least 40–60 mg/day of prednisone, and continued after the diagnosis is confirmed. Symptoms as well as ESR should determine the tapering schedule. Clinicians also should start appropriate therapies, such as calcium and vitamin D, to lessen the toxicity of corticosteroids. To date, steroid-sparing agents such as methotrexate have not been shown to be useful in lowering the dose of steroids.

6. What are the characteristic features of elderly-onset rheumatoid arthritis?

Rheumatoid arthritis (RA) is a chronic inflammatory disease involving the synovium that may be accompanied by systemic manifestations of fever, malaise, fatigue, and weight loss. The etiology of the disease is unknown. Typically, it affects patients during the third to fifth decades of life with a prevalence rate of 0.3–3%. Women are affected more often than men with a ratio of 2:1 to 3:1. The prevalence of RA increases with age. The proportion of affected men also rises with age. Patients with long-standing RA often have more severe disease with extraarticular manifestations, joint deformities, and comorbidities.

Patients who develop RA after age 60 generally have been perceived to have milder arthritis, lack rheumatoid nodules, and are rheumatoid factor-positive in only 32–58%, unlike disease seen in younger patients. Patients with RA gradually develop symmetric pain, swelling, and stiffness in peripheral joints, sparing the distal interphalangeal joints. Occasionally, RA presents acutely. In hemiplegic patients, the paralyzed side is not affected by the disease. In the elderly patient, large joints, such as shoulders, are more frequently affected and may be mistaken for polymyalgia rheumatica. In general, the features of polymyalgia rheumatica and remitting seronegative symmetric synovitis with pitting edema and rheumatoid arthritis overlap. Often an immediate response to low-dose steroids help to distinguish polymyalgia rheumatica from other disorders. Studies evaluating the prognosis of elderly-onset RA have been contradictory. Most early studies describe a rapid decline, whereas more recent reports describe a more benign course. Other diagnostic considerations in the elderly patient who develops an acute symmetric polyarticular synovitis include pseudogout, polyarticular gout (especially in women on diuretics), systemic lupus erythematosus, and paraneoplastic disease.

7. How often does systemic lupus erythematosus occur in older adults?

Systemic lupus erythematosus (SLE) may present in 15–20% of elderly patients with women being more frequently affected. Unlike the female-to-male ratio of 5–8:1 that is found in the younger population, the ratio is 2:1 in the elderly. The disease in the elderly also is milder, with manifestations of serositis, joint pain, interstitial lung disease, and sicca symptoms being more common. Central nervous system (CNS) involvement and renal disease are less frequent. Laboratory tests may include a positive antinuclear antibody (ANA), low complement levels, and positive antibodies to ds-DNA, SS-A, SS-B or Sm. Healthy older adults may have a low-titer positive ANA present in their serum without evidence of any systemic disease.

Drug-induced SLE occurs more commonly in the elderly and should alert the physician to detect the causative agent. Inciting drugs include procainamide, hydralazine, and isoniazid. Anti-histone antibodies, in addition to a positive ANA, are found in 70–95% of patients. Symptoms resemble those seen in older-onset SLE.

8. What are the features of primary Sjögren's syndrome?

Primary Sjögren's syndrome is a frequent diagnosis in elderly patients who present with sicca symptoms. Patients often complain of grittiness in their eyes and dryness of their mouth associated with odynophagia. Polyarthritis, arthralgias, myalgias, fever, and fatigue may be accompanying symptoms. Systemic manifestations of vasculitis, interstitial nephritis, Raynaud's phenomenon, interstitial lung disease, hypothyroidism, and central and peripheral nervous system involvement occur infrequently.

9. What is rheumatism?

Many elderly patients complain of having "rheumatism" when they describe generalized musculoskeletal pain. Rheumatism refers to painful, nondeforming, nonsystemic musculoskeletal conditions that arise from soft tissue, bursa, ligaments, and tendons rather than bone or joints. Rheumatism may be localized to a bursa or tendon or to a region such as the neck or back or may be generalized as in fibromyalgia syndrome.

10. Which conditions are associated with nonarticular or soft-tissue rheumatism?

Soft-tissue rheumatism is another entity frequently reported in the elderly. It refers to conditions such as fibromyalgia, bursitis, tendinitis, low back pain, and cervical spine pain syndromes. It is important to realize that low back pain may be due simply to back strain but also may have more serious causes, including compression fractures secondary to osteoporosis or primary or secondary malignancies such as multiple myeloma and metastatic cancer. Other common soft-tissue conditions in the elderly include rotator cuff tendinitis, which may result in severe shoulder pain that radiates to the elbow and impairs range of motion of the shoulder. Elderly men and women may develop adhesive capsulitis that results following a period of inactivity of the shoulder. The presentation is that of progressive stiffness and discomfort of the shoulder with limitation of motion. Pain often occurs with movement.

11. Describe the fibromyalgia syndrome.

Fibromyalgia syndrome (FMS) is a noninflammatory musculoskeletal disorder manifested by chronic widespread pain and dysregulation of neuroendocrine function and sleep. Associated symptoms include stiffness, fatigue, memory and concentration difficulties, subjective hand puffiness, dizziness, headaches, Raynaud's phenomenon, paresthesias, sicca symptoms, irritable bowel and bladder syndrome, and disrupted sleep. Criteria for diagnosis of FMS have been established by the American College of Rheumatology and include widespread pain present for at least three months and pain on digital palpation in 11 of 18 tender point sites. Laboratory and radiographic studies frequently are unremarkable. FMS has not been well studied in the elderly, although recent estimates have demonstrated a rising prevalence rate among the elderly. Wolfe demonstrated rates of 2% among 30- to 39-year-olds, 5.6% among 50- to 59-year-olds, and 7.4% among 70-year-olds. Fibromyalgia was found to be 6 times more prevalent among women over the age of 50 years than men. The increased frequency seen in the elderly may be due to the rising presence of other musculoskeletal pain disorders contributing to persistent nociceptive input and sustained hyperalgesia. Fibromyalgia may coexist with other rheumatologic disorders including osteoarthritis, rheumatoid arthritis, systemic lupus erythematosus, Sjögren's syndrome, and psoriatic arthritis. It also has been described in patients with chronic fatigue syndrome, hypothyroidism, and conditions associated with the administration or withdrawal of steroids.

12. How does reflex sympathetic dystrophy syndrome present?

Reflex sympathetic dystrophy occurs commonly in the elderly with diabetes or following trauma, cerebrovascular events, or peripheral nerve pathology. It presents with severe burning pain and swelling of an extremity, hand, or foot. Signs of vasomotor instability are often present, manifested by temperature changes, edema, sweating, and trophic changes of hair, skin, and nails. As the disorder progresses, skin and muscle atrophy occurs with the development of contractures and restricted motion. During the later stages of the disorder, radiographs of the extremity often reveal diffuse osteoporosis.

13. What are the common rheumatic manifestations of endocrinopathies and malignancies?

Endocrinopathies such as hypothyroidism may be associated with joint and muscle pain and stiffness. Weakness is not a prominent feature. Hyperthyroidism can present as a painless proximal myopathy or, infrequently, with soft-tissue swelling, clubbing, and periostitis called thyroid acropathy. Acromegaly frequently produces degenerative changes of cartilage. Carpal tunnel syndrome may be a manifestation of diabetes, hypothyroidism, and acromegaly. Diabetes also has been associated with diffuse idiopathic skeletal hyperostosis, Charcot joints, and limited joint mobility. Pseudogout has been associated with hypothyroidism and hyperparathyroidism.

Primary **malignancies** and metastatic tumors may present with polyarticular joint pain, and these diagnoses should be considered in patients with an abrupt onset of a rheumatologic condition. Lymphomas and leukemias may present in the elderly with synovitis that resembles rheumatoid arthritis or polymyalgia rheumatica. Hypertrophic osteoarthropathy may be seen with pulmonary malignancies and other cancers. Neoplasms have been associated with the development of polymyositis and dermatomyositis. In one series, 25% of cases were associated with neoplasia of the breast, lung, ovary, colon, stomach, and uterus.

14. What are the features of remitting seronegative symmetric synovitis with pitting edema?

This disorder primarily occurs in older men, with a male-to-female ratio of 2:1. It presents as an acute symmetric polyarthritis involving the wrists, flexor digitorum tendon sheaths, metacarpophalangeal joints, tarsal and metatarsophalangeal joints, and interphalangeal joints. Associated pitting edema of the hands, soft tissue swelling of the distal upper and lower limbs, and morning stiffness are present.

Constitutional symptoms are often absent. This disease may be closely related to seronegative rheumatoid arthritis. Synovial fluid is mildly inflammatory, and the ESR is often elevated. The disease occurs more often in autumn but can occur throughout the year. The overall prognosis is good, and response to treatment with low-dose prednisone is often immediate.

BIBLIOGRAPHY

1. Evans JM, Hunder GG: Polymyalgia rheumatica and giant cell arteritis. Clin Geriatr Med 14:455–473, 1998.
2. Lawrence RC, Helmick CE, Arnett FC, et al: Estimates of the prevalence of arthritis and selected musculoskeletal disorders in the United States. Arthritis Rheum 41:778–799, 1998.
3. McCarty DJ: Perspective syndrome of remitting seronegative symmetric synovitis with pitting edema. J Clin Rheumatol 1:203–204, 1995.
4. McGuire JL: The endocrine system and connective tissue disorders. Bull Rheum Dis 39(4):1–8, 1990.
5. Michet CJ, Evans JM, Fleming KC, et al: Common rheumatologic disease in elderly patients. Mayo Clin Proc 70:1205–1214, 1995.
6. Salvarani C, Gabriel S, O'Fallon WM, Hunder GG: Epidemiology of polymyalgia rheumatica in Olmsted County, Minnesota, 1970–1991. Arthritis Rheum 3:369–373, 1995.
7. Van Schaardenburg D: Rheumatoid arthritis in the elderly. Prevalence and optimal management. Drugs Aging 7:30–37, 1995.
8. Van Schaardenburg D, Breedveld F: Elderly-onset rheumatoid arthritis. Semin Arthritis Rheum 23:367–368, 1994.
9. Wolfe F, Ross K, Anderson J, et al: The prevalence and characteristics of fibromyalgia in the general population. Arthritis Rheum 38:19–28, 1995.

42. ARTHRITIS AND MUSCULOSKELETAL PAIN IN THE ELDERLY

Edna P. Schwab, M.D.

1. What changes occur in the aging joint and how are they related to the development of osteoarthritis?

Aging is a risk factor for the development of osteoarthritis. There are distinctions in the pathogenesis of the aging joint and the joint affected by osteoarthritis. Cartilage matrix is composed of predominantly type II collagen, proteoglycans consisting of a protein core, and side chains of the glycosaminoglycans chondroitin sulfate and keratan sulfate. Sixty percent of this tissue is composed of water. With aging one sees decreased strength and stiffness of this organized network. Tissue damage may occur secondary to the inability of cartilage to accommodate increased mechanical loading and result in increased fibrillations, erosions, and permeability to fluids. The increased water content within cartilage may predispose the joint to development of osteoarthritis. Aging also is associated with chondrocyte senescence, a state in which chondrocytes can no longer replicate. Although these cells remain metabolically active and respond to cytokines such as IL-1, as senescent cells accumulate their rate of synthesis and degradation appears to be reduced even among growth factors and cytokines. Currently, it is not clear if these changes predispose to osteoarthritis. Less is known about the aging changes found in subchondral bone and its association with osteoarthritis.

Periarticular muscles are the major shock absorbers protecting the joint. When a load occurs unexpectedly, damage can occur to the articular cartilage and subchondral bone rather than the load being absorbed by the muscle. Joint trauma has been linked to the development of osteoarthritis in this manner. As muscle mass and strength diminish with age, the joint may be predisposed to increased loads and joint injury. Quadriceps strengthening in the elderly may retard the rate of muscle loss, diminish pain, and improve gait and knee strength as well as decrease joint trauma.

In the joint affected by osteoarthritis, the dominant feature is cartilage loss. The water content of cartilage is increased, and inflammatory mediators, either derived from chondrocytes or synovial fluid, decrease proteoglycan composition and synthesis while degrading proteoglycans and collagens.

2. How prevalent are arthritic conditions in the elderly?

Arthritis and musculoskeletal disorders are two of the most prevalent chronic conditions among the elderly and are important public health problems among adults of working age. As the population ages, the prevalence of arthritis, with its negative impact on function, is expected to rise. In a study by Hughes, the most frequent musculoskeletal conditions diagnosed among a sample of elderly persons over age 60 were osteoarthritis (83%), old fractures (32%), and soft-tissue rheumatism (13%). Joint impairment was most frequently observed in the upper and lower spine (92%), hands (58%), feet (55%), knees (35%), and hips (20%). Joint impairment, pain, and psychological status all had an effect on predicting future disability.

3. What is the impact of pain?

Pain and limitation in motion from arthritis can restrict the independence of older persons by impairing their performance of activities of daily living (ADLs). Upper extremity impairment is more pronounced in men and significantly related to inability in performing ADLs, whereas lower extremity impairment is more common in women and is significantly related to impairment in instrumental ADLs. Both upper and lower extremity impairments occur in increased frequency in both sexes over the age of 80.

The National Health Interview Survey revealed that elderly persons in the community with arthritis represent 70% of the population with 1 or more limitations in physical activity and represent one-third of those persons with 5 or more ADL impairments. Data from the Longitudinal Study on Aging indicate that the extent of arthritis-related disabilities increases with time. These impairments were found to be strong risk factors for predicting adverse outcome. Elderly people with 1 or more ADL impairments were 2.5 times more likely to die and 5 times more likely to end up in a nursing home when compared to those without any limitations. In the nursing home, pain as a result of musculoskeletal disorders is extremely common, often limiting the patient's ability to function.

Prevention by the identification of risk factors preceding the development of musculoskeletal disorders, early diagnosis, and implementation of appropriate treatment will help to prevent or retard disability associated with arthritis and enhance an older person's quality of life. Symptoms in the elderly, however, may not be as apparent as in younger persons due to multiple coexisting conditions and cognitive impairment. A decline in function may not be perceived by a patient, family member, or staff members until impairment or disability is significant.

4. What are the causes of musculoskeletal symptoms in the elderly?

Symptoms of joint pain, limitation of motion, swelling, and morning stiffness are features of various arthritides. A thorough history with a review of systems and physical examination will help to differentiate the various rheumatic conditions in the elderly, such as those with articular or soft-tissue involvement (i.e., osteoarthritis, crystal arthropathies, periarthritis, tendinitis, bursitis, and entrapment neuropathies) from conditions that also have systemic manifestations. These conditions include infectious arthritides, polymyalgia rheumatica, giant cell arteritis, elderly-onset rheumatoid arthritis, and other connective tissue disorders. Appropriate radiographs and laboratory tests including synovial fluid analysis help to establish an early and accurate diagnosis.

5. Which is the most common form of chronic arthritis?

By far, the most common and disabling rheumatic condition in patients over 55 years of age is **osteoarthritis**. Radiographic changes often precede symptoms and frequently may not correlate well with symptoms until marked progression and cartilage loss occur. Approximately 65% of elderly patients have symptoms of joint pain, stiffness, and limitation in range of motion (ROM). Studies have demonstrated that 12% of elderly patients cannot perform ADLs as a result of pain and limitation from osteoarthritis. About half of these individuals end up confined to the bed or wheelchair. Predictors of disability include the severity of other coexisting diseases, visual or hearing impairment, functional capacity, social support, education level, income, and availability of social and home-care services. Anxiety, depression, and coping mechanisms also influence the development and severity of disability.

6. Describe the common symptoms and findings characteristic of osteoarthritis.

Joints that are commonly involved in osteoarthritis include areas of weight-bearing, such as the lumbar spine, hips, and knees. Hands (especially the first carpometacarpal joint), cervical spine, and feet (primarily the first metatarsophalangeal joints) are also commonly involved. Early morning stiffness, when present, characteristically lasts 10–30 minutes. Stiffness may occur following periods of inactivity, whereas pain often increases with activity and improves with rest. Patients may complain of buckling or instability as well as loss of motion. Musculoskeletal examination may reveal swelling, deformities, bony overgrowth (referred to as Heberden's and Bouchard's nodes when involving the distal and proximal interphalangeal joints of the hands, respectively), crepitus, limitation of motion, and synovial effusions. Muscle spasm, tendon contractures, and capsular contractures also may be observed depending on the site of involvement.

Cervical and lumbar pain may result from arthritis of the apophyseal joints, osteophyte formation, pressure on surrounding tissue, and muscle spasm. Radicular symptoms are caused by nerve root impingement. Cervical and lumbar stenosis develops when facet joints and the ligamentum flavum hypertrophy as a result of disc degeneration, which narrows the spinal canal causing compression of the cord. Anterior vertebral osteophytes also may contribute to cord compression. Patients may develop localized pain, extremity weakness, gait ataxia, or abnormal neurologic findings. Pseudoclaudication is a characteristic feature of lumbar stenosis and is described as pain in the buttocks or thighs occurring with ambulation and relieved by rest or lumbar flexion. Hip pain is usually felt in the groin or the lateral or medial aspects of the thigh; however, it can be referred to the knee or buttocks and may be misdiagnosed as lumbar stenosis.

Pain from osteoarthritis may develop from any part of the involved joint or tissue. Ischemia and interosseous pressure from subchondral bone, inflammation of the synovium, distention of the joint capsule, inflamed ligaments and bursae, cartilage destruction, and nerve terminal release of enzymes and inflammatory mediators, as well as increased volume of synovial fluid and muscle spasm, all contribute to pain. Sleep disruption as a result of pain may exacerbate the pain cycle, contributing to further disability and depression.

7. What are the laboratory and radiographic findings in osteoarthritis?

Laboratory findings in osteoarthritis are usually normal. Radiographs classically reveal the presence of joint-space narrowing with subchondral sclerosis as an early finding. As arthritis progresses, the development of marginal osteophytes, subchondral bone cysts with sclerosis, and subluxation occurs. In advanced disease, loose bodies and subchondral bone collapse may be evident. Synovial fluid analysis reveals noninflammatory fluid (< 500 cells/ml).

8. What risk factors are associated with the development of osteoarthritis?

• Age (although not everyone develops pain and immobility)
• Genetic predisposition
• Female sex and menopausal status
• Obesity
• Ethnic/racial background
• Prior trauma
• Occupational knee bending/physical labor
• Abnormal biomechanics and physical loading (soccer players and weight lifters)
• Increased bone mineral density
• Quadriceps weakness (also implicated in the pathogenesis of the disease)
• Congenital abnormalities (Perthes' disease and congenital dislocation of the hip)
• Inflammatory conditions (crystal arthropathies, septic arthritis)
• Chondrocalcinosis
• Metabolic disorders (acromegaly and hemachromatosis)

9. How is osteoarthritis best managed?

Realistic goals need to be established with the patient. Pain often leads to deconditioning, loss of ROM and disability. The physician should educate the patient about arthritis prevention, exercise, joint protection, knee bracing, and incorporation of rest periods in order to alleviate pain and delay disease progression. Preventive techniques include identification of risk factors such as obesity and behavioral modification for weight loss, diminishing injury during exercise, and altering job demands in those who experience repetitive trauma and joint injury. The patient should be made aware of the various treatment options available for the management of osteoarthritis. The suggested course of management might include a combination of the following:

Nonpharmacologic Therapies

Exercise and Rehabilitation: Resting the joint for prolonged periods, especially in the elderly, may result in deconditioning, muscle atrophy, contractures, and osteoporosis. A supervised exercise program with a physical therapist and occupational therapist will help to strengthen weakened muscles and improve range of motion. An evaluation for appropriate assistive devices and appliances should be performed. Aerobic exercise, resistive exercise, and aquatic therapy have been demonstrated to improve function and disability in addition to decreasing pain. The application of **heat or cold packs** following exercise is often helpful. Acute inflammation responds to the application of cold, whereas chronic pain improves with heat. **Acupuncture** has been used for treatment, especially in Asian countries; however, controlled trials have not demonstrated significant improvement. **Transcutaneous electrical nerve stimulation, low-power laser therapy**, and **pulsed electric and electromagnetic fields** have not been extensively studied.

Psychological counseling: Relaxation techniques and biofeedback may be effective in diminishing the degree of pain in some affected patients. The older patient may require psychological counseling, especially if depression is evident. Persistent pain, disability, deformity, decline in function, and limited independence can often lead to depression. This depression can be exacerbated if the patient has sexual difficulties and/or is unable to work as a result of arthritis. The patient should receive psychiatric, sexual, or financial counseling if any of these situations arise.

Pharmacologic Therapy

Initiation of drug therapy should take into account the side effect profile of the drug, comorbidities of the patient, and potential drug interactions.

Analgesics

Acetaminophen is an effective analgesic agent used to treat osteoarthritis. It has fewer side effects than nonsteroidal anti-inflammatory drugs (NSAIDs) when used in therapeutic doses (4.0 gm/day) and is as effective as NSAIDs in many patients. Use in patients with liver disease or alcohol-induced cirrhosis should be monitored closely, and renal function should be assessed in chronic users of analgesics.

Opioids such as codeine, hydrocodone, and oxycodone may be used when conservative therapies are ineffective or when contraindications exist to the use of traditional NSAIDs. These are frequently used when there is bony collapse, as in avascular necrosis, or in situations involving nerve impingement.

Tramadol, a centrally acting analgesic, has also been found to be useful in controlling symptoms.

The practitioner using these agents should monitor for common adverse effects including delirium, dizziness, somnolence, and constipation, especially when used in patients who also take other centrally acting agents (i.e., antidepressants).

Analgesic/Anti-inflammatory Agents

NSAIDs are the most commonly prescribed agents to treat arthritis, but the elderly are at increased risk of adverse effects from these drugs, including acute renal failure, gastric ulceration and bleeding, cardiovascular effects, hepatotoxicity, and cognitive impairment. Patients using NSAIDs should be monitored closely for evidence of adverse reactions. Risk factors identified for the development of gastrointestinal complications include increasing age, history of peptic ulcer disease, concomitant corticosteroid or anticoagulant use, cigarette smoking or alcohol use, and ingestion of multiple NSAIDs. H_2 blockers or misoprostol, a prostaglandin E2 inhibitor, should also be prescribed in patients at high risk for gastrointestinal complications.

Cyclooxygenase-2 inhibitors (COX-2) may provide protection from gastrointestinal side effects, but further trials need to be conducted in order to assess their safety in the elderly.

Antidepressants have been found to control chronic pain with some success when used in low doses. The blockage of serotonin reuptake augments the inhibitory pathways of the spinal tract, thereby inhibiting pain perception.

Intraarticular corticosteroid injections may be used to alleviate the pain from arthritis. These agents should not be used more than 3–4 times a year because of possible deleterious effects on cartilage. **Viscosupplementation with hyaluronic acid** derivatives also have been shown to provide superior relief when compared to intraarticular corticosteroids and NSAIDs.

Topical analgesic creams such as methylsalicylate or capsaicin, an inhibitor of the release of substance P from nerve terminals, have been helpful in alleviating joint pain. Side effects frequently encountered include burning at the site of application.

Alternative remedies have become increasingly popular among patients as a result of limited pain relief with the traditional agents available. **Glucosamine sulfate** and **chondroitin sulfate** have demonstrated improved symptom relief but not structure modification in European trials. The mechanism of action for glucosamine is not yet known. Both are available in health food stores. Compared to ibuprofen, however, the effects of glucosamine were not statistically different. The role of antioxidants such as **vitamin C**, **vitamin E**, and **beta carotene** in preventing disease progression require further investigation.

Investigational agents used to modify disease have yet to be established. These agents include enzyme inhibitors, growth factors, and cytokine inhibitors. Osteochondral grafts of chondrocytes and/or stem cells are in various stages of development.

Patients who have not benefited from conservative measures may benefit from invasive therapies, such as arthroscopy with joint debridement or lavage. The efficacy of lavage may result from the removal of debris and inflammatory mediators. Arthroplasty should be reserved for patients who continue to have persistent pain, loss of motion, and loss of function despite maximal medical management. The complication rate of this procedure is 2.5–3.5 times higher in the elderly than in younger patients. Thirty percent of older patients who are cognitively impaired experience a prolonged course of rehabilitation.

10. Which rheumatologic conditions can present with an acute monarthritis in the elderly?

When a joint becomes acutely inflamed and painful, it requires an immediate evaluation. Several arthritides can present with a single acutely swollen and painful joint:

Infectious arthritis	Neurogenic arthropathy (Charcot's joint)
Bacteria	Avascular necrosis
Mycobacteria	Tumor
Fungi	Systemic disease with monarticular flare
Spirochetes	(much less common)
Viruses	Rheumatoid arthritis
Crystal-induced arthritis	Systemic lupus erythematosus
Gout	Psoriatic arthritis
Pseudogout	AIDS
Hydroxyapatite disease	Inflammatory bowel disease
(Milwaukee shoulder)	Behçet's disease
Osteoarthritis	Reiter's syndrome
Foreign-body reaction	Reactive arthritis

11. What are the complications and mortality rate associated with septic arthritis?

Septic arthritis is the most life-threatening and destructive form of arthritis in all age groups. Joint destruction can occur in 1–2 days if the infection is unrecognized or inadequately treated. Approximately 25–40% of patients diagnosed with a septic arthritis are over age 60. Among the elderly, the mortality rate has been reported to be between 19 and 33%, as compared to 10% in the general adult population. Complications such as osteomyelitis, loss of joint motion and function, and osteoarthritis arise in the elderly. Three factors predicting poor outcome include old age, preexisting joint disease, and infected prosthetic joints.

12. Describe the clinical and diagnostic features of septic arthritis.

Physical findings include fever, joint swelling secondary to fluid distending the joint capsule, warmth, loss of motion, and severe pain. Constitutional symptoms may or may not be present. An investigation for an extraarticular site of infection should always be pursued.

Diagnosis is made by arthrocentesis of the involved joint. The presence of organisms on synovial fluid Gram stain or culture and evidence of an inflammatory synovial fluid help to confirm the diagnosis. Synovial fluid cell counts are often > 50,000 cells/mm^3 with > 80–90% neutrophils on the differential. Low white cell counts have also been reported, in the range of 6,000 cells/mm^3, but this is less frequent. Stains will be positive for organisms in approximately 75% of gram-positive infections and 50% of gram-negative infections. Other diagnostic tests include blood cultures, which may be positive in 25–78% of patients with nongonococcal bacterial arthritis but frequently negative in gonococcal arthritis. Appropriate imaging techniques, such as radiographs or MRI, should be obtained to evaluate for joint destruction and osteomyelitis. Antibiotic treatment should be started to cover organisms usually involved in septic arthritis. Treatment can be altered once culture results are available.

13. Which organisms are most commonly found in a septic arthritis?

Gram-positive aerobes cause infection in approximately 85% of cases; *Staphylococcus aureus* accounts for 67%, *Streptococcus pneumoniae* for 3%, and non-group A, β-hemolytic streptococci for 15%. *Staphylococcus epidermidis* is frequently found in prosthetic joint infections. Gram-negative bacteria account for 18% of infections but also have been reported to occur in up to 30% of geriatric patients. Gram-negative and anaerobic infections are more commonly seen in parenteral drug users, immunocompromised hosts, and those with extremity wounds and GI cancers.

Although not considered common in the elderly, *Neisseria gonorrhoeae* can cause migratory arthritis, tendinitis, and an acute monarthritis. This form of infectious arthritis is less destructive than that caused by nongonococcal organisms. *N. gonorrhoeae* needs to be considered in the elderly when appropriate clinical features are present. Tenosynovitis is the most frequent clinical presentation, although skin lesions in the form of pustules and macules also may be seen in two-thirds of the patients with disseminated gonococcal infection. In only 25% of patients with disseminated gonococcal infection will synovial fluid culture be positive.

Other agents, including fungi, viruses, spirochetes (Lyme disease), mycobacteria, and parasites, also have been reported to cause septic arthritis but usually have a more insidious course.

Microbiology of Septic Arthritis

ORGANISM	FREQUENCY
Gram-positive organisms	85%
Staphylococcus aureus	67%
Streptococcus pneumoniae	3%
Non-group A, b-hemolytic streptococci	15%
Gram-negative organisms	18%
Other agents	
Fungi	
Viruses	
Spirochetes	
Mycobacteria	
Parasites	

14. Discuss the pathogenesis of septic arthritis.

Septic arthritis most commonly occurs by hematogenous spread. Less frequent causes of infection include joint surgery, intraarticular injections, or penetrating trauma. The most common sites of infection involve the large joints, such as the knee and hip, but smaller joints also may be involved.

Risk factors predisposing the elderly patient to septic arthritis include:

Preexisting joint disease (rheumatoid arthritis and osteoarthritis)

Trauma

Intraarticular joint injection with glucocorticoids (infrequent; < 1/10,000 injections)

Concurrent extraarticular infection (skin, soft tissue, urinary tract, subacute bacterial endocarditis)

Illnesses or medications that impair host defenses:

Diabetes mellitus	AIDS
Chronic renal failure	Corticosteroid therapy
Cirrhosis	Cytotoxic agents

15. What are the common crystal-induced diseases in the elderly?

Crystal-induced arthritis often presents as a monarticular arthritis. **Gout** is a metabolic disease characterized by recurrent attacks of arthritis affecting one or more joints of the extremity and is caused by deposition of monosodium urate crystals in the cartilage of synovial membrane, thereby provoking an inflammatory response. The prevalence of gout increases with age and approaches 4% among patients in the 50–74-year-old range. It frequently occurs in the first metatarsophalangeal (MTP) joint, ankle, metatarsals, or knee, although any joint may be involved. The involved joint is often extremely tender, hot, swollen, and red, resembling an acute infection. Initial attacks are monarticular, but subsequent flares may be polyarticular and accompanied by fever. Tophaceous gout often occurs in elderly men, whereas diuretic-induced gout has been observed in elderly women. Diagnosis is made by demonstrating urate crystals in synovial fluid with a polarizing light microscope. Radiographs in early disease are usually normal, but in chronic disease they may demonstrate classic erosions with overhanging edges.

The prevalence of **calcium pyrophosphate deposition** (CPPD) disease, also called **pseudogout**, increases with age. Between the ages of 65 and 75 years, 10–15% of individuals have evidence of CPPD. This rate increases to 30–60% after age 85. Joints most commonly affected include the wrists and knees, but other joints also may be involved. The typical presentation is that of an acute self-limiting monarticular arthritis; however, asymptomatic disease with evidence of chondrocalcinosis on radiographs and a subacute chronic destructive arthropathy may develop. Radiographic changes often reveal the presence of chondrocalcinosis in the meniscus of the knee, the triangular ligament of the wrist, and occasionally the cartilage of the shoulder. Other findings resembling osteoarthritis include joint-space narrowing, bony sclerosis, subchondral cysts, and osteophyte formation. One should keep in mind that both gout and pseudogout also can present with a bursitis and tendinitis. Pseudogout has been associated with other conditions, including hypothyroidism, hyperparathyroidism, hemochromatosis, hypomagnesemia, and hypophosphatasia.

Apatite-induced arthritis, either secondary to hydroxyapatite (a component of bone) or other apatites, can cause an acute arthritis or periarthritis in joints affected by osteoarthritis. A rapidly destructive arthritis due to hydroxyapatite has been found in the elderly and is called **Milwaukee shoulder syndrome**, typically seen in women over age 70. Other joints, including the knee, also may be involved. The synovial fluid is often bloody with evidence of apatite crystals.

Common Crystal-Induced Arthritis

TYPE	CRYSTAL	PREVALENCE	PRESENTATIONS
Gout	Monosodium urate crystals	4% of 50–70 year olds	Most commonly affects first MTP joint, metatarsals, ankle, knee. Other joints may be affected. May be monarticular or polyarticular
CPPD	CPPD crystals	10–15% of 65–75-year-olds 30–60% after age 85	Commonly affects wrists, knees, but other joints may be affected Usually monarticular but can be polyarticular
Apatite-induced arthritis	Hydroxyapatite or other apatite	Most common in 65–75-year-olds	Acute arthritis or periarthritis Rapidly destructive arthritis called Milwaukee shoulder

16. How do you treat a crystal-induced arthritis?

Treatment of gout, pseudogout, and apatite disease is very similar. The first line of therapy is often an NSAID, which should be used cautiously in the elderly person, especially if other coexisting diseases are present. Prostaglandin analogs should be considered for gastric protection.

Colchicine is used less often for the acute flare of crystal-induced arthritis but may be used for prophylaxis for gout and pseudogout. Systemic glucocorticoids also may be used in the acute attack, especially if polyarticular joint involvement is present or contraindications to NSAID use are present. Intraarticular corticosteroid injection is an alternative treatment if a single joint is involved. In chronic arthritis, treatment modalities are similar to those used for osteoarthritis. Allopurinol and probenecid are reserved for use in chronic gouty arthritis.

17. Define osteonecrosis and discuss its features.

Osteonecrosis is another possible cause of pain in elderly patients. Pain develops as a result of impaired circulation to the affected bone, resulting in bony necrosis. Commonly involved sites include the knee, hip, or shoulder, but small joints also may be affected. Osteonecrosis is associated with a wide range of disorders, including systemic lupus erythematosus, systemic corticosteroids, trauma, alcoholism, cigarette smoking, and osteoarthritis, but it also may be idiopathic.

18. What risk factors are associated with the development of Charcot's joint?

Charcot's joint or neurogenic arthropathy may occur in patients who have peripheral sensory neuropathies, such as in diabetes mellitus, tabes dorsalis, pernicious anemia, and leprosy. Joint destruction occurs as a result of loss of pain perception. Other sensations also may be compromised, such as proprioception, touch, and temperature perception. Foot, ankle, and metatarsal joints are most commonly affected in diabetics, whereas larger joints are involved in those with tabes dorsalis.

BIBLIOGRAPHY

 1. Baker DG, Schumacher HR: Acute monoarthritis. N Engl J Med 329:1013–1020, 1993.
 2. Bridwell KH: Lumbar spinal stenosis: Diagnosis, management, and treatment. Clin Geriatr Med 10: 677–701, 1994.
 3. Chang CC, Greenspan A, Gershwin ME: Osteonecrosis: Current perspectives on pathogenesis and treatment. Semin Arthritis Rheum 23:47–69, 1993.
 4. Creamer P, Flores R, Hochberg M: Management of osteoarthritis in older adults. Clin Geriatr Med 14:435–454, 1998.
 5. Hamerman D: Aging and the musculoskeletal system. Ann Rheum Dis 56:578–585, 1997.
 6. Hughes SL, Dunlop D: The prevalence and impact of arthritis in older persons. Arthritis Care Res 8:257–267, 1995.
 7. Lawrence RC, Helmick CG, Arnett FC, et al: Estimates of arthritis and selected musculoskeletal disorders in the United States. Arthritis Rheum 41:778–799, 1998.
 8. McAdam PF, Ratella-Laawson F, Mardini IA, et al: Systemic biosynthesis of prostacyclin by cyclooxygenase (cox)-2: The human pharmacology of selective inhibitor of cox-2. Proc Natl Acad Sci USA 96:272–277, 1999.
 9. Norman DC, Yoshikawa TT: Infections of the bone, joint, and bursa. Clin Geriatr Med 10:703–718, 1994.
10. Schumacher HR: Osteoarthritis and crystal deposition disease. Curr Opin Rheumatol 10:244–245, 1998.
11. Towhead TE, Hochberg MC: A systmatic review of randomized controlled trials of pharmacological therapy of the knee with an emphasis on trial methodology. Semin Arthritis Rheum 26:755–770, 1997.
12. Yelin E, Callahan LF: The economic cost and social and psychological impact of musculoskeletal conditions. Arthritis Rheum 38:1351–1362, 1995.

43. HIP FRACTURES

John Bruza, M.D.

1. Who is at risk for hip fracture?

Over 90% of hip fractures result from falls, and the majority occur in people over 70-years-old. Nevertheless, only a small minority of falls (around 5%) result in a hip fracture. Independent risk factors for hip fracture include osteoporosis, female sex (across all ethnic subgroups but especially white and Asian women), chronic corticosteroid use, urban residence, residence in a nursing home, and dementia.

2. What morbidity and mortality rates are associated with hip fracture?

Functional dependence and death are important consequences of hip fracture. Over 250,000 hip fractures occur annually in the United States. This number is projected to double by the year 2000 as the elderly population expands. Mortality among elderly 1 year after hip fracture ranges from 14% to 36%. Mortality data from the Medicare population are probably the most reliable and demonstrate rates of 7% at 1 month, 13% at 3 months, and 24% at 12 months after fracture.

Approximately 35–50% of patients with a fractured hip do not regain their previous level of ambulating, and up to 20% may become nonambulatory. Rates of returning home after hip fracture vary widely from 40% to 90% and probably reflect regional differences in availability of home care services, skilled nursing facilities, and the value placed on returning home. At 6 months after hip fracture, 60% of patients regain walking ability, about 50% recover prefracture activities of daily living (ADLs), and about 25% recover prefracture instrumental activities of daily living (IADLs). Since the advent of the prospective payment system, which has shortened the in-hospital length of stay, the rate of institutionalization at 1 year after hip fracture has increased significantly.

3. What factors are associated with death after hip fracture?
- Advanced age
- Male sex
- Poorly controlled medical illness (especially cardiac, pulmonary, and cerebrovascular disease)
- Psychiatric illness
- Poor preoperative stabilization
- Postoperative complications

4. What factors predict recovery of walking after hip fracture?
- Male sex
- Younger age
- Absence of dementia
- Use of assistive device before injury (brings previously learned skills to therapy)

5. What factors are associated with nursing home placement after hip fracture?
- Age over 80 years
- Delirium or dementia
- Need for assistance with ADLs prior to fracture
- Lack of family involvement
- Inadequate physical therapy at skilled nursing facility

6. How do you evaluate a patient with a painful hip and a reportedly normal hip radiograph?

Think of a hip fracture until proven otherwise. Occult fracture should be suspected in patients with painful hip and difficulty in standing or walking despite normal anteroposterior (AP) pelvis and lateral hip radiographs. Other diagnoses to consider include acetabular fracture, pubic ramus fracture, isolated trochanteric fracture, and trochanteric bursitis or contusion. Try repeating the AP view with the leg internally rotated 15–20°. If the radiograph is still normal, consider magnetic resonance imaging of the hip. Bone scanning is also a possibility but is more costly and may require that the fracture be 2 or 3 days old to appear on scan.

7. What are important perioperative considerations for hip fracture patients?

The medical consultant plays an important role in clearance for hip surgery. Because patients often are brought to medical attention many hours or days after the injury, identifying the time of injury helps to guide the evaluation for dehydration, rhabdomyolysis, and delirium. Medical stabilization of fluid and electrolyte imbalances, cardiovascular stabilization (especially congestive heart failure), identification of delirium and comorbid infections (pneumonia, urinary tract infections [UTIs]), and assessment of nutritional status should be completed before surgery.

Early repair within 24–48 hours after admission is associated with a reduction in 1-year mortality. Hence prompt identification and treatment of medical problems may prevent surgical delay and the attendant risks of immobilization (deep venous thrombosis, atelectasis, pneumonia, UTIs, deconditioning, and skin breakdown). However, some patients may have medical conditions such as unstable angina that clearly benefit from delay for further stabilization and subsequent surgery in a timely manner.

Thorough evaluation of preinjury functioning in ADLs and IADLs assists in deciding the type of surgical repair and the plan for rehabilitation. As the treatment goal of all hip fractures is the return to prior level of functioning, establishing that prior level guides all treatment decisions. For example, a nonambulatory nursing home resident with advanced dementia and minimal discomfort after hip fracture may have no significant change in level of functioning and may best be treated with nonoperative management.

Successful return to premorbid functioning depends on good fracture reduction, maintaining range of motion in the hips, preventing weakness and muscle atrophy, adequate pain control, nutritional support, and preventing complications.

8. What are the considerations for a femoral neck fracture?

Femoral neck fractures account for 30% of hip fractures and can be treated by internal fixation with multiple screws or prosthetic replacement. Femoral neck fractures are intracapsular and risk disruption of the blood supply to this region. Some controversy exists over the best surgical procedure; bone quality, patient age, prior level of functioning, displacement, comminution, and risk of delayed ambulation should be taken into consideration. Incomplete to minimally displaced fractures may be treated with internal fixation. Displaced fractures pose a greater risk (up to 40%) of avascular necrosis and nonunion and generally require prosthetic total hip replacement in the elderly population. Prosthetic replacement allows weight-bearing, usually on the following morning, and thus a more rapid return to full function.

9. What are the considerations for an intertrochanteric fracture?

Intertrochanteric fractures are most common, accounting for up to two-thirds of hip fractures in the elderly. Standing falls deliver their impact most commonly in this region. Bleeding into the soft tissue is common and sometimes severe, requiring close following of blood counts and monitoring for hypotension. Treatment is less controversial and consists of internal fixation with a sliding nail or screw mechanism. Ambulation begins soon after surgery but is often more gradual with higher demands for pain management. Return to full unassisted ambulation may take a few months.

10. Is antibiotic prophylaxis necessary?

Prophylactic antibiotics reduce postoperative deep wound infections by 44%. First- and second-generation cephalosporins are most commonly used and should be dosed 0–2 hours before surgery and continued for 24 hours. Most studies have shown no added benefit for longer routine courses of antibiotics.

11. Which type of deep venous thrombosis (DVT) prophylaxis should be used?

The answer is somewhat controversial. Most studies support the use of low-dose heparin infusion or low–molecular-weight heparin injections, starting upon admission. The following table summarizes the various regimens.

DVT Prophylaxis for Hip Fracture

Low-dose heparin	Inexpensive and proved effective in numerous studies.
Low–molecular-weight heparin	May be slightly more effective than regular heparin but also higher bleeding risk and much more expensive.
Low-dose warfarin	Effective but more likely to be over- or underdosed and requires regular monitoring. Goal for INR is 1.5 times control.
Aspirin	Not as effective as above three. May be suitable alternative for patients with high bleeding risk that contraindicates heparin and warfarin.
Pneumatic compression stockings	Of added benefit to all above regimens and should be used routinely.

INR = international normalized ratio.

12. What is the most important postoperative consideration?

Early mobilization. The first day after surgery the patient should be moving from bed to chair and standing or walking during the first or second day. Some difficult surgical fixations may warrant an exception to limited weight-bearing but should be avoided as much as possible because much higher complication rates are associated with immobilization and delay in rehabilitation participation.

13. What are the common complications of hip fracture?

Delirium	Urine retention and incontinence
DVT	Unsuccessful fracture union, instability, or dislocation
Pain	Pneumonia or atelectasis
Functional decline	Malnutrition
Catheter-associated UTI	Surgical infection (wound, joint, or bone)

14. Discuss the use of urinary catheters.

Indwelling urinary catheters are best removed within 24 hours after surgery to reduce the common problems of urinary infections, retention, and incontinence and to assist in early mobilization. Periodic straight catheterization may be necessary after removal but is preferable to continued use of indwelling catheters.

15. How common is delirium? What are the risk factors?

Delirium is a common complication of hip fractures (about 60% of cases). Older age, history of dementia, history of heavy alcohol use, and severe medical illness are common risk factors.

16. What are the causes of delirium? How is it treated?

Few studies have examined the causes of delirium specifically in hip fracture patients. Looking at combined medical and surgical patients, common causes include fluid and electrolyte imbalances, adverse drug reactions (especially among opioids, sedative-hypnotics, and anticholinergics), infection, metabolic disorders, and decreased brain perfusion. Goals of treatment include early recognition, identification of cause, prompt treatment of reversible causes, and anticipating safety concerns for the patient. In addition, supportive reorientation and control of the sensory environment (increasing stimuli for the sensory-impaired and decreasing sensory stimuli for those who appear agitated) can be beneficial.

17. Discuss specific orthopedic complications.

Specific orthopedic complications include infection of the wound, joint, or bone; problems of fracture union (delayed union, malunion, nonunion); avascular necrosis; compartment syndrome of the leg; and posttraumatic arthritis. Infection occurs in up to 5% of patients and is treated mainly with antibiotic therapy but may require surgical irrigation, debridement, or replacement. Loss of internal fixation occurs in up to 15% and usually requires additional surgery. Compartment syndrome occurs shortly after injury or repair and results from increasing pressure (from edema, bleeding, infection, or an external brace or cast) within a confined anatomic compartment causing uncontrollable pain out of proportion to the injury and sensory deficits followed by motor deficits. The threatened leg may require fasciotomy to relieve the pressure. Nonunion, avascular necrosis, and posttraumatic arthritis occur months to years after injury.

18. How common is malnutrition?

Severe malnutrition is identified in up to 20% of patients with hip fracture. Improving nutrition with oral protein supplementation has been shown to reduce minor complications, preserve body protein stores, and significantly reduce length of hospital stay.

19. How is the risk of recurrent fracture assessed?

Assessing fall risk in patients with hip fracture may help to reduce the high risk for recurrent fracture. Exercise and balance training help to reduce fall risk. See Chapter 34 for assessment of fall risk and prevention treatment.

44. OSTEOPOROSIS

Michael Pazianas, M.D., and Edna P. Schwab, M.D.

1. What is osteoporosis?

Osteoporosis is a systemic disease characterized by low bone mass and microarchitectural deterioration of bone tissue, with a consequent increase in bone fragility and susceptibility to fracture.

2. Discuss the economic and functional impact of osteoporosis.

Osteoporosis is a major health problem as a result of the high morbidity and mortality rates associated with fractures. It affects 25 million people and accounts for 1.5 million fractures annually, including 240,000 hip fractures. The costs associated with the complications of osteoporosis were $13.8 billion in 1995 and are projected to reach $240 billion by the year 2040 as a result of the expanding aging population.

Osteoporosis is associated with a great deal of functional loss as well as skeletal deformities, pain, dependence, and depression. Vertebral fractures occur more frequently than hip fractures. Compared with women without fractures, women with a history of vertebral or hip fractures have more difficulty with bending, lifting, reaching, walking, and ascending and descending stairs and experienced impairment in dressing, cooking, shopping, and housework. Approximately 40% of hip fracture survivors were able to return to their prior level of performance for activities of daily living (ADLs), whereas only 25% returned to their prefracture level for instrumental activities of daily living (IADLs). The ability to perform ADLs and IADLs, along with social supports, often determines whether a person can return to independent living. Approximately 15–25% of patients with hip fractures require institutionalization.

3. What is the mechanism of bone loss in osteoporosis?

Bone is composed of two types of tissue: trabecular bone, which is metabolically more active, and cortical bone, which is less active. Bone remodeling is a tightly organized process consisting of bone formation closely coupled to bone resorption. Systemic humoral factors, such as parathyroid hormone, growth hormone, estrogens, and testosterone, and local humoral factors (e.g., IGF-1, TNF, IL-1, and IL-6) contribute to proper functioning. The majority of adult bone mass is laid down during adolescence; however, peak bone mass is not obtained until the fourth decade. Peak mass is determined by numerous genetic and environmental factors, including sex, family history, body type, and activity level. By age 40 years there is a slow decline in bone mass in both men and women. Aging alters the tight coupling between bone resorption and formation, resulting in augmented osteoclastic resorption and diminished osteoblastic activity. Estrogen deficiency accelerates the rate of bone loss. Total lifetime bone loss in men may be 20–30% of peak bone mass, whereas in women it may amount to 40–50%.

4. List the risk factors associated with osteoporosis.

- Increasing age
- White or Asian ancestry
- Thin body frame
- Early menopause (< 45 years old)
- Calcium/vitamin D-deficient diet
- Sedentary lifestyle
- Cigarette smoking
- Heavy ethanol use
- Family history of osteoporosis
- Late menarche (> 16 years old)
- Amenorrhea or irregular menstrual periods
- Immobilization

5. Which disorders should be considered in evaluating a patient for low bone density?

Osteoporosis is a diagnosis of exclusion. Secondary causes of low bone density need to be excluded before a diagnosis of osteoporosis is made.

Secondary Causes of Low Bone Density

- Hyperthyroidism
- Hyperparathyroidism
- Rheumatoid arthritis
- Eating disorders (anorexia, bulimia)
- Idiopathic hypercalciuria
- Cushing's syndrome
- Diabetes mellitus
- Prolactinoma
- Hemolytic anemia
- Gastrointestinal dysfunction (malabsorption)
- Mastocytosis
- Hepatobiliary dysfunction
- Hypogonadism (men)
- Vitamin D deficiency
- Paget's disease
- Corticosteroid therapy
- Estrogen deficiency
- Malignancy
- Multiple myeloma
- Renal insufficiency
- Transplant therapy
- Vitamin D receptor allele anomaly

6. **Which pharmacologic agents are associated with low bone density?**
   - Anticonvulsants
   - Glucocorticoids
   - Lithium
   - Antacids (chronic use of phosphate-binding antacid)
   - Heparin
   - Methotrexate
   - Gonadotropin-releasing hormone agonist or antagonist
   - Warfarin (Coumadin)
   - Excessive thyroid supplementation
   - Phenothiazines

7. **Which laboratory tests help to evaluate a patient with low bone density?**
   Unfortunately, questionnaires and a detailed clinical history often identify less than 50% of patients with low bone mass. However, before making a diagnosis of osteoporosis, metabolic diseases of different pathology (e.g., osteomalacia, hyperparathyroidism) should be excluded by obtaining a thorough history, physical examination, and appropriate laboratory studies. Risk factors, diet, exercise, and medications should be reviewed. Initial laboratory studies include complete blood count, liver and renal function tests, alkaline phosphatase, calcium, phosphorus, albumin, total protein, thyroid-stimulating hormone, vitamin D level, 24-hour urine calcium, and urinalysis. These tests are normal when bone loss is due to primary osteoporosis. Depending on clinical suspicion, further studies, such as parathyroid hormone, bone specific alkaline phosphatase, serum protein and urine protein electrophoresis, testosterone levels, and erythrocyte sedimentation rate may be obtained.

   Measurements of fragments of bone collagen in urine and blood, such as pyridinoline and deoxypyridinoline, may determine the rate of bone loss; either of the two terminals released by procollagen in its transformation to collagen indicates the rate of bone formation.

   All of these measurements provide only a snapshot of bone dynamics at the time of the test and no information about the actual bone mass of the patient. Therefore, they may be useful only for monitoring changes of bone activity after treatment. The clinician should keep in mind that inter- and intraassay variability frequently exceeds 20%.

   The most commonly used bone markers are procollagen type 1 C-terminal peptide (PICP), immunoreactive free deoxypyridinoline (iFDpd), and N-terminal cross-linked telopeptides of type 1 collagen (NTx).

8. **Name the various methods used to measure bone density.**
   - Skeletal radiographs are not a sensitive test because osteopenia becomes evident on radiographs only after more than one-third of bone mass has been lost.
   - Quantitative computed tomography (QCT) estimates the amount of minerals in the bone. Although it can analyze the bone in three dimensions and even distinguish trabecular from compact bone tissue, it has a number of practical disadvantages: it is available at a small

number of centers; it is expensive; the radiation dose is not negligible; the error around re-
peated measurements may be high; and it evaluates only small volumes of bone.
- Peripheral quantitative computed tomography (pQCT) offers some advantages over QCT.
  It is portable and can measure the forearm, which is a relatively large bone area.
- Bone densitometry (dual energy x-ray absorptiometry [DXA]). Bone mineral density
  (BMD) measurement of the spine and hip has become the standard test for assessing the
  risk of osteoporosis. The lower the result, the higher the risk of fracture. The test is highly
  accurate and reproducible (less than 2% error, depending on the site measured). The scan
  time is short (less than 5 minutes; with the latest technology, less than 1 minute) at each site
  (i.e., spine and hip), and the radiation dose to which the patient is exposed is extremely low
  (one-twentieth that of a chest radiograph). DXA requires lying on a table (fully clothed)
  while the arm of the machine swings over the torso. Portable x-ray peripheral densitome-
  ters are available, and a new portable ultrasound device scans the heel (calcaneus).
  Readings correlate well with the risk of fracture.

9. What does the DXA report reveal?

Before you read the report, remember that the terms *osteopenia* and *osteoporosis* were introduced to label different levels of bone density and do not mean that the patient has osteoporosis
for the following reasons:
- Low BMD may be due to a number of metabolic bone diseases other than osteoporosis; osteomalacia and hyperparathyroidism are the most common examples.
- Osteoporosis is a diagnosis by exclusion.

BMD is estimated in gm/cm^2 and then compared with prestored data from two groups of normal
individuals of the same gender and race. One group consists of individuals of the same age and the
other of young adults. Comparison with the first group produces a Z-score, which is the number of
standard deviations (SD) above or below the normal BMD for the same age. Comparison with the
second group produces a T-score, which is the number of SD above or below the normal BMD of
young adults. The T-score is the more important result because it shows how much bone is left compared with the peak bone mass of a normal young adult. According to the World Health
Organization, a BMD of 1–2.5 SD below that of a normal young adult classifies the patient as os-
teopenic and below 2.5 SD as osteoporotic. Generally, a drop of 1 SD doubles the risk of fracture.

10. What are the indications for bone density studies?

Postmenopausal women under the age of 65 with identifiable risk factors should be screened
for osteoporosis as should women over 65, regardless of risk factors. BMD can confirm the diagnosis of osteoporosis, evaluate a woman's risk for osteoporosis, and assess efficacy of treatment.

Indications for Bone Density Screening
- Estrogen-deficient women
- Patients with history of fractures
- Persons taking long-term corticosteroids
- Persons with endocrinopathy (hyperthyroidism, hyperparathyroidism, Cushing's disease/
  syndrome)
- Patients with significant risk factors, regardless of age
- Hypogonadal men
- Assessment of treatment efficacy
- Postmenopausal women considering therapy for osteoporosis when BMD will facilitate
  treatment decisions
- Age > 65 years

11. What strategies help to prevent osteoporosis?

Osteoporosis is preventable during the early stages of bone loss. Unfortunately, bone loss
of a degree that causes hip or vertebral fracture is largely irreversible. Preventive measures are
required during all three skeletal phases:

1. Genetic factors determine the optimal bone mass that we can acquire (peak bone mass) by the time we reach the early thirties. However, high calcium intake and exercise may increase the bone mass up to 15%. At periods when the skeleton is under stress, such as pregnancy and lactation, a diet adequate in calcium, vitamin D, and other nutrients is essential.

2. Until women reach menopause and men their 50s, adequate calcium and physical activity contribute the most to preserve skeletal strength. Women of all ages should be counseled about achieving peak bone mass, including education about appropriate diet, calcium intake, regular weight-bearing exercise, and avoidance of factors that have a negative impact on bone turnover (e.g., smoking, excessive alcohol and caffeine, sedentary lifestyle). Girls aged 11–24 years should consume 1200–1500 mg of calcium/day. Premenopausal women and women between the ages of 50 and 65 years on hormone replacement therapy should consume 1000 mg/day of calcium. In women > 65 years, 1500 mg calcium/day is recommended along with vitamin D, 800 IU/day. The risks vs. benefits of hormone replacement therapy in prevention and treatment of osteoporosis should be reviewed and individualized for all peri- and postmenopausal women based on risk factors and BMD.

3. Finally, at any time during menopause or in men over 50, the following drug and nondrug treatments should be considered if the bone mass is low (T-score < –1.5): estrogen, bisphosphonate therapy, calcitonin, raloxifene, and fall prevention.

12. What medications are available to treat established osteoporosis?

The Food and Drug Administration (FDA) has approved four drugs for treatment of established osteoporosis and three for prevention. The best treatment is not the same in all individuals and should be determined by the physician. Drugs used to treat osteoporosis decrease bone resorption (antiresorptive drugs). Drugs that encourage bone formation and restore its structural integrity are still in the experimental stage. The most commonly used agents include estrogen (hormone replacement therapy), bisphosphonates, calcitonin, and raloxifene. Raloxifene, although not yet approved by the FDA for treatment, is a selective estrogen receptor modulator (SERM) that has been shown to improve bone density in women by decreasing the risk of fractures. It is not known to have any adverse effects on breast or endometrial tissues.

TREATMENT	MECHANISM OF ACTION	INDICATION	OTHER BENEFITS	ADVERSE EFFECTS
Estrogens Premarin, 0.625 mg or transdermal patches; combined treatment with progesterone indicated in nonhysterectomized women	Inhibit bone resorption	Treatment of choice for prevention and postmenopausal osteoporosis Estrogen replacement reduces rate of bone loss and reduces risk of fractures of spine up to 80% and hip by as much as 50%	May reduce risk of ischemic heart disease up to 50%, but HERS trial indicated estrogen plus progestin was not effective for secondary prevention of coronary heart disease in postmenopausal women Suggestions that estrogen may reduce risk of colon cancer, improve cognitive function, and delay onset or prevent Alzheimer disease (not well established)	Vaginal bleeding Breast tenderness Bloating Thromboembolism (with family history of DVT or history of pulmonary embolus, severe varicose veins, obesity, surgery, trauma, prolonged bed rest) Risk of breast cancer may increase, especially in women receiving estrogen for more than 10 years

Table continued on facing page

TREATMENT	MECHANISM OF ACTION	INDICATION	OTHER BENEFITS	ADVERSE EFFECTS
Bisphosphonates Alendronate, 10 mg/day for treatment and 5 mg/day for prevention (the only bisphosphonate approved by FDA)	Inhibit osteoclast function Analogs of pyrophosphate (Pi-O-Pi) resistant to enzymatic hydrolysis	After 3 years of treatment, average increase in spinal bone density is 8% and 6% in hip Reduction in vertebral, wrist, and hip fractures is approximately 50% Poorly absorbed by GI tract; must be ingested in morning before food or drink except water		GI problems such as esophagitis and gastritis Absolute contraindication: upper GI disease, including achalasia or esophageal stricture Relative contraindication: gastroesophageal reflux
Calcitonin Injection form Nasal spray administered daily in alternating nostrils	Inhibits bone resorption by directly inhibiting osteoclast function	May reduce risk of fracture by 40% without increasing bone mineral density	Analgesic properties in patients with vertebral fractures	Injection form is inconvenient with side effects of local reaction and pain at injection site Nasal spray may cause nasal irritation
Raloxifene (selective estrogen receptor modulator)	Antiestrogen with estrogenic effect on bone	Approved by FDA for prevention/treatment of osteoporosis Reduces risk of vertebral fracture by 40–50%	Positive effects on lipids No effect on breast or endometrium	Increased risk of DVT Increases incidence of hot flashes
Vitamin D, 800 IU	Increases calcium absorption Ameliorates secondary hyperparathyroidism, a common complication of aging		May reduce risk of fracture in men and women over age of 65 Useful in institutionalized patients, in whom vitamin D deficiency is common	
Calcium supplements Calcium carbonate contains greatest proportion of elemental calcium (40%) Calcium gluconate contains 9% elemental calcium		Timing not of therapeutic significance; best to divide daily dose to improve absorption	Studies suggest that calcium with or without vitamin D can reduce bone loss and fractures in older adults Amount of calcium necessary depends on age, sex, and diet NIH established appropriate daily calcium requirement for general population at various ages and stages of life	

DVT = deep venous thrombosis.

13. What is the role of exercise?

Weight-bearing exercise is important in maintaining and building bone mass. It also helps to strengthen muscles and reduces the risk of falls. Resistance and flexibility exercises, such as weight-training and tai chi or yoga, also strengthen muscles and help maintain bone mass.

BIBLIOGRAPHY

1. Cosman F, Lindsay R: Is parathyroid hormone a therapeutic option for osteoporosis? A review of the clinical evidence. Calcif Tissue Int 62:475–480, 1998.
2. Eastell R: Treatment of postmenopausal osteoporosis. N Engl J Med 338:736–746, 1999.
3. Eastell R, Boyle IT, Compston J, et al: Management of male osteoporosis: Report of the UK Consensus Group. Q J Med 91:71–92, 1998.
4. Eastell R, Reid DM, Compston J, et al: A UK Consensus Group on management of glucocorticoid-induced osteoporosis: An update. J Intern Med 244:271–292, 1998.
5. Fleisch H: Bisphosphonates in Bone Disease: From the Laboratory to the Patient. New York, Parthenon, 1997.
6. Hulley S, Grady D, Bush T, et al: Randomized trials of estrogen plus progestin for secondary prevention of coronary heart disease in postmenopausal women. Heart and Estrogen/progestin Replacement Study (HERS) Research. JAMA 280:605–613, 1998.
7. Kanis J: Osteoporosis. Oxford, Blackwell Science, 1994.
8. Scheiber LB, Torregrosa L: Evaluation and treatment of postmenopausal osteoporosis. Semin Arthritis Rheum 4:245–261, 1998.
9. WHO Study Group: Assessment of fracture risk and its application to screening for postmenopausal osteoporosis. WHO Technical Report Series 843. Geneva, World Health Organization, 1994.
10. Zaidi M, Pazianas M: Therapy of Osteoporosis. Cell Biology, Pharmacology and Drug Development. London, Derwent Science, 1995.

45. RENAL DISEASE

Ray Townsend, M.D.

1. What changes in kidney function occur with aging?

Concentrating ability of the kidney declines with age. As a result, solute loads such as salt and protein are not excreted as quickly or as efficiently. Older patients are at greater risk for hypernatremia and hyperosmolality if they are deprived of adequate water intake. The higher risk of hypernatremia is in part worsened by a reduction in thirst sensation with advancing age. Drugs such as lithium (which impairs thirst and also results in a nephrogenic diabetes insipidus), osmotic diuretics (mannitol and radiology contrast media), and high protein feedings should be used and monitored cautiously in the elderly.

Diluting ability also declines with advancing years, leading to a substantial prevalence of hyponatremia in the elderly. Thiazide diuretics and older antihyperglycemic medications (chlorpropamide) may produce severe hyponatremia in some elderly patients.

In dealing with disorders of sodium and water, which are common in the elderly, it is important to distinguish between disorders of hydration (in which the serum sodium itself is abnormal) and disorders of volume depletion (in which the serum sodium may be perfectly normal, but the patient may have a volume excess [e.g., edema] or deficiency [e.g., orthostatic vital sign findings] as manifested by clinical examination).

2. In older people, does a serum creatinine within the normal range mean that kidney functions are normal?

Not necessarily. After age 40, kidney function decreases an average of 1% per year, or roughly 10% per decade. However, the serum creatinine does not increase by 10% per decade; this is due to the fact that at the same time kidney function declines, creatinine production declines proportionately because of a progressive decrease in body muscle mass. Creatinine is produced by a nonenzymatic dehydration of muscle creatine, and the amount of creatinine produced each day is proportional to the size of the muscle mass. Kidney function is generally measured by a creatinine clearance derived from a 24-hour urine collection and a serum creatinine measurement using a standard clearance formula. For example, if a 25-year-old man who is 6'2" tall, weighs 220 pounds, and has an obviously well-developed muscle mass collects a 24-hour urine sample and undergoes a blood test, the lab may report the following: 24-hour urine volume of 2750 ml, urine creatinine concentration of 85 mg/dl, and serum creatinine of 1.6 mg/dl. To calculate his creatinine clearance:

1. Determine the amount of creatinine excreted: [(2750 ml/24 hr) × (85 mg/dl)]/(100 ml/dl) = 2337.5 mg/24 hr.

2. Determine the minute excretion of creatinine (since clearance is expressed in the amount of blood cleared of a substance per minute) by dividing the total excreted by 1440 minutes in a day: [(2337.5 mg/24 hr)/(1440 min/24 hr)] = 1.62 mg/min.

3. To determine the clearance, divide the minute excretion of creatinine by the serum concentration: [(1.62 mg/min)/(1.6 mg/dl)] × (100 ml/dl) =101.5 ml/min.

An average creatinine clearance is about 100 ml/min. If the young man's 185-pound, 5'10" grandfather performed a similar collection, the following results may be expected: 24-hour volume of 2750 ml, urine creatinine concentration of 45 mg/dl, serum creatinine of 1.4 mg/dl; to determine creatinine clearance:

1. Calculate mg of creatinine excreted in 24 hours:

$$\frac{2750 \text{ ml/24 hr} \times 45 \text{ mg/dl}}{100 \text{ ml/dl}} = 1237.5 \text{ mg/24 hr}$$

2. Calculate the minute excretion of creatinine:

$$\frac{1237.5 \text{ mg/24 hr}}{1440 \text{ min/24 hr}} = 0.86 \text{ mg/min}$$

3. Calculate the creatinine clearance:

$$\frac{0.86 \text{ mg/min}}{1.4 \text{ mg/dl}} \times 100 \text{ ml/dl} = 61.4 \text{ ml/min}$$

Despite a lower serum creatinine level, the older patient actually has less kidney function because the daily creatinine production is less. When a 24-hour urine collection is not available or not practical, a useful formula to estimate kidney function—one that takes into account age, weight, and gender (women tend to have proportionately less muscle mass)—is that of Cockcroft and Gault:

$$\text{Creatinine clearance} = \frac{[(140 - \text{age in years}) \times (\text{weight in kg})]}{[(72) \times (\text{serum creatinine in mg/dl})]}$$

The result is multiplied by 0.85 for women. In the example given, if an elderly man is 71-years-old, the formula predicts his creatinine clearance as follows:

$$[(140 - 71) \times (185 \text{ lb}/2.2 \text{ lb/kg})]/[(72) \times 1.4 \text{ mg/dl})] = 57.6 \text{ ml/min}$$

This result is acceptably close to the 61.4 ml/min actually measured. The (72) in the formula is a constant factor for the units that, after division, result in the final value of ml/min for the calculation. For an elderly woman of the same age and weight, the result would be $57.6 \times 0.85 = 48.9$ ml/min. This formula is particularly useful for dosing guidelines in hospitalized elderly renal patients when there is not enough time to collect a 24-hour urine.

The Cockcroft and Gault formula, however, is not as useful in obese patients. For patients more than 25–30% above ideal body weight, the following formulas of Salazar and Corcoran should be used:

Male creatinine clearance =

$$\frac{(137 - \text{age in yr} \times [(0.285 \times \text{weight in kg}) + (12.1 \times \text{height in meters}^2)]}{(51 \times \text{serum creatinine in mg/dl})}$$

Female creatinine clearance =

$$\frac{(146 - \text{age in yr}) \times [(0.287 \times \text{weight in kg}) + (9.74 \times \text{height in meters}^2)]}{(60 \times \text{serum creatinine in mg/dl})}$$

Try the Cockcroft formula on an 80-year-old woman who weighs 110 pounds and has a "normal" creatinine of 1.3 mg/dl (do not forget to multiply by 0.85). Then run the same calculation for the 25-year-old man used as the first example.

3. When should an elderly patient be referred to a nephrologist?
There are no strict guidelines; however, consider referring an older patient to a nephrologist when he or she has:
- Unexplained proteinuria (dipstick $\geq$ ++ or $\geq$ 1.0 gm/24 hr)
- Unexpected or unexplained decline in renal function (increase in serum creatinine by > 20% from baseline and confirmed by rechecking)
- Hematuria (gross or microscopic)
- Late onset of hypertension (age > 55 years)
- Refractory or unexplained electrolyte disorders (e.g., hyponatremia, hypo/hyperkalemia, hypomagnesemia)
- Noncardiac peripheral edema

In general, elderly patients with a creatinine $\geq$ 3.0 mg/dl should be considered for nephrologic evaluation, in part to address unapparent renal problems (such as renal osteodystrophy), in part to establish a relationship for future dialysis or transplant care, and in part to address subtleties of divalent ion metabolism (such as decreases in serum calcium and increases in serum phosphorus), which tend to occur early in renal insufficiency.

4. Which kinds of medications are particularly troublesome in elderly patients with renal disease?

Drug/Class	Clinical Effect
Digoxin	Accumulates more readily due to less renal excretion (digitalis toxicity)
Aminoglycosides	May impair renal function through tubular toxicity
NSAIDs	Sodium retention, loss of blood pressure control; impair kidney function by interfering with renal blood flow
Lithium	Hypernatremia—through impaired thirst and impairment of urinary concentration mechanisms
Thiazides	Hyponatremia—through impaired renal diluting mechanisms and water retention

5. Is there anything special I need to know about proteinuria in older patients?

The main causes of nephrotic syndrome (characterized by ≥ 3 gm of protein excreted in the urine over 24 hours and usually attended by a low serum albumin, peripheral edema, and increases in triglyceride and/or cholesterol) differ in old and young patients. In the elderly, the most common cause of proteinuria is diabetes mellitus. In the absence of diabetes, membranous glomerulopathy is the most common idiopathic form of nephrotic syndrome in the elderly (about $\frac{1}{3}$ of cases), followed by minimal change disease (about $\frac{1}{5}$–$\frac{1}{4}$ of cases). The finding of membranous glomerulopathy on a kidney biopsy is an important observation, because about 1 of 5 patients has a malignancy associated with membranous glomerulopathy. A thorough history and physical, a chest x-ray, rectal and prostate exam (including a stool for occult blood), and a gynecologic exam with mammography are usually adequate screening procedures for malignancy when membranous glomerulopathy is found.

6. Which kinds of renal disease are more common in the elderly? How do I recognize them?

Acute glomerulonephritis (AGN) occurs in older patients. The most common form of AGN in elderly patients is a rapidly progressive glomerulonephritis (RPGN): roughly one-fifth of patients have anti–glomerular basement membrane (GBM) antibodies, two-fifths have a different form of immune-complex mediated disease, and two-fifths have no detectable immune deposits (pauci-immune). The typical presentation is hematuria, some proteinuria (often *not* in nephrotic range), edema, and hypertension. The specific diagnosis is aided indirectly by elevated titers of anti-GBM antibodies (in anti-GBM disease) or antineutrophil cytoplasmic antibodies (ANCA) in the pauci-immune varieties. The specific diagnosis is made by a renal biopsy.

Obstructive uropathy due to prostate hyperplasia or neoplasia is clearly more common in elderly men as opposed to women or younger men. The history is helpful in that older men may have noticed a decrease in the size or force of the urine stream, hesitancy in starting urine stream, straining, dribbling, and a feeling that the bladder is not empty after voiding. In addition, some elderly men may develop an acute worsening of underlying prostate problems when they take an anticholinergic or antihistaminic drug. A rectal exam confirms prostate enlargement and/or neoplasia.

Cholesterol embolization is a clinically challenging condition to recognize. In older patients it results from atheroma in the arterial circulation. It typically becomes manifest after an arteriogram with or without an angioplasty or after anticoagulant therapy. The clinician may see livedo reticularis, cyanosis, or (ultimately) gangrene in the toes; fever; eosinophilia; a progressive rise in serum creatinine concentration; and a loss of blood pressure control. A skin or renal biopsy showing typical cholesterol clefts in the arterioles confirms the clinical diagnosis.

Ischemic renal disease is characterized by progressive atherosclerotic obliteration of the main renal arteries and their branches, with a loss in kidney volume and function over time. It is increasingly recognized as more older patients undergo arteriographic procedures, and it may be responsible for 10–15% of renal failure leading to dialysis in elderly patients. Important clues are a smoking history, known coronary artery disease, bruits (anywhere, but especially in the flank areas), and an increase in the serum creatinine concentration after the use of an angiotensin-converting enzyme inhibitor, especially in patients who are also on a diuretic. Another clue is repeated episodes of pulmonary edema. Magnetic resonance angiography, Doppler ultrasound, spiral computed tomography, and angiography are useful procedures in making the diagnosis.

Clues to Ischemic Renal Disease

HISTORY	PHYSICAL	LABORATORY
Cigarette use	Bruits (anywhere)	Increase in serum creatinine following angiotensin-converting enzyme inhibitor therapy (especially with diuretic)
Angina	Pulmonary edema	

7. Is acute renal failure more common in elderly patients? How do I recognize which older patients are at risk for a sudden decline in renal function?

Although intuitively one may think that older patients frequently have a loss of kidney function after surgery or a hypotensive episode, in fact older patients typically do well after elective or emergent surgical procedures. The most common identifiable risk factor that predisposes to acute renal failure (often defined simply as a doubling of the serum creatinine concentration over 1–2 days) is volume depletion, either as a consequence of intentional diuretic usage or as a result of unrecognized osmotic diuresis or diarrhea in patients who receive parenteral or enteral nutrition that is high in protein or who are hyperglycemic. A daily weight (unarguably one of the least expensive in-hospital procedures) can help to identify an older patient who is becoming volume depleted. Other situations that should be kept in mind include:

- Aminoglycoside antibiotic usage—doses that are well tolerated by younger patients are more likely to cause a fall in renal function in elderly patients
- Obstructive uropathy, especially when induced by medications that may impair bladder emptying in older patients
- Usage of the histamine-blocking agent cimetidine or the antibiotic trimethoprim, both of which compete with creatinine for secretion in the proximal tubule of the kidney and may functionally elevate the serum creatinine (not by reducing filtration but by impairing secretion)
- Intravenous contrast usage—the risk of acute renal failure depends on the initial level of kidney function and the presence of other disorders (e.g., diabetes, myeloma, preexisting renal disease from any cause, and volume depletion).

8. What are the main causes of kidney failure leading to dialysis in the elderly?

Diabetes and hypertension, as in younger patients. The incidence of older patients who begin dialysis as a result of ischemic renal disease is also increasing. In older patients, type 2 diabetes is more common than type 1 diabetes as a cause of end-stage renal disease (ESRD). Unlike younger patients, hypertension is more commonly considered the cause of ESRD in older compared with younger patients, and is equal in incidence with diabetes in older patients as the cause of ESRD. In patients 65 years and older, diabetes (all types) accounts for 36% of all new elderly dialysis patients, and hypertension accounts for 37% of all new elderly dialysis patients. Together, diabetes and hypertension account for about 75% of ESRD in the elderly.

9. Should age be a barrier to starting a patient on dialysis?

Age alone is not a barrier to dialysis. In patients with dementia (but not uremic encephalopathy), malignancy, and advanced hepatic failure, however, its use should be carefully reviewed.

Initiation of dialysis is not a mandate for its continuance in patients who tolerate dialysis poorly or who fail to thrive. Dialysis, an expensive resource, should be used to maintain life rather than to prolong death. If it is clear that a patient is continuing to fail despite adequate dialysis, a dialogue between the patient and his or her family and the medical team should remain open, and the option to stop dialysis should be a topic of continued discussion.

10. Do elderly patients do poorly on dialysis compared with younger patients?

Elderly patients often do quite well on dialysis. Both hemodialysis and peritoneal dialysis have been used in the care of end-stage renal disease in the elderly, and patient survival is similar between the two dialysis modalities. Compared with younger patients, elderly patients on hemodialysis are at greater risk for hypotension during dialysis, malnutrition, dialysis-associated amyloidosis, gastrointestinal bleeding, depression, subdural hematoma, voluntary withdrawal from the hemodialysis program, and inadequate dialysis (either because of limitations imposed by poor access—i.e., poor blood flow in the arteriovenous connection in the patient—or because of problems such as nausea, muscle cramping, or hypotension during dialysis, which reduce blood flow rates and thus impair efficiency). Elderly patients on peritoneal dialysis may become volume-depleted, develop peritonitis, or experience metabolic consequences such as hyperglycemia and hyperlipidemia (hypertriglyceridemia) from the high glucose concentrations in the peritoneal dialysate.

11. What are the main causes of death in elderly patients on dialysis?

The main causes of death depend in part on the modality used, but in general they are as follows (in descending order):

Hemodialysis	Peritoneal dialysis
Heart disease and stroke	Heart disease and stroke
Infection	Peritonitis
Voluntary discontinuation	Other infections

Voluntary discontinuation is not uncommon in hospitalized patients dying from multisystem organ failure; withdrawal of dialysis sets up a terminal event.

12. Should older patients in renal failure be considered for a kidney transplant?

Although roughly 40% of patients with end-stage renal disease (including both dialysis and transplant patients) are > 65 years old, < 3% of patients in this age range receive a kidney transplant. Contributing factors include cadaver-kidney shortage (more potential recipients than donors), poor results with prior immunosuppressive regimens (i.e., past experience with antirejection drugs), and the idea that age alone is a barrier to transplantation. However, with careful patient selection and particular attention to the immunosuppressive regimen (e.g., recognizing that the P450 enzyme system that metabolizes cyclosporine is less active in the elderly and may allow use of a lower dose), elderly patients should not be refused transplantation on the basis of age alone. Transplanted kidneys are lost in the elderly mostly because of patient death (about 50%, with the chief causes being heart disease, infection, and malignancy, in that order). In younger patients, death accounts for only about 15% of graft loss, with acute and chronic rejection accounting for most of the remainder. In evaluating an older patient for transplant, the following procedures are commonly used:

- Exercise stress test with thallium and coronary angiogram for patients with coronary symptoms or diabetes
- Careful evaluation of peripheral pulses, because the transplanted kidney may "steal" blood flow from the leg
- Ultrasound of gallbladder, because cholelithiasis is a problem in the elderly, especially those with diabetes
- Barium enema (although its value is debatable in some patients) is considered useful because of the poor outcome in transplant patients with a colon perforation (usually from underlying diverticular disease) and the possible masking of bowel symptoms when a patient

is on immunosuppressive drugs. Many authorities strongly consider a barium enema in patients with polycystic kidney disease.
• Mammography and prostate evaluations

13. What other factors affect the treatment of elderly patients with acute renal failure?

1. Recovery from acute renal failure in the elderly is no different from recovery in younger patients, and the patient's ultimate prognosis, not his or her age, should weigh heavily in the decision to use renal replacement therapy (dialysis).

2. Maintain a reasonable index of suspicion for ischemic renal disease, which may be responsive to angioplasty or arterial bypass, thus prolonging the renal life span.

3. Recognize that elderly patients are more prone to dialysis-related events such as hypotension and hemodialysis access problems, but these events are usually manageable. Many elderly patients do quite well on dialysis.

4. Do not rule out transplantation in an older patient with failing kidney function on the basis of age alone.

Bear in mind, however, that a transplant evaluation committee is more likely to approve older patients as potential transplant recipients if they appear in good health, with reasonably stable weight, no claudication, and a low index of suspicion for coronary artery and gastrointestinal diseases (gallstones and diverticulosis).

14. How does renal function in the elderly affect prescription of medications?

Elderly patients frequently consume a great number and remarkable variety of medications. Drug interaction, which is difficult to predict in normal patients with healthy kidneys and livers, becomes impossibly difficult in patients with compromised renal function. The following guidelines may be helpful:

1. Start with low doses, titrate slowly, and be willing to consider discontinuing drugs with marginal benefit.

2. Expect normal electrolytes and acid-base metabolism in older patients and look for precipitating drugs and intercurrent illnesses when abnormalities occur.

ACKNOWLEDGMENT

The research reported in this chapter was supported in part by NIH grants DK-07006, DK-45191, and by administrative/educational funds from the DCI RED Fund.

SUGGESTED WEB SITES: NEPHROLOGY

http://www.med.umich.edu/usrds/   Contains the text of the yearly U.S. Renal Data Systems report and summaries on dialysis and transplantation in the elderly.
http://nephron.com   Contains a variety of links to CME, quizzes, and general kidney information.
http://www.ajkdjournal.org/atlas/31/1/atlas31_1.htm   One of several sites from Vanderbilt University School of Medicine with pictures/slides of renal pathology.
http:www.sin-italia.org/imago/sediment/sed.htm   Italian site with English text. Urinary sediment is reviewed completely.

BIBLIOGRAPHY

1. Abrass CK: Glomerulonephritis in the elderly. Am J Med 5:409–418, 1985.
2. Cockcroft DW, Gault MH: Prediction of creatinine clearance from serum creatinine. Nephron 16:31–41, 1976.
3. Ismail N, Hakim R, Helderman JH: In-depth review. Renal replacement therapies in the elderly. Part II: Renal transplantation. Am J Kidney Dis 23:1–15, 1994.
4. Ismail N, Hakim R, Oreopoulos DG, Patrikarea A: In-depth review. Renal replacement therapies in the elderly. Part I: Hemodialysis and chronic peritoneal dialysis. Am J Kidney Dis 22:759–782, 1993.
5. Lye WC, Cheah JS, Sinniah R: Renal cholesterol embolic disease. Case report and review of the literature. Am J Nephrol 13:489–493, 1993.

6. Mange K, Matsura D, Cizman B, et al: Language guiding therapy: The case of dehydration versus volume depletion. Ann Intern Med 127:848–853, 1997.
7. Novick AC: Atherosclerotic ischemic nephropathy. Epidemiology and clinical considerations. Urol Clin North Am 21:195–200, 1994.
8. Salazar D, Corcoran G: Predicting creatinine clearance and renal drug clearance in obese patients from estimated fat-free body mass. Am J Med 84:1053–1060, 1988.
9. U.S. Renal Data System: USRDS 1998 Annual Data Report. Bethesda, MD, National Institutes of Health, National Institute of Diabetes and Digestive and Kidney Diseases, 1998.

46. DEHYDRATION

John D. Cacciamani, M.D., and Edna P. Schwab, M.D.

1. Is dehydration a significant cause of illness in the elderly?
Dehydration is a significant cause of mortality in the elderly. Studies have demonstrated that the mortality rate may exceed 50% in hospitalized dehydrated patients if they remain untreated. Other clinical studies have shown that as many as 50% of patients admitted with a primary diagnosis of dehydration die within 1 year after discharge. In addition, the incidence and social costs are significant. Data from the National Hospital Discharge Survey indicate that in 1991 189,000 elderly patients were discharged from short-stay hospitals with the primary diagnosis of dehydration; the average length of stay was 9.8 days. The cost to Medicare was estimated at $1,158,125,000.

2. Why are the elderly at greater risk for dehydration?
• Many elderly people have functional deficits that hinder access to water.
• Elderly patients generally have less total body water than younger patients and therefore less intracellular reserve.
• As one ages, many of the normal hormonal responses to dehydration are depressed.
• Many elderly people have an impaired central thirst mechanism.
• Elderly people are more likely to take medications that exacerbate or even cause dehydration.

3. What are the common signs of dehydration?
The most common physical findings of dehydration include dry mucus membranes, tachycardia, decreased skin turgor, constipation, and orthostatic hypotension. Confusion and disorientation also may be present. In elderly patients, such symptoms are generally more difficult to interpret, and confusion due to dehydration frequently is superimposed on a baseline dementia. Therefore, if dehydration is suspected, a thorough investigation to identify the possible underlying cause is justified.

4. How does one determine whether orthostatic hypotension is present?
Orthostatic hypotension is calculated by measuring the blood pressure and heart rate while the patient is sitting and standing. Wait at least 1 minute between each measurement. A drop in systolic blood pressure of 20 mmHg or a drop in diastolic blood pressure of 10 mmHg represents a positive test. An increase in heart rate of > 10 bpm also indicates a positive test. One must be cautious in interpreting this test for several reasons. Many elderly patients take medications that impair the natural compensatory response. Examples include most antihypertensive medications, particularly beta blockers, which usually diminish heart rate and vasoconstrictive response. Of note, several studies have indicated that 20–30% of community-dwelling elderly have orthostatic changes based on neurologic illness or prolonged bedrest—not on volume depletion.

5. Is there a difference between the normal extracellular volumes of young and elderly adults?
Extracellular volume levels are not significantly different in young and elderly adults of similar sizes. However, the total body water of elderly adults is lower because they have a higher percentage of fat than younger adults. The higher percentage of fat results in a lower percentage of intracellular water. When elderly patients experience dehydration, therefore, they have less intracellular water reserve and become dehydrated more quickly.

6. What are the hormonal differences in young and elderly adults?
Elderly patients have decreased renin activity and decreased aldosterone secretion. In addition, studies have shown that a pure volume stimulus results in lower vasopressin levels

compared with younger adults, yet hyperosmolar stimuli of vasopressin are elevated. Despite the varied response of vasopressin, almost all elderly people demonstrate a relative end-organ resistance to vasopressin. This resistance is believed to have significant consequences, including decreased renal free water retention and impairment of thirst mechanisms. In general, dehydrated elderly adults take longer to correct volume depletion because they are unable to resorb free water and frequently are not thirsty.

7. How is dehydration most frequently categorized?

Dehydration frequently is divided into categories based on sodium status and osmolarity. Differentiating among these forms of dehydration is essential for appropriate treatment. Many clinicians believe that it is best not to simplify the presence of hypovolemia into the general category of dehydration but rather to describe the condition accurately. All forms of dehydration are found in elderly patients, but hypernatremic hypovolemia is more common than hyponatremic hypovolemia.

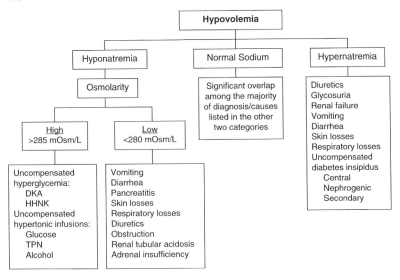

General conditions and causes associated with hypovolemia. DKA = diabetic ketoacidosis; HHNK = hyperglycemic hyperosmolar nonketotic coma; TPN = total parenteral nutrition.

8. What common medical conditions may cause hypernatremic dehydration?

The many causes of hypernatremic dehydration include renal failure, uncompensated diabetes insipidus, and gastrointestinal losses. But the most common cause in the elderly is insensible losses through the skin and lungs, which frequently are exacerbated by fever. If this condition is accompanied by inability to increase oral intake, dehydration results.

9. How should one correct the free water deficits of the elderly hospitalized hypernatremic patient?

The answer requires significant understanding of the patient's clinical condition and medical history. If a patient is in shock and hypotensive, pressure support with normal saline for volume repletion is the highest priority. If the patient is not in shock, other points need to be considered before volume repletion. A patient who has been hypernatremic for some time is at risk for cerebral edema if volume status and sodium status are corrected too quickly. The brain synthesizes idiogenic osmoles to help maintain intracellular volume. These intracellular osmoles counteract the high intravascular osmolarity caused by hypernatremia. Secondary cerebral edema occurs

when the intravascular osmolarity is corrected too quickly, and fluid consequently moves into the cells of the central nervous system. This occurrence is rare, but congestive heart failure in elderly patients after rapid volume repletion is common. As a general rule of thumb for elderly patients, 30–50% of the free water deficit may be repleted in the first 24 hours. The key points:
- Treat symptomatic volume depletion with normal saline.
- Replete ongoing losses with the type of fluid lost.
- Continue to give fluid to cover normal daily requirements.
- Replete 30–50% of the free water deficit in the first 24 hours—no faster.
- Monitor the physical exam and serum sodium to confirm accurate and timely volume repletion.

10. When an elderly patient is dehydrated and has hypernatremia, how do you calculate the free water deficit?

$$FWD = (\text{baseline weight} \times 0.45) - (\text{baseline weight} \times 0.45 \times [140/\text{serum sodium}])$$
$$= (70 \times 0.45) - (70 \times 0.45 \times 140/160)$$
$$= 31.5 - 27.6$$
$$= 3.9 \text{ L}$$

where FWD = free water deficit, baseline weight = 70 kg, and serum sodium = 160. For elderly adults, 0.45 is used as the percentage of free water in the body, whereas in younger adults the percentage is 0.60. As mentioned before, this difference is due to the higher percentage of fat in older adults.

11. What conditions are most commonly associated with hypovolemic hyponatremia?

Hyponatremic dehydration frequently is associated with low serum osmolarity and often coincides with medical conditions such as renal tubular acidosis, adrenal insufficiency, partial renal obstructions, and, most commonly, diuretic effects. Other factors that may result in hyponatremic dehydration are diarrhea, vomiting, and skin losses. The last three also may present as hypernatremic dehydration and isotonic dehydration with normal serum sodium.

12. Is urine osmolarity a good measure for dehydration in elderly adults?

The normal renal response to dehydration is to retain water and thus to concentrate urine. This results in higher urine osmolarity, especially compared with plasma osmolarity. Yet in elderly adults, the kidney's response to vasopressin is often impaired. Thus the concentrating capacity is diminished. Therefore, the increase in urine osmolarity frequently underestimates the degree of dehydration.

13. Is measuring the blood urea nitrogen useful in measuring the volume status of elderly adults?

Measuring blood urea nitrogen helps to determine prerenal azotemia. In younger patients a ratio > 20:1 suggests prerenal azotemia. In general, the elderly have a decreased glomerular filtration rate and increased protein turnover; therefore, a ratio > 28:1 suggests dehydration. Other causes of an elevated ratio include renal vascular disease, gastrointestinal bleeding, obstructive uropathy, and steroid-induced catabolism, which may or may not be associated with concomitant dehydration.

14. Does incontinence contribute to dehydration?

Incontinence can indirectly result in dehydration. Because many elderly adults are fearful of having an incontinent episode in public, they severely restrict their fluid intake. Care should be taken to identify such patients. Encourage water intake; then diagnose and treat the incontinence.

15. What medications put patients at risk of dehydration?

The most common medications that cause dehydration are diuretics. Several psychiatric medications may result in dehydration. Lithium, in particular, may cause diabetes insipidus. Pain medications that alter mental status, such as opiates, ares notorious for resulting in decreased oral intake and secondarily cause dehydration. In addition, the osmolarity and malabsorption associated with enteral tube feedings may result in diarrhea and dehydration.

16. What is hypodermoclysis (HDC)?

HDC is rehydration therapy in which fluid is infused directly into the subcutaneous tissue. This method usually is used for patients who are dehydrated but have poor IV access or are in a nursing home where IV access is not an authorized procedure. HDC was used more frequently in the 1950s and 1960s. During the 1960s a high incidence of infection and sepsis was noted; therefore, the practice was almost abolished. Since the advent of improved sterile methods and the creation of disposable catheters, the incidence of infection has decreased significantly. HDC is performed by inserting a catheter into the subcutaneous tissue of the abdomen, leg, or gluteal region and then infusing fluids. Normal saline is best tolerated, but 5% dextrose in water also may be given if it is supplemented with sodium. Maximal infusion rate is 1500 ml/day per site. No more than two concurrent sites are recommended. In the past hyaluronidase was added to the infusion solution to decrease pain and augment fluid resorption, but recent studies have shown that it does neither. Its use is no longer recommended.

17. Do patients with Alzheimer's disease have a greater risk of dehydration than other elderly patients?

Some studies suggest that patients with Alzheimer's disease have depressed vasopressin levels compared with age-matched controls. This finding was not always statistically significant and has not been directly associated with an increase in the incidence of dehydration. Nevertheless, this finding in combination with impaired mental status should alert the physician to monitor this type of patient carefully for dehydration.

18. Is the normal fluid volume of tube feedings adequate for most elderly patients?

In most cases enteral tube feedings do not have adequate amounts of free water. Free water needs to be supplemented to meet daily free water requirements. In general, total daily free water requirements range from 1.5–2 L/day.

19. What simple methods help to prevent dehydration during periods of extreme heat?

The most important factors are to drink at least 8 glasses of water per day during hot weather and to stay out of direct sunlight as much as possible. Because the elderly have diminished hormonal and central nervous system response to dehydration and temperature changes, they are at extreme risk for dehydration during hot and humid days. The best way to stay cool is to stay within an air-conditioned home. If this is not possible, fans should be used liberally. In addition, dampening clothes or adding moistened towels onto or over a fan can help to keep a room cool.

BIBLIOGRAPHY

1. Albert S, Nakra B, Grossberg GT, Caminal ER: Vasopressin response to dehydration in Alzheimer's disease. J Am Geriatr Soc 37:843–847, 1989.
2. Ferry M, Dardaine V, Constans T: Subcutaneous infusion or hypodermoclysis: A practical approach. J Am Geriatr Soc 47:93–95, 1999.
3. Lavizzo-Mourey R, Johnson J, Stolley P: Risk factors for dehydration among elderly nursing home residents. J Am Geriatr Soc 36:213–218, 1988.
4. Leaf A: Dehydration in the elderly. N Engl J Med 311:791–792, 1984.
5. Phillips PA, Rolls BJ, Ledingham JG, et al: Reduced thirst after water deprivation in elderly men. N Engl J Med 311:791–792, 1984.
6. Snyder N, Feigal DW, Arieff AI: Hypernatremia in elderly patients: A heterogeneous, morbid, and iatrogenic entity. Ann Intern Med 107:309–319, 1987.
7. Weinberg AD, Minaker KL: Dehydration: Evaluation and management in older adults. JAMA 274:1552–1556, 1995.

47. PRESSURE ULCERS

Robert Goldman, M.D.

1. What are pressure ulcers? Where and how do they occur?

Pressure ulcers are areas of skin disruptions consisting of focal necrosis of epidermis, dermis, subdermis, fascia, muscle, or joint capsule. They are caused by excessive, prolonged pressure that produces ischemia to soft tissue over bony prominences (hot spots) such as the greater trochanter of the femur, sacrum, ischial tuberosity, or calcaneus. Injury may occur from prolonged sitting or lying without transient relief of pressure. Although commonly observed on patients that are bed-bound or bedfast, the term *pressure ulcer* is preferable to "bedsores" or "decubitus ulcers." Pressure ulcer better describes the cause, and because ulcers also occur on sitting patients, the other terms are not accurate descriptors.

2. What is the relationship of pressure to ulcer formation?

Unrelieved axial pressure of 4–6 times systolic blood pressure causes necrosis in as short as 1 hour, but pressure similar to systolic requires 12 hours to cause a similar lesion. Shear, defined as force tangential to the skin surface, causes ulceration at markedly lower axial pressure. Skin moisture aggravates both axial and shear forces and predisposes to breakdown; ischemic change occurs in response to compromised capillary perfusion. Periodic pressure relief increases resistance of tissue to breakdown. Therefore, sitting patients should be instructed to lift their buttocks from the seat at least 15 seconds every 30 minutes. Supine patients should be turned every 2 hours.

3. How are pressure ulcers assessed and classified?

The National Pressure Ulcer Advisory Panel (NPUAP) classification, which is partially based on the well-known Shea system, is recommended:

Stage I	Nonblanchable skin erythema (difficult to assess in patients with heavily pigmented skin)
Stage II	Breakdown into dermis, but not subcutaneous tissues (i.e., subdermis)
Stage III	Ulcer extends from subcutaneous depth to fascia
Stage IV	Ulcer extends from depth of the fascia to bone

Serial reassessments of area and depth, at no longer than weekly intervals, quantify healing and assess the success of current treatment strategies. The simplest method is to measure the length along major and minor axes. A more quantitative technique is to trace the ulcer margin onto an acetate sheet (i.e., for photocopying transparencies) with a laundry marker, placing polyethylene film (e.g., Saran Wrap) between the ulcer and the sheet. Photography assesses the ulcer's appearance and size. Depth should be documented with swabs.

4. What interventions relieve pressure and shear?

- Placing pillows or other cushioning between trochanteric prominences and bed for side-lying patients
- Keeping the bed as horizontal as possible
- Using heel protectors
- Using special beds and mattresses

There is a wide spectrum of choice, with maximal efficiency of pressure and shear relief correlated with maximal cost. For patients with stage IV ulcers or stage III ulcers with spinal cord injury, low air loss (e.g., SAR Low Air Loss Mattress System) or air fluidized systems (e.g., Clinitron) are suggested. Less effective for pressure reduction and much lower in price are foam mattresses (e.g., "Sof-care" mattress). Seating systems for wheelchairs are issued to many patients who lack protective sensation or cannot shift weight. Examples are air-filled vinous (e.g., Roho), contoured foam with a gel insert (e.g., Jay), or contoured foam (e.g., polyurethane) with or without protective cover. A solid seat (rather than the usual sling seat) may be prescribed for stability. Doughnut-shaped air cushions are not recommended, because pressure at the margin of the cushion exceeds the safe limit.

5. Which patients are most likely to develop pressure ulcers?

The mnemonic **DECUBITUS** is suggested as a learning aid.

D **D**elirium, **d**ementia, **d**ependence. Only a patient with a clear mind can act purposefully to relieve a noxious stimulus. Therefore, patients with altered mental status, such as coma or severe dementia, are at risk for skin breakdown. Patients at risk of pressure ulcers are partially or completely dependent on others. Patients who require one or two persons to assist them in getting into bed are at high risk for ulceration.

E **E**lderly. Seventy percent of pressure ulcers occur in the elderly. Frailty, dependence, incontinence, chronic illness, and degenerative neurologic disease increase with age. Associated with aging are diminished pain perception and blunting of the inflammatory response. Histologic changes in skin include flattening of the dermal-epidermal junction and reduced elastin content, both of which increase susceptibility to shear and minor laceration. Ulcer closure is delayed because of reduced rates of both reepithelialization and contraction.

C **C**ontractures. If severe, contractures prevent routine turning and positioning on most mattress types. Thus they contribute to delayed healing and increased incidence.

U **U**rinary incontinence. Wet skin is easily macerated. If the urine is infected, the skin and any ulcers will be contaminated.

B **B**owel incontinence. Soiling may lead to bacterial colonization or local infection. The wet skin associated with diarrhea also contributes to ulcer formation.

I **I**mmobility. Chronic bed rest leads to a decrease in lean muscle mass of 5% per week and contributes to osteoporosis and contractures through collagen remodeling within tendons and joint capsules. Immobility feeds a vicious cycle of wasting, contractures, pressure "hot spots," and worsening ulceration.

T **T**ension O_2 low. Ischemia is related to ulcer formation. Anemia should be corrected (e.g., by iron supplementation). Edema impairs gas and nutrient exchange between healing tissue and the blood supply.

U **U**ndernourishment. Inadequate caloric or protein intake may result in malnutrition and impaired ulcer healing. (See question 10.)

S **S**pasticity, **s**ensory loss, **s**pinal cord injury. By several mechanisms, neurologic injury predisposes to pressure ulcer formation:

  • Spasticity (increased muscle tone) predisposes to contracture formation and poor mobility.
  • Lack of protective sensation, which leads to pressure ulcer formation, may be dermotomal with spinal cord injury or hemisensory with stroke.
  • Spinal cord injury, especially above T6, is related to sympathetic nervous system dysfunction and impaired skin perfusion at sites of pressure.

6. What are occlusive or semiocclusive dressings? How are they used in pressure ulcer care?

Occlusive dressings create a barrier against moisture loss and a seal with normal skin around the ulcer. A moist environment results, with (semiocclusive) or without (occlusive) oxygen exchange. This moist milieu promotes formation of granulation tissue. The concern that an occluded environment brings about infection has not been substantiated for ulcers that do not appear clinically infected. The choice to use one or the other is more a matter of personal preference than influence on wound-healing kinetics. Occlusive dressings form a better seal with skin outside the ulcer margin and thus resist contamination more effectively. Examples of occlusive dressings include polyurethane film (e.g., Tegaderm, OpSite), hydrocolloid (e.g., Duoderm), and hydrocolloid gel (e.g., Vigilon). The following treatment examples must be confirmed by experienced practitioners for specific cases:

Stage I: Cover with an occlusive dressing to prevent continued shear. Change weekly, when the dressing becomes dislodged, or when the ulcer seal is broken.

Stage II, III or IV: Treatment depends on appearance of ulcer base.
- Clean ulcers have beefy red granulation tissue without fibrinous material.
  - Use wet-to-wet dressings. Examples are saline-soaked gauze and calcium alginate (e.g., Sorbsain) or hydrocolloid gel (both covered by polyurethane film). The surrounding skin should be kept dry, if possible, to avoid maceration.
- Ulcers with a white to yellow film (i.e., fibrinous exudate) require debridement (see question 7).
  - Black, hard eschar (most often found on the heel), according to the Pressure Ulcer Advisory Panel, should be covered with dry gauze for protection and not debrided if "clean and dry."

7. What types of debridement are used for ulcer care? What are their indications?

Devitalized tissue promotes infection and is a barrier to reepithelialization. Therefore, it should be debrided by mechanical, enzymatic, or autolytic means. Examples of **mechanical methods** include (1) manual (i.e., surgical or "sharps") debridement, (2) wet-to-dry dressings, and (3) irrigation. Sharps debridement is usually reserved for thick or adherent eschar or infected ulcers. Eschar (and, unfortunately, viable tissue) adheres to wet-to-dry dressings during removal; hence, the method is slower to work. Prepare by soaking gauze pads in saline, wringing out the liquid, completely unraveling, loosely packing all cavities of the ulcer, covering with dry gauze, and securing with paper tape. Hydrotherapy is usually performed by physical therapists for fibrinous stage III or IV ulcers (or locally infected ulcers; see question 11). Irrigation can also be done at the bedside with, for instance, a 50-ml syringe, 19-gauge Angiocath, and normal saline. **Enzymatic debridement** (e.g., Elase) uses collagenase and other protease to break down eschar. It works slowly and is therefore used mostly in institutional or home settings. **Autolytic debridement** depends on proteolytic enzymes in ulcer fluid and is the slowest acting.

8. Should topical antiseptics, such as Betadine, peroxide, or sodium hypochlorite (i.e., Daken's) solution, be used routinely?

No, according to current guidelines. Overall, these agents retard epithelialization in animal models and are toxic to fibroblasts in vitro. However, this point is controversial. Some researchers point to animal studies suggesting that short-term, low-dose treatment may not delay healing. Some of the discrepancy may lie in how the agent is applied to the wound and the definition of healing. Animal studies that use daily application of topical agents and measure the time to 50% healing demonstrate reductions in healing rate. Studies that apply single doses of topical agent or measure time to 100% healing show no difference.

9. What is the role of adjunctive treatment?

- **Electrotherapy:** Both decubitus and leg ulcers reportedly heal more rapidly with electrotherapy. Short "high-voltage" pulsed electrotherapy, such as high volt pulsed galvanic stimulation (HVPGS), has been sanctioned to "promote local blood flow" by the Food and Drug Administration (FDA). However, the FDA has not specifically sanctioned electrotherapy for wound healing. This disparity has led to inconsistencies in Medicare reimbursement for this service.
- **Growth factor therapy:** Important wound healing phenomena include wound cell proliferation, extracellular matrix formation, and neoangiogenesis, which are all controlled by ubiquitous soluble proteins called growth factors. One of the best studied growth substances is platelet derived growth factor (PDGF). Rh-PDGF-BB (recombinant PDGF, BB isoform) has recently been FDA-approved for treatment of neuropathic, diabetic foot ulcers under the trade name Regranex®. Beyond foot ulcers, pressure ulcers

of the buttocks respond to PDGF-BB in limited clinical trials, but the FDA has yet to approve use of growth factors on pressure ulcers. Therefore, pressure ulcers are treated with growth factors in only a few specialized centers.

10. What is the role of nutrition in the prevention and treatment of pressure ulcers?

A pressure ulcer may be a sign of malnutrition. Indicators of poor nutrition include a serum albumin of < 3.5 mg/dl, total lymphocyte count of < 1,800 mm^3, and body weight decrease of > 15%. Determining that the prealbumin is low is a sensitive measure of malnutrition, if available. Goals of nutrition therapy are correction of the above indices as well as a positive nitrogen balance (1.25–1.5 gm of protein/kg/day). Important vitamins for ulcer healing include vitamin C, vitamin A, and zinc. Supplementation of these substances is of questionable benefit if serum levels are normal.

11. How is an infected ulcer diagnosed and managed?

A foul smell, greenish or copious drainage, scant granulation, and dull whitish or pink base (rather than bright red granulation tissue) indicate local infection. Cellulitis is an invasion of organisms beyond ulcer margins, marked by erythema, warmth, swelling, or tenderness. Signs of bacteremia or systemic invasion include fever, elevated white count, change of mental status, or increasing insulin requirements in diabetics.

The surfaces of all ulcers are colonized by bacteria; therefore, ulcer cultures should not be performed routinely. An indication for culture is abscess, freshly exposed. Surface swabs are misleading, because they do not isolate the causative organism. However, qualitative culture of tissue below the ulcer surface, collected under sterile conditions, is more definitive. It is routinely performed in hospital microbiology laboratories. Quantitative culture is most definitive, and results are described as colony-forming units (CFU) per gram of tissue. At levels above 10^5 CFU, ulcers heal poorly. However, quantitative culture may not be available in community hospitals.

Clinical infection is almost always polymicrobial, including both facultative aerobes and strict anaerobes. Aerobic organisms are usually found in surface swabs, whereas anaerobes are more often isolated from deep tissue and blood. In one study deep tissue isolates included *Proteus mirabilis,* group D streptococci, *Escherichia coli, Staphylococcus aureus, Pseudomonas aeruginosa, Bacteroides fragilis,* and *Peptostreptococcus* species. Anaerobes are associated with ulcers having necrotic material and foul odor.

For locally infected ulcers, start a course of frequent ulcer inspection and mechanical debridement (e.g., wet-to-dry dressings and hydrotherapy). The Pressure Ulcer Advisory Panel recommends application of topical bactericidal agents only if infection does not resolve within 1 week. For systemic signs of infection, such as chills or sweats, fever or drop in body temperature, hypotension, or glucose intolerance (in diabetics), broad-spectrum coverage is recommended, because infection is usually polymicrobial. Urgent surgical debridement is required, because bacteremia doubtless will not clear without removal of necrotic material or drainage of abscess.

12. How is osteomyelitis in a pressure ulcer diagnosed and treated?

Osteomyelitis should be suspected in stage IV decubiti. However, the gold standard, a bone biopsy, is usually not done except as part of aggressive debridement. There is much controversy about the best noninvasive test for osteomyelitis. An elevated erythrocyte sedimentation rate, elevated white blood cell count, and positive plain x-ray, taken together, are 88% specific and 89% sensitive for osteomyelitis. (A plain film is positive in the presence of reactive bone formation and periosteal elevation.) For difficult cases, imaging studies with optimum diagnostic power include magnetic resonance imaging (MRI) and indium 111 leukocyte scanning. Indium leukocyte scanning has a sensitivity and specificty of 88% and 85%, respectively; in a review of 11 studies MRI has a sensitivity and specificity of 95% and 88%, respectively. In addition, MRI provides pathoanatomic detail (e.g., on location of sinus tracts or abscesses). In the presence of an infected ulcer and positive plain film, bone biopsy should be performed with needle aspiration through intact skin. The biopsy is positive if it shows a chronic inflammatory infiltrate (plasma cells, lymphocytes) and positive quantitative culture > 10^3 organisms/gm of bone.

13. When should surgical closure be considered?

Surgical closure should be done when the patient does not progress with optimal care, including available adjunctive care. In addition, the patient must agree to and be able to tolerate surgery, which may involve extensive blood loss, and osteomyelitis must be adequately treated. Frequently, stage IV ulcers require surgical evaluation. Musculocutaneous flaps are usually the treatment of choice. However, for the flap to be successful, pressure relief must be addressed; if inadequate pressure relief was the original cause of the ulcer, the skin is likely to break down again.

14. Should the goal of ulcer care always be complete healing?

Not all ulcers will heal, even with optimal care. Motivation of the patient and compliance with therapies are critical for a successful outcome. Factors associated with a high risk of non-healing include:

- Bacterial colonization by $> 10^5$ CFU/gm of tissue
- Osteomyelitis (25% of nonhealing ulcers)
- Chronic granulation for > 30 years (may indicate malignancy, with biopsies consistent with epidermoid cancer [Marjolin's ulcer])

15. What is the differential diagnosis for pressure ulcers?

Skin conditions that cause erythema around perianal, perineal, or gluteal skin folds may be confused with stage I and stage II pressure ulcers. Examples include dermatophytosis (tinea cruris), *Candida albicans* (often associated with vaginal monilia), and intertrigo. Contact dermatitis also should be considered. Herpes zoster classically presents with vesicles and crusts and may occur around sacral dermatomes. Skin ulceration has a long differential diagnosis. However, subcutaneous and dermal ulcers at bony prominences at the ischium, gluteal fold, or sacrum usually are caused by pressure. In contrast, ulceration of the lower extremities may be vascular, arterial, or infectious.

16. Can a pressure ulcer be a marker for abuse?

Yes. A pressure ulcer is likely to occur in a neglected, bed-bound patient. Unintentional abuse may result from inexperience, excessive caregiver burden, or lack of motivation. Elder abuse should be considered in the following settings:

- The caregiver has a history of mental illness or alcohol or drug abuse, is socially isolated, or has undergone recent stressful life events.
- The dependent patient presents with signs of dehydration, malnutrition, or poor personal hygiene in addition to the ulcer.

BIBLIOGRAPHY

1. Clinical Practice Guideline: Treatment of Pressure Ulcers. Rockville, MD, U.S. Department of Health and Human Services, Agency for Health Care Policy and Research, 1994, AHCPR publicatioin 950652.
2. Harding KG: Methods for assessing change in ulcer status. Adv Wound Care 8:37–42, 1995.
3. Kertesz C, Chow AW: Infected pressure and diabetic ulcers. Clin Geriatr Med 8:835–852, 1992.
4. Kosiak M: Etiology and pathology of ischemic ulcers. Arch Phys Med Rehabil 40:62–68, 1959.
5. Makleburst J: Pressure ulcer staging systems. Adv Wound Care 8:11–13, 1995.
6. Margolis DJ: Definition of a pressure ulcer. Adv Wound Care 8:8–10, 1995.
7. Ruan CM, Escobedo E, Harrison S, Goldstein B: Magnetic resonance imaging of nonhealing pressure ulcers and myocutaneous flaps. Arch Phys Med Rehabil 79:1080–1088, 1998.
8. Salcido R, Hart D, Smith AM: The prevention and management of pressure ulcers. In Braddom RL (ed): Physical Medicine and Rehabilitation. Philadelphia, W.B. Saunders, 1996, pp 630–647.
9. Yarkony GM: Pressure ulcers: A review. Arch Phys Med Rehabil 75:908–917, 1994.

48. URINARY INCONTINENCE

Grace A. Cordts, M.D., M.S., M.P.H.

1. What is urinary incontinence?

Urinary incontinence (UI) is a significant cause of disability and dependency, especially among the elderly. It is estimated that 15–30% of community-dwelling older people and 50% of institutionalized older people suffer from UI. UI is defined as the involuntary loss of urine, severe enough to cause social or hygienic problems. Potential adverse effects include social isolation, depression, stress, skin breakdown, recurrent urinary tract infections, falls, and high economic costs.

2. How do you identify patients with UI?

At least one-half of older patients with incontinence can improve without extensive evaluations and interventions. The problem arises in identifying people with UI. Because of the long-held belief that UI is a normal part of aging, many patients do not seek help from their primary care provider. Even if patients complain of UI, many health care professionals are reluctant to discuss the problem or to offer adequate evaluation and treatment. The importance of identifying and treating UI is reflected in the fact that UI was one of the first clinical guidelines to be tackled by the Agency for Health Care Policy and Research (AHCPR).

Questions about UI should become a part of the health care provider's initial and ongoing evaluation. Health care providers should ask elderly patients and, if appropriate, their family and caregivers about UI. Questions such as "Do you have trouble holding your urine?" are effective ways to open discussion of UI. They can be followed with specific questions, such as, "Do you ever lose urine when you don't want to?," "Do you ever have difficulty getting to the bathroom?," and "Do you ever wear a pad to collect your urine?" If the answer to any of these questions is yes, further evaluation should be undertaken.

3. How is UI classified?

The initial clinical classification consists of two categories: acute reversible forms and persistent incontinence. Acute reversible UI has a sudden onset and is usually associated with an acute medical illness or an iatrogenic cause. Persistent UI occurs over time and is unrelated to acute events. Acute reversible factors may contribute to and worsen persistent UI.

4. What can cause acute reversible UI?

D **D**elirium
R **R**estricted mobility, retention
I **I**nfection, inflammation, impaction
P **P**olyuria, pharmaceutics

Patients with delirium may become unaware of the urge to void or be unable to get themselves to a toilet. When the delirium resolves, urinary continence returns.

Any condition that acutely restricts mobility can precipitate functional incontinence or worsen persistent incontinence. Such conditions include fractured hip, stroke, Parkinson's disease, use of restraints, or exacerbation of arthritis.

Urinary retention due to medication or anatomic obstructions can cause overflow incontinence.

Acute urinary tract infections can cause new onset of UI. Inflammatory conditions such as atrophic vaginitis and urethritis may precipitate incontinence. Fecal impaction is a common cause of acute UI.

Any condition that causes polyuria can precipitate UI. Glucosuria and calciuria are common metabolic problems. Congestive heart failure and venous insufficiency cause edema and nocturia, precipitating nocturnal urinary incontinence. The list of medications that precipitate incontinence is long. Examples include alcohol, calcium channel blockers, beta-adrenergic agonists, alpha-adrenergic agonists, alpha-adrenergic blockers, narcotic analgesics, psychotropics, anti-cholinergics, and diuretics. Medications are implicated in acute urinary incontinence if urinary incontinence develops soon after the drug is started. Medications should be stopped when possible.

5. How is persistent UI classified?

Persistent UI can be classified in several ways, including anatomic, pathophysiologic, and clinical. The clinical classification is most useful for practicing physicians because it helps direct clinical evaluation and intervention. The clinical categories include the following:

1. **Stress incontinence**—involuntary loss of urine when intra-abdominal pressure increases, as during coughing, sneezing, or exercising. A common cause is relaxation of pelvic floor musculature. It is the most common cause of UI in people under the age of 75 years. It is more common in women but may occur in men if the anatomic sphincters are damaged after transurethral surgery or radiation therapy. Patients complain of losing urine when laughing, coughing, or standing. The amount of urine lost varies from a small amount that requires no intervention to large amounts that require intervention.

2. **Urge incontinence**—involuntary loss of urine associated with the sensation of the desire to void. Urge incontinence is usually, but not always, associated with involuntary detrusor contractions (detrusor overactivity). Neurologic problems are often associated with this type of incontinence, including stroke, dementia, Parkinson's disease, and spinal cord injury. If a neurologic disorder is present, it is called detrusor hyperreflexia; if no neurologic disorder is present, it is called detrusor instability. Patients complain that they do not have enough time to get to the bathroom after they have the urge to void. It is the most common cause of incontinence in people over 75. One variation of urge incontinence is detrusor hyperactivity with impaired contractility. Patients have involuntary contractions but do not empty the bladder completely. They have symptoms of urge incontinence and high postvoid residuals. They may also have symptoms of obstruction, stress incontinence, and overflow incontinence. It is important to identify this condition because it can mimic other types of incontinence and may be treated inappropriately.

3. **Overflow incontinence**—involuntary loss of urine associated with overdistention of the bladder. It is caused by an anatomic obstruction, such as prostate enlargement; neurogenic factors, such as diabetes, detrusor areflexia, or multiple sclerosis, that result in an underactive or acontractile bladder; or medications, such as anticholinergics, narcotics, or antipsychotics.

4. **Functional incontinence**—involuntary loss of urine secondary to factors outside the lower urinary tract. Common causes are severe dementia, severe musculoskeletal problems, neurologic problems, psychological problems, and environmental factors that make access to a bathroom difficult. This is a diagnosis of exclusion; even frail elderly patients with significant dementia and physical impairments can have treatable causes of UI.

Frequently, UI in elderly patients presents with a variety of symptoms and a urodynamic picture of more than one type of UI. Correct treatment requires identification of all components.

6. Discuss the neurophysiology and anatomy of continence.

To be continent, a person must be able to recognize that his or her bladder is full and to get to a bathroom. Although this sounds easy, it is a complex physiologic process involving autonomic reflexes and volitional control. It involves the bladder, urethra, and pelvic floor musculature as well as their neural pathways.

Anatomically, the lower urinary tract consists of the bladder, urethra, internal sphincter, and external sphincter. The bladder is made up of a smooth muscle, called the detrusor muscle, that can contract in all directions. The urethra is 4 cm in women and 20 cm in men. The urethral mucosa in women is maintained by estrogen. The mucosa atrophies in estrogen-deficient states. There is a 90° angle between the bladder and urethra. Normal pelvic geometry allows intra-abdominal pressure to be distributed equally to the urethra and bladder. Therefore, when intra-abdominal pressure increases from coughing or laughing, urinary leakage is prevented. The internal sphincter is located at the base of the bladder and consists of smooth muscle. The external sphincter, which is made up of smooth muscle and striated muscle, allows voluntary interruption of voiding.

The lower urinary tract is innervated by parasympathetic, sympathetic, and somatic nerves. Parasympathetic cholinergic nerves from the sacral micturition center innervate the bladder. Stimulation causes the bladder to contract. The bladder base, neck, and internal sphincter are supplied by alpha-adrenergic sympathetic nerves from the hypogastric plexus. Stimulation of these nerves causes contraction of the bladder neck and urethra. Beta-adrenergic fibers from the hypogastric plexus connect to the detrusor muscle. Stimulation causes bladder relaxation. In addition, sympathetic nerve fibers inhibit parasympathetic tone. Stimulation of the pudendal nerve, which innervates the pelvic floor musculature, results in increased tone of the pelvic floor muscles. (See figure below.)

Thus, urine storage can be considered primarily a sympathetic process. Stimulation of the sympathetic fibers causes relaxation of the bladder and contraction of the bladder neck and urethra. Urination can be viewed as primarily a parasympathetic process with stimulation of the nerves causing contraction of the bladder.

Higher centers in the brainstem, cerebral cortex, and cerebellum can influence the lower urinary tract and thus affect voiding. (See figure, next page.) As the bladder fills, sensory impulses are sent to the detrusor motor nucleus in the pons. This nucleus fires, causing the detrusor to contract and the sphincter to relax, allowing urination (Loop II). Neurons in the frontal lobe can inhibit the pontine nucleus and thus stop urination. Disorders of the cerebral cortex, such as stroke, Parkinson's disease, or dementia, and disorders of the brainstem can cause incontinence (Loop I). There are involuntary controls over the pelvic floor musculature (Loop III). Neurons in the frontal lobe can control voluntarily the external urethra and pelvic floor musculature (Loop IV). Knowledge of the anatomy and physiology helps to elucidate the cause of incontinence and possible treatment modalities.

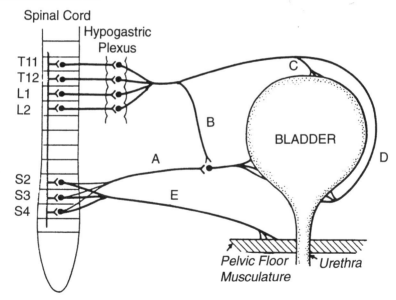

TYPE OF NERVE	FUNCTION
A PARASYMPATHETIC CHOLINERGIC (Nervi Erigentes)	Bladder contraction
B SYMPATHETIC	Bladder relaxation (by inhibition of parasympathetic tone
C SYMPATHETIC	Bladder relaxation (β-adrenergic)
D SYMPATHETIC	Bladder neck and urethral contraction (α-adrenergic)
E SOMATIC (Pudendal nerve)	Contraction of pelvic floor musculature

Parasympathetic, sympathetic, and somatic innervation of the bladder. (From Ouslander JG: Geriatric urinary incontinence. Dis Mon 38:67–149, 1992, with permission.)

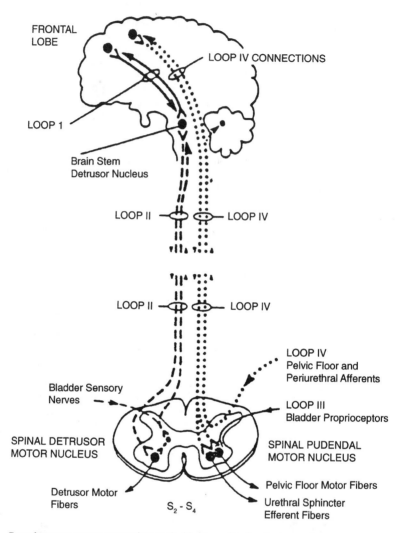

Central nervous system connections to the bladder and periurethral musculature.

7. What normal changes in the urinary tract are associated with aging?

As with all systems of the body, age-related changes affect the lower urinary tract. Such changes predispose an elderly person to incontinence but do not cause incontinence per se. Thus, incontinence is not a normal part of aging. Aging involves decreases in estrogen, bladder capacity, urethral pressure, and urinary flow rate and increases in uninhibited detrusor contractions, postvoid residuals, nocturnal urine production, and prostate size. Despite these predisposing factors, usually an added insult precipitates incontinence. Such insults are typically reversible causes outside the lower urinary tract. Treating the added insult often cures the incontinence.

8. What is the goal of the basic evaluation of UI?

The goal of the initial evaluation is to confirm UI and to identify transient causes, patients who need further evaluation, and patients who can begin treatment without extensive testing. This goal can be accomplished with a careful history, a complete physical exam, simple bedside testing, and a few laboratory tests.

9. What is the focus of the history in a UI evaluation?

A thorough history begins the work-up, as in any other medical evaluation. The history should focus on details of the symptoms, looking for clues to determine the type, pathophysiology, and precipitating factors:

- Duration and characteristics of UI
- Timing and amount of both continent and incontinent urination
- Fluid intake; type and amount—caffeine, alcohol
- Other symptoms, such as nocturia, dysuria, frequency, hematuria, pain
- Associated events—cough, surgery, new diabetes, new medications
- Alterations in bowel or bladder function
- Use of absorbent pads or other protective devices
- Previous treatment of UI and its effects

The medical history should focus on problems such as diabetes, congestive heart failure, venous insufficiency, cancer, neurologic problems, stroke, and Parkinson's disease. The genitourinary history should include any abdominal or pelvic surgery, childbirth, or urinary tract infections. A review of medications, both prescribed and over-the-counter, is important. Many classes of drugs are particularly associated with UI, including sedative-hypnotics, diuretics, anticholinergic agents, adrenergic agents, and calcium channel blockers. There is usually a time connection between the use of these medications and onset of incontinence or worsening of chronic incontinence.

10. What should the physical exam include?

The goals of the physical exam are to identify causes precipitating incontinence and to help establish pathophysiology. In addition to a complete general physical exam, the physician should concentrate on the abdomen, genitalia, rectum, neurologic function, and, in women, the pelvis.

Key Aspects of the Physical Exam

Abdominal exam	Identify bladder fullness, tenderness, masses, surgery
Rectal exam	Identify stool impaction, sphincter tone, perineal sensation, bulbocavernous reflex, prostate nodules, rectal masses
Genital exam	Identify anatomic abnormalities, skin condition
Pelvic exam	Identify muscle atrophy, genital atrophy, masses, pelvic organ prolapse, muscle tone
Neurologic exam	Identify treatable disorders, spinal cord compression, stroke Evaluate cognitive status
Functional status	Identify ability to use bathroom, dress and undress, ambulate

11. Which simple bedside evaluation should be done?

Simple urodynamic testing can be done at the bedside without the use of expensive technical equipment. Postvoid residual (PVR) should be estimated by physical exam. A specific measurement can be made with ultrasound or urinary catheterization. Bladder ultrasound is commonly used to test for PVR. It is noninvasive and therefore does not involve the risk of introducing infection as urinary catheterization does. It requires equipment costing from $6,000 to $10,000. Stress-induced leakage can also be evaluated at the bedside with direct visualization. This evaluation should be done when the patient has a full bladder with the urge to void. The patient is asked to cough while in the lithotomy and standing positions. Leakage can easily be seen. Bladder filling can be evaluated by a simple technique outlined by Ouslander,[3] although interpretation of the data involves potential errors. Information can be obtained on first urge to void, presence or absence of involuntary bladder contractions, and bladder capacity.

12. Which laboratory studies should be done?

Urinalysis should be done for all patients to evaluate hematuria, pyuria, bacteriuria, glyco-suria, and proteinuria. Serum electrolytes, blood urea nitrogen, creatinine, glucose, and calcium are assessed to determine baseline renal function and conditions causing polyuria.

13. Are voiding records useful?

Voiding records track voiding patterns. They are used to record the timing and amount of continent and incontinent voids and symptoms associated with UI. They can clarify symptoms or identify factors contributing to UI. They can be used in an ambulatory or institutional setting. They are kept for 1–3 days. The records can also be used to monitor therapeutic response. Keeping the records can be a therapeutic intervention because it makes patients aware of precipitating factors associated with incontinent episodes.

14. Who should be referred?

Most geriatric patients with UI can be helped by health care professionals without invasive testing. Patients should be referred to specialists for more invasive evaluation and testing in the following settings:

- Hematuria without infection
- UI with recurrent symptomatic urinary tract infections
- PVR > 200 ml
- Prostate nodule
- Diagnosis is unclear and a rational plan cannot be developed from bedside evaluation
- Failure to respond to adequate therapeutic trial
- Symptomatic pelvic prolapse
- Other symptoms that indicate a more serious underlying problem
- Recent history of lower urinary tract surgery, pelvic surgery, or radiation treatment

15. What are the mainstays of treatment?

Treatment of UI consists of behavioral, pharmacologic, and surgical interventions. The rule of thumb in choosing a therapeutic option is that the least invasive and least dangerous should be used first. A combination of surgical, behavioral, and pharmacologic treatment may help. The optimal treatment strategy depends on the patient, type of UI, and risk-benefit ratio of each intervention. The success of each modality depends on the accurate identification of the cause of UI.

16. Describe the behavioral techniques.

Behavioral techniques present little risk to the patient and may provide a decrease in UI frequency. General strategies include education of the patient or caregiver and positive reinforcement when progress is made. Specific techniques include bladder training, habit training, prompted voiding, and pelvic muscle exercises. High-tech techniques that can supplement and enhance behavioral methods include biofeedback, electrical stimulation, and vaginal cone retention.

Bladder retraining involves progressive increases in the intervals between mandatory voiding with distraction or relaxation techniques. It requires that the patient resist or inhibit the sensation to void. It has been shown to be helpful in urge and stress incontinence.

Habit training requires scheduled toileting. It is most successful when the timed toileting is matched with the patient's natural voiding pattern. It is best used with functional incontinence and requires staff or caregiver involvement.

Prompted voiding attempts to teach patients to recognize their continence status and to request toileting. It has been used successfully in patients with cognitive impairment in nursing homes.

Pelvic muscle or Kegel exercises involve repetitive contraction of the pelvic floor muscles. By strengthening the pelvic floor, these exercises help to increase closing pressure on the urethra and support of the pelvic structures. They are helpful for stress and urge incontinence.

An adjunct to behavioral techniques is evaluation of the **physical and social environment**, including toilet access, clothing that makes disrobing easier, chairs that are easy to rise from, and accessible call system.

17. How do you instruct a patient to do Kegel exercises?

Women are instructed to contract the muscles of the pelvic floor by contracting the muscles used to stop the stream of urine. This approach can be tricky because many women recruit abdominal muscles and perform a Valsalva maneuver without contracting the pelvic floor muscles. Women can be taught to contract the correct muscles during a pelvic exam. The examiner should palpate the pelvic floor muscles and instruct the patient to contract the muscles around the examiner's finger by using the muscles that she would use to stop a stream of urine. Care should be taken that the patient is not contracting the abdominal, buttock, or thigh muscles. The patient can practice at home by trying to stop a stream of urine or by placing her finger intravaginally and contracting the pelvic floor muscles.

The ideal intensity and number of repetitions are not known. A reasonable approach is to suggest that the patient begin holding contractions for 4 seconds and eventually work up to 10 seconds. One set of 10 contractions should be done 3 time daily. The patient should be instructed that this, like any exercise, takes time to work.

18. Which medications are helpful in treating UI?

Several drugs can be helpful in UI; they are used to increase bladder storage and to facilitate bladder emptying. The initial dose of any of these drugs should be low. The patient must be monitored closely for side effects and urinary retention. The drug is titrated slowly to maximize benefit and minimize side effects.

Drugs beneficial in **urge incontinence** have anticholinergic and smooth muscle-relaxant properties. Examples include propantheline, oxybutin, imipramine, calcium channel blockers, and flanoxate. Low-dose oxybutin seems to be the most useful for elderly patients. The starting dose of oxybutin should be 2.5 mg in the evening.

Drugs effective for **stress incontinence** have alpha-adrenergic agonist properties because of the high number of alpha-adrenergic receptors in the bladder neck and base and proximal urethra. Estrogen is also beneficial because of its direct effect on urethral mucosa. The drugs most often used are phenylpropanolamine and estrogen. Both are more helpful in patients with mild-to-moderate stress incontinence and no major anatomic abnormalities.

Drugs for **overflow incontinence** stimulate bladder contractions or relax the sphincter. These agents include cholinergic agents, such as bethanechol, and alpha-adrenergic blockers, such as terazosin, prazosin, and tamsulosin. Alpha-adrenergic agents are used in men with prostate enlargement because of the number of alpha-adrenergic receptors in the capsule of the prostate. These agents cause the prostate capsule to contract and can decrease the symptoms of prostate hypertrophy.

19. When is surgical intervention appropriate?

Surgical intervention for UI should be considered in patients with stress or overflow incontinence and in patients with pathology in the lower urinary tract that contributes to UI. Successful surgical intervention requires careful assessment of the cause of UI and careful correlation of anatomic and physiologic findings with the surgical procedure. Age alone should not be a deterrent to indicated surgery, but estimation of surgical risk is extremely important. Patients with mixed causes of UI need to be assessed carefully to determine how much the surgical procedure will affect the outcome. For instance, patients with stress and urge incontinence may not benefit from surgery for stress incontinence if detrusor instability is present. There are various types of surgical procedures for restoring continence. Of interest, recently available procedures include injection of collagen or Polytef paste into periurethral tissue to provide increased resistance to urine outflow in patients with sphincter weakness. The long-term efficacy is not yet known.

20. What other measures or devices can be used for the management of UI?

Absorbent pads and garments are available in wide variety. They should be used only after evaluation of UI and trial of proper treatment. Early use of absorbent pads can lead to difficulty in achieving continence. When used improperly, they also contribute to skin breakdown.

Penile clamps can be useful in stress incontinence in elderly men. If they are not properly used, complications such as penile erosion and edema can occur.

Pessaries are useful in incontinence associated with pelvic prolapse. Patients require frequent monitoring. The pessaries must be changed every 3 months. Complications include fistula formation and ulcerations of the vagina (see figure, below).

External catheters are preferable to indwelling catheters, but they are associated with urinary tract infections. Again, they must be properly used to avoid mechanical irritation, contact dermatitis, and penile obstruction.

Intermittent catheterization involves insertion of a catheter into the bladder every 4–6 hours for drainage. This option is preferable to indwelling catheters because of its lower incidence of

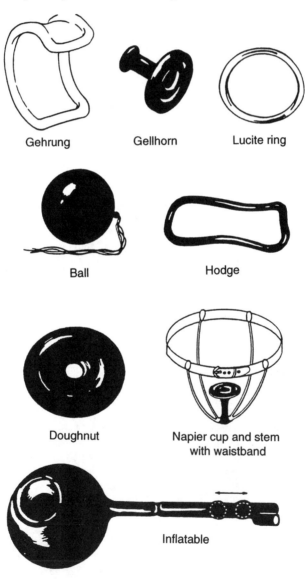

Gehrung   Gellhorn   Lucite ring

Ball   Hodge

Doughnut   Napier cup and stem
with waistband

Inflatable

Types of pessaries.

symptomatic UTIs and stone formation. Frail elderly patients and caregivers are able to use this technique.

Indwelling catheters should not be used in the routine management of UI. Complications include sepsis, stone formation, epididymitis, abscess formation, and leakage. Indwelling catheters should be used only when persistent urinary retention causes symptomatic infections or renal compromise that cannot be treated surgically or medically and intermittent catheterization is not feasible. Indwelling catheters may be appropriate in patients with a terminal illness when frequent clothing and bed changes are painful; in patients with significant skin problems that are made worse by UI; and in patients who have not responded to specific treatments and prefer a Foley catheter. Indwelling catheters can be changed monthly. When a urine culture is indicated in a catheterized patient, the catheter is changed and the culture obtained from the new catheter.

21. What community resources are available to the patient and primary care practitioner for UI?

The increase in awareness of UI and its consequences has led to an abundance of information for both practitioner and patient. The Clinical Practice Guidelines on Urinary Incontinence in Adults can be obtained by calling the AHCPR Clearinghouse at 1-800-358-9295. The guidelines are also available in a format suitable for patients and their families. Continence clinics using nonsurgical techniques for UI are becoming more common. Contacting medical centers or aging clearinghouses can identify these clinics. The following national organizations also can help people with incontinence:

Help for Incontinent People   Simon Foundation for Continence
P.O. Box 544   P.O. Box 835
Union, SC 29379   Wilmette, IL 60091
(864) 579-7900   (800) 23-SIMON

BIBLIOGRAPHY

1. Baum N, Suarey G, Appel RA: Urinary incontinence: Not a "normal" part of aging. Postgrad Med 90:99–109, 1991.
2. Burgio KL, Goode PS: Behavioral interventions for incontinence in ambulatory geriatric patients. Am J Med Sci 314:257–261, 1997.
3. Du Beau CE, Resnick NM: Evaluation of the causes and severity of geriatric incontinence: A critical appraisal. Urol Clin North Am 18:243–256, 1991.
4. Ouslander JG: Geriatric urinary incontinence. Dis Mon 38:67–149, 1992.
5. Pannell FC: Urinary incontinence for the primary care physician. Ct Med 57:299–308, 1993.
6. Resnick NM, Yalla SV: Management of urinary incontinence in the elderly. N Engl J Med 313:800–805, 1985.
7. Urinary Incontinence Guideline Panel: Urinary Incontinence in Adults: Clinical Practice Guidelines. Rockville, MD, Agency for Health Care Policy and Research, Public Health Service, U.S. Department of Health and Human Services, 1992, AHCPR publication 92-0038.
8. Vernon MS: Urinary incontinence in the elderly. Primary Care 16:515–528, 1989.

49. COMMON GASTROINTESTINAL DISORDERS

Joyann A. Kroser, M.D.

GENERAL GASTROENTEROLOGY

1. What age-related physiologic events affect gastrointestinal and hepatobiliary functioning?

In elderly patients, age-related physiologic events should be differentiated from problems that result from disease. Numerous pathologic disorders affect primarily older people and should be given more serious consideration than in younger people. Vascular diseases (e.g., mesenteric ischemia) affect older people with well-documented atherosclerosis. Atrophic gastritis and its sequelae rarely occur in young people. Aging leads to poorer T-cell function and decreased intraepithelial lymphocytes, both of which impair gut-associated immunity. Hepatic blood flow also is reduced with age, leading to decreased clearance of drugs that are metabolized by the liver.

2. How may the differential diagnosis and presentation of acute abdominal pain differ in elderly and younger patients?

1. Presenting signs and symptoms in the elderly may be altered by central nervous system disease, depression, or delay in seeking medical care.

2. The differential diagnosis of acute abdominal pain is different in the elderly. Biliary tract disease is responsible for 25% of all cases of acute abdominal pain in elderly patients requiring hospitalization. Bowel obstruction and incarcerated hernia are the next most common causes, followed by appendicitis, malignancy, and diverticulitis. In younger patients appendicitis is the most common cause of acute abdominal pain, followed by pelvic inflammatory disease, peptic ulcer disease, and cholecystitis.

3. Acute abdominal pain in some conditions (e.g., appendicitis) is muted by age. Pain is often minimal, fever mild, and leukocytosis unreliable.

4. Myocardial infarction also should be in the differential diagnosis of abdominal pain in a patient over 50 years of age. An electrocardiogram should be part of the evaluation.

5. Pain localization may be atypical in persons older than 60 years. The initial diagnostic impression in older patients with acute abdominal pain may be wrong in up to two-thirds of cases. The evaluation of symptoms in older patients requires more care and patience and should encompass a broader range of complaints than in the young.

3. Should endoscopic or surgical procedures be avoided in the elderly?

Diagnostic endoscopic or radiographic studies should *not* be avoided in the elderly. These procedures usually are well tolerated unless severe cardiopulmonary disease is present, although sedative dosages may be reduced. The site of gastrointestinal bleeding does not differ greatly with age and should be managed aggressively in older persons. Abdominal surgery should not be avoided solely on the basis of age; surgical risk correlates more closely with associated morbidities than with age.

ESOPHAGUS

4. What causes disorders of swallowing and food intake in the elderly?

- Anorexia
- Dementia
- Depression
- Physical inability to prepare food or to eat
- Dental problems
- Ill-fitting dentures

- Diseases that impair bolus transfer to the esophagus
  - Cerebral vascular accident
  - Parkinson's disease
  - Amyotrophic lateral sclerosis
  - Myasthenia gravis
  - Muscular dystrophies
  - Polymyositis
  - Amyloidosis
- Diseases of esophageal transfer
  - Motility disorders
    - Achalasia
    - Scleroderma
    - Diffuse esophageal spasm
  - Intrinsic mechanical lesions
    - Benign stricture
    - Schatzki's ring
    - Carcinoma
    - Esophageal webs
  - Extrinsic mechanical lesions
    - Vascular compromise
    - Mediastinal abnormalities
    - Cervical osteoarthritis

5. Discuss age-related pharyngeal problems.

The muscles of the mouth and pharynx may weaken, altering mastication. Pharyngeal muscle discoordination may result from neuromuscular disorders (e.g., Parkinson's disease, cerebrovascular accidents, polymyositis, dermatomyositis, myasthenia gravis). Altered pharyngeal sensation and proprioception can change taste perception and alter discrimination of bolus size and consistency. Lip closure may be impaired with advanced age. The cumulative result of such age-related changes are slowed tongue function, food spills, prolonged swallowing, and drooling. Although the number of taste buds decreases with age, taste disturbances more commonly result from medication effects, inadequate oral hygiene, or denture problems. In addition, the sense of smell is important in taste perception, and considerable olfactory impairment has been demonstrated in persons older than 70 years. Certain primary pharyngeal problems (e.g., Zenker's diverticulum and cricopharyngeal achalasia) occur mainly in elderly people.

6. What physiologic changes in esophageal function occur in the elderly?
- Dyssynchrony of deglutition and respiration
- Prolonged swallowing
- Decreased upper esophageal sphincter (UES) pressure
- Altered UES relaxation
- Increased tertiary contractions (little or no pathophysiologic significance)

7. Which esophageal disorders deserve special consideration in the elderly?
- Pill-induced esophagitis
- Achalasia
- Esophageal carcinoma

8. Which medications are associated with esophageal ulceration?
- Doxycycline hydrate
- Tetracycline hydrochloride
- Clindamycin
- Potassium chloride
- Ferrous sulfate
- Quinidine
- Aspirin
- Theophylline
- Alendronate

9. Which studies help to evaluate swallowing disorders?

A barium swallow is a useful first study because it helps to exclude structural esophageal lesions. It is important to communicate that a swallowing evaluation is also desired so that the radiologist will interpret the study with dynamic images using different consistencies of barium. The study also alerts the endoscopist to any potential anatomic difficulties, such as large Zenker's diverticulum, that may pose a perforation risk during upper endoscopy. Upper endoscopy can diagnose neoplasms, pill-induced esophageal injury, and ulcer disease. Esophageal manometry helps to diagnose esophageal motility disorders (e.g., achalasia, diffuse esophageal spasm, nutcracker esophagus). This diagnostic algorithm does not differ from that used for younger patients.

10. Is the management of gastroesophageal reflux disease (GERD) different in elderly and younger patients?

Diagnosis of GERD is more difficult because the elderly often present with less typical or few symptoms. GERD should be considered in the differential diagnosis of unexplained wheezing, persistent nonproductive cough, noncardiac chest pain, persistent dysphonia, or recurrent pneumonia. The elderly tend to underreport and tolerate symptoms that younger people find less tolerable. Symptoms are not particularly helpful in predicting the severity of esophageal mucosal disease. In a large prospective study, the presence of moderate or severe pyrosis in the elderly did not correlate with the presence or degree of esophageal mucosal disease (erosive esophagitis or Barrett's esophagus). Many clinicians empirically reduce the dosage of antisecretory medication in the elderly, in part based on an impression that basal gastric acid secretion decreases with age. Compelling data, however, show that GERD in geriatric patients is associated with more severe mucosal disease that requires aggressive diagnosis and treatment. It is prudent to perform at least one screening endoscopy in any patient older than age 60 with suspected GERD in order to assess the degree of mucosal damage and to exclude Barrett's esophagus, esophageal carcinoma, and other complications. If erosive esophagitis is present, proton-pump inhibitors (PPIs) are the drugs of choice, although high-dose H_2 blockers also may be effective. A definite subset of patients requires high-dose PPI therapy (> 1 tablet twice daily).

STOMACH/DUODENUM

11. Why may the incidence of peptic ulcer disease be increased in the elderly?
- Increased use of nonsteroidal anti-inflammatory drugs (NSAIDs)
- Smoking
- Poor nutrition
- Increased prevalence of *Helicobacter pylori* infection

12. What physiologic changes of the stomach are associated with aging?

Gastric acid secretion does *not* decrease in the majority of older persons; only 25–30% show acid hyposecretion. Duodenal secretion of bicarbonate may decrease in the elderly, but gastric emptying, intrinsic factor secretion, and other physiologic functions of the stomach do not change.

13. What sequelae are associated with hypochlorhydria?

Hypochlorhydria, caused by chronic atrophic gastritis, is a disorder of the elderly. Gastric polyps develop in atrophic gastritis, but the long-term risk of gastric cancer development is increased only three- to fourfold. Gastric hypochlorhydria increases the proximal duodenal pH, predisposing the patient to infection with *Salmonella* species, *Vibrio cholera*, and *Giardia* species and increasing the risk of bacterial overgrowth in the small intestine. Hypochlorhydria also may cause malabsorption of iron, calcium, and vitamin B_{12}.

14. How are the evaluation and management of ulcer disease different in elderly and younger patients?

The symptoms of peptic ulcer disease (PUD) are more variable and subtle in older persons and often are reported only as anorexia and vague discomfort that does not radiate. Substernal chest pain may mimic angina. One-third of patients report no pain at all. Complications from ulcer hemorrhage are common in older patients, including more frequent rebleeding after initial control of hemorrhage, more severe hypotension as a result of blood loss, and significant cardiopulmonary compromise as a result of fluid resuscitation. The mortality rate for ulcer perforation is high in the elderly. The management of PUD does not differ significantly from that in younger patients. Early endoscopy, acid-suppressive therapy, *H. pylori* testing and eradication, avoidance of NSAIDs, and surgery (if necessary) are principles of management regardless of age.

15. How is *H. pylori* infection diagnosed?

Various diagnostic methods with high sensitivity and specificity have been developed for the detection of *H. pylori*. Each has its own advantages and disadvantages.

TESTS	SENSITIVITY	SPECIFICITY	DESCRIPTION
Nonendoscopic			
Office-based rapid serology	88–99%	86–95%	Rapid, qualitative, in-office tests that measure presence of antibodies to *H. pylori*
Lab-based ELISA	98.7%	100%	Quantitative test sent to central lab; more costly
Urea breath test	90–100%	98–100%	Urease of *H. pylori* breaks down ingested C-urea; patient exhales labeled CO_2
Endoscopic			
Histology	93–99%	95–99%	Microscopic examination of biopsied tissue
Culture	77–92%	100%	Culture of biopsy
Rapid urease test	89–98%	93–98%	Urease of *H. pylori* generates ammonia and color change

ELISA = enzyme-linked immunosorbent assay.

16. Which tests for *H. pylori* are best-suited to common clinical settings?

Clinical setting	Diagnostic test
New, recurrent, or history of PUD	Serology or urea breath test
Complicated PUD	Esophagogastroduodenoscopy (EGD) with rapid urease test and/or histology
Follow-up (wait ≥ 4 weeks)	Urea breath test
Patient having EGD	Rapid urease tests with or without histology
Adherent patient with several treatment failures	EGD, histology, culture and susceptibility testing

One approach to using diagnostic tests for evaluation and follow-up of patients with suspected or proven *H. pylori* infection is suggested above. It is not necessary to reconfirm the presence of peptic ulcer in patients with ulcer documented in the past. Endoscopy is generally indicated in patients with complicated ulcer disease to plan the best strategy for management and to deal directly with the complication (i.e., endoscopic hemostasis). Confirmation of eradication is generally indicated only in patients who have had a complicated course. The urea breath test is preferred because it is noninvasive and cost-effective.

17. Which patients should be tested for *H. pylori* and treated if positive?

Testing for *H. pylori* should be performed only in patients for whom therapy is contemplated. Any patient who tests positive should be offered treatment. Do not test asymptomatic people. Definitely test and treat patients with active PUD or documented history of uncomplicated or complicated duodenal or gastric ulcer, patients who have undergone resection of early gastric cancer, and patients with low-grade mucosa-associated lymphoid tissue lymphoma. At this time it is uncertain whether testing and treatment of patients with dyspepsia are beneficial.

18. What are the commonly accepted regimens for eradication of *H. pylori*?

Regimens for Eradication of H. Pylori

TREATMENT	DURATION	DOSING	EFFICACY	PROS	CONS	NOTES
Bismuth triple therapy (BMT)	14 days	Bismuth, 2 tablets qid Metronidazole, 250 mg qid Tetracycline, 500 mg qid	> 90%	Least expensive	16-pill regimen; Metronidazole resistance reduces efficacy	Add 28 days acid suppression therapy for active ulcer
Tritec triple therapy	14 days	Ranitidine, bismuth, and citrate (RBC): 400 mg bid Clarithromycin, 500 mg bid Amoxicillin, 1000 mg bid	> 90%	Twice-daily dosing Few side effects	Limited clinical data	More clinical studies needed Not FDA-approved
Amoxicillin triple therapy	10–14 days	Lansoprazole, 30 mg bid *or* Omeprazole, 20 mg bid *and* Amoxicillin, 1000 mg bid Clarithromycin, 500 mg bid	85–95%	Twice-daily dosing Few side effects	Resistance to clarithromycin may reduce efficacy	
Metronidazole triple therapy	10–14 days	As above, except metronidazole, 500 mg bid, substituted for amoxicillin, 1000 mg bid	85–95%	Twice-daily dosing Few side effects	Resistance to either antibiotic may reduce efficacy	Not FDA-approved
PPI clarithromycin (PC)	14 days	Omeprazole, 40 mg qd *or* Lansoprazole, 60 mg qd *plus* Clarithromycin, 500 mg tid	70–75%	Simpler regimen	Lower eradication rate	Add 14 days of PPI with active ulcer
RBC clarithromycin (RC)	14 days	RBC, 400 mg bid Clarithromycin, 500 mg tid	80–85%	Simpler regimen	Lower eradication rate	28 days RBC with active ulcer

qid = 4 times/day, bid = 2 times/day, qd = each day, tid = 3 times/day, PPI = proton pump inhibitor, FDA = Food and Drug Administration.

19. What are the major advantages and disadvantages of detecting and treating *H. pylori* infection in older persons?

H. pylori infection is a health problem for elderly patients. The prevalence of infection in the 70–80-year-old cohort is 70–80%, which probably reflects acquisition of infection in childhood. The overall prevalence in the U.S. is approximately 35%. Major issues of concern include the overall effects on general health of atrophic gastritis caused by infection, such as development of stomach cancer or increased risk of enteric infections. In addition, potential interactions between *H. pylori* and NSAIDs may lead to increased morbidity and mortality from ulcer disease. Treatment is relatively easy, but adding three medications for elderly patients already taking several other prescription drugs is likely to increase the chance of serious side effects. In addition, the incidence of gastric cancer in the U.S. has fallen about fivefold since the early part of the century; thus, a screening program for *H. pylori* cannot be recommended. Overtreatment of the infection produces antibiotic resistance, making the selection of appropriate patients critical.

SMALL INTESTINE

20. What is the differential diagnosis of malabsorption in older patients?
- Pancreatic disease
- Celiac sprue
- Bacterial overgrowth
- Ischemic bowel

21. List the common causes of bacterial overgrowth.
- Stricture due to:
  Crohn's disease
  Radiation therapy
  Surgery
  Malignancy
- Diverticula of the small intestine
- Coloenteric fistula
- Gastric achlorhydria
- Decreased intestinal IgA and lysozyme production

COLON

22. What are the common causes of diarrhea in older persons?

In contrast to constipation, diarrhea is not a common gastrointestinal problem in the elderly. New-onset diarrhea may result from medication side effects, fecal impaction (paradoxical response), abuse of laxatives, diabetic neuropathy, and, rarely, infection with *Escherichia coli, Clostridium difficile, Clostridium jejuni,* or other organisms. Fecal incontinence is frequently misreported as diarrhea.

23. What initial diagnostic and therapeutic maneuvers are recommended for evaluating diarrhea?
1. Withdraw offending medications, if possible:
   - Laxatives
   - Sorbitol-containing dietetic products
   - Selective serotonin reuptake inhibitor antidepressants (e.g., sertraline)
   - Antibiotics
2. Rule out fecal impaction
3. Send stool samples for *C. difficile* toxin assay and culture and sensitivity studies
4. Flexible sigmoidoscopy or colonoscopy if diarrhea persists more than 2–4 weeks

24. What are the causes of fecal incontinence?
1. Normal pelvic floor
   - Diarrheal states
     Infectious diarrhea
     Inflammatory bowel disease
     Short gut syndrome
     Laxative abuse
     Radiation enteritis*

- Overflow
  Impaction*
  Encopresis
  Rectal neoplasm
- Neurologic conditions
  Congenital anomalies   Dementia, strokes, tabes dorsalis
     (e.g., myelomeningocele)   Neuropathy (e.g., diabetes)*
  Multiple sclerosis   Neoplasms of brain, spinal cord, cauda equina
2. Abnormal pelvic floor
  - Congenital anorectal malformations
  - Trauma
    Accidental injury
    Anorectal surgery*
    Obstetric injury*
  - Pelvic floor denervation (idiopathic neurogenic incontinence)
    Vaginal delivery   Rectal prolapse*
    Chronic straining at stool   Descending perineum syndrome
* Most common causes.

25. What are the treatment options for fecal incontinence?

Treatment must be individualized. Patients with rectal prolapse or fecal impaction may respond best to treatment of underlying constipation. Rare patients may respond to surgical resection of the anorectal angle. Anal repair surgery has limited success in patients with anal sphincter dysfunction. Conversely, biofeedback retraining of the external anal sphincter may be successful in some elderly patients, although bed-bound patients are unlikely to benefit from this technique.

26. How does inflammatory bowel disease (IBD) differ in older patients?

IBD is more common in elderly patients than generally recognized. Two-thirds of older patients with Crohn's disease are women who have predominantly colonic involvement, often in a left-sided distribution similar to that found in diverticular disease. Ulcerative colitis restricted to the rectum and sigmoid colon occurs more commonly in older patients. Surgery is necessary less often in elderly patients than in young patients, and disease recurrences are less frequent. Extraintestinal complications of IBD occur less frequently in the elderly. Nevertheless, the mortality of IBD is 2–3 times higher in the elderly than in younger patients. Specifically, mortality from the *first* attack of IBD is significantly higher in the elderly, primarily because delays in diagnosis result in the need to perform risky emergency surgery.

27. What is Ogilvie's syndrome?

Ogilvie's syndrome, also known as acute colonic pseudoobstruction (ACPO) or ileus, is acute nontoxic megacolon. The typical presentation is a postoperative patient who develops a distended abdomen. Abdominal pain is generally minimal in the early stage of disease. Nausea and vomiting occur in about two-thirds of patients. Bowel sound are usually present. Peritoneal signs are absent unless perforation occurs. The syndrome carries a 20–30% mortality rate, due, in part, to associated conditions. Perforation of the cecum (in accordance with Laplace's law) occurs in 14%. Abdominal radiographs are essential to the diagnosis and reveal massive segmental dilation of the right colon, especially the cecum. ACPO should be distinguished from mechanical causes of obstruction, such as sigmoid or cecal volvulus, and from toxic megacolon with underlying inflammation or infection of the bowel.

28. What factors contribute to acute colonic ileus?

1. Recent surgery
2. Recent general anesthesia

3. Medications
  - Nonsteroidal analgesics
  - Opiate analgesics
  - Antidepressants
  - Antipsychotics
  - Antiseizure drugs
  - Calcium antagonists
  - Antiparkinson drugs
  - Monoamine oxidase inhibitors
  - Antacids (e.g., sulcralfate, aluminum/calcium antacids)
  - Cationic agents (e.g., iron/calcium supplements, barium sulfate, bismuth salts)
4. Congestive heart failure
5. Electrolyte abnormalities
  - Hypokalemia
  - Hypocalcemia
  - Hypomagnesemia
  - Hypophosphatemia
  - Hyponatremia
6. Chronic obstructive lung disease
7. Underlying neurologic disorders
8. Diabetes
9. Uremia
10. Hip fracture

29. What is the treatment of ACPO?
- Discontinue all medications that may be contributing factors (see above).
- Place nasogastric tube for suctioning.
- Instruct nurse to roll patient from side to side hourly to assist in mobilizing colonic gas.
- Correct electrolyte imbalances.
- Obtain serial abdominal radiographs every 6–8 hours to assess progression of cecal dilation.
- Do frequent physical examinations of the abdomen.
- Consider rectal tube placement if left colon is also distended.
- Decompressive colonoscopy is needed if conservative measures fail (50–75% of patients may respond to conservative therapy).
- If the patient does not respond to colonoscopy or if dilation recurs, surgical cecostomy should be performed.
- Avoid enemas and oral laxatives.
- Recent reports suggest that intravenous neostigmine may be helpful. More studies are forthcoming.

30. Classify the types of intestinal ischemia.
1. Acute mesenteric ischemia
  - Nonocclusive mesenteric ischemia
  - Superior mesenteric artery (SMA) embolus
  - SMA thrombosis
  - Superior mesenteric vein thrombosis
  - Focal segmental ischemia
2. Chronic mesenteric ischemia (abdominal angina)
3. Colonic ischemia
  - Reversible ischemic colopathy
  - Transient ulcerating ischemic colitis
  - Chronic ulcerating ischemic colitis
  - Colonic strictured
  - Colonic gangrene
  - Fulminant universal ischemic colitis

31. What are the major clinical differences between colonic ischemia and acute mesenteric ischemia?

COLONIC ISCHEMIA	ACUTE MESENTERIC ISCHEMIA
90% of patients over age 60	Most patients over age 50
Acute precipitating cause is rare	Acute precipitating event usual (e.g., myocardial infarction, hypotensive episodes, cardiac arrhythmias, congestive heart failure)
Associated predisposing lesion in 20% (e.g., colon carcinoma, stricture, diverticulitis, fecal impaction)	Predisposing lesion uncommon
Patients do not appear ill	Patients usually appear seriously ill
Mild abdominal pain with tenderness and guarding usual	Pain more severe; abdominal findings minimal early in course
Moderate rectal bleeding or bloody diarrhea	Rectal bleeding and diarrhea not common until late in course
First diagnostic procedure should be gentle flexible sigmoidoscopy or colonoscopy	First diagnostic procedure should be angiography
Usually noncatastrophic; usually does not require surgery	Catastrophic emergency with high mortality rate; surgical intervention usually required
Involves inferior mesenteric distribution	Super mesenteric distribution
Presentation after ischemic episode is complete and blood flow to the segment of colon has has returned to normal	Presentation during ischemic episode as a result of hemodynamic and metabolic problems
Good prognosis	Generally poor prognosis

32. Classify the spectrum of diverticular disease of the colon.
   1. Uncomplicated diverticular disease (found in about 75% of people by age 80)
      • Asymptomatic
      85% sigmoid colon
      Right-sided diverticulosis more common in Asians and young people
      • Symptomatic (painful diverticular disease)
      Treat with fiber supplement with or without antispasmodics for symptom relief
   2. Complicated diverticular disease (10–20% of patients)
      • Diverticular hemorrhage: brisk, painless
      • Diverticulitis (CT scan is the test of choice for diagnosis and assessment of complications)
      • Peridiverticulitis
      • Bowel obstruction
      • Fistula: colovesicular, colovaginal, coloenteric, colocutaneous
      • Abscess
      • Peritonitis

33. How is diverticulitis treated?
   1. Mild (nontoxic appearance, able to tolerate oral intake)
      • Outpatient management
      • Oral antibiotics (ampicillin/sublactam or ciprofloxacin/metronidazole)
      • Low fiber diet
   2. Moderate or severe (more toxic, presence of complications or comorbidities)
      • Inpatient management
      • Parenteral antibiotics

- Bowel rest
- Drainage of large abscesses (either percutaneously or surgically)
- Surgery
  Emergent/urgent for peritonitis, medically unresponsive patient
  For fistula or stricture (timing of surgery based on clinical status)
  Elective for chronic pain, recurrences

34. What are the current guidelines for colon cancer screening?

In the United States it is currently recommended that people with average risk begin screening at age 50 with annual fecal occult blood testing and flexible sigmoidoscopy every 4–5 years. People with above average risk include those with a family history of colorectal carcinoma or adenomatous polyps in a first-degree relative under 50 years of age or a personal history of inflammatory bowel disease. Such patients should have surveillance with colonoscopy. No guidelines relate to stopping screening in the very old. The decision to defer screening based on advanced age or other comorbidities should be made on an individualized basis.

HEPATOBILIARY DISORDERS

35. What is the approach to an elderly patient with abnormal liver-associated tests?

Liver structure and function change little with age, and liver chemistry abnormalities strictly referable to advanced age are not reported. Elevations of alkaline phosphatase levels occur in 27% of geriatric patients; they are caused by bone disease in 50% and liver disease in 25%. Unsuspected hyperbilirubinemia usually is related to underlying congestive heart failure. Hepatitis in elderly patients may be milder but often produces more severe complications. Drug-induced hepatotoxicity should be considered in elderly patients with new liver chemistry abnormalities.

36. Discuss the important general points about biliary disease in the elderly.

The prevalence of gallstones increases with age, reaching 35% by age 80. Juxtapapillary duodenal diverticula are most common in the elderly and are associated with gallstones in 65–85% of patients. Postcholecystectomy bile duct stones may occur. The common clinical presentations of cholelithiasis include biliary colic, cholecystitis, cholangitis, and pancreatitis. Cholangitis may present as a vague discomfort or altered mental status, whereas cholangitis may produce hypotension. Gallbladder empyema has a high mortality rate but may produce only mild symptoms. Gallstone pancreatitis is potentially fatal. The clinical scoring systems to predict disease severity are less accurate in patients older than 75 years. Obstructive jaundice from choledocholithiasis is common in the elderly and may mimic the presentation of pancreatic carcinoma.

BIBLIOGRAPHY

1. Brown K, Peura D: Diagnosis of *Helicobacter pylori* infection. Gastroenterol Clin North Am 22:105–116, 1993.
2. Dorudi S, Berry AR, Kettlewell MGW: Acute colonic pseudo-obstruction. Br J Surg 79:99–103, 1992.
3. Ferzoco LB, Raptopoulos V, Silen W: Acute diverticulitis. N Engl J Med 338:1521–1526, 1998.
4. Freeman SR, McNally PR: Diverticulitis. Med Clin North Am 77:1149–1167, 1993.
5. Holt PR: Approach to gastrointestinal problems in the elderly. In Yamata T, Alpers DH, Owyang C, et al (eds): Textbook of Gastroenterology, 2nd ed. Philadelphia, J.B. Lippincott, 1998, pp 968–987.
6. Hunt RH: Eradication of *Helicobacter pylori* infection. Am J Med 100:42S–51S, 1996.
7. Lander SM, Karki S, Mathew LM: Usage patterns of gastrointestinal antisecretory medications in an academic nursing home. Ann Long-Term Care 5:436–443, 1997.
8. Ott DJ, Chen MYM: Specific acute colonic disorders. Radiol Clin North Am 32:871–884, 1994.
9. Ponec RJ, Saunders MD, Kinney MB: Neostigmine for the treatment of acute chronic pseudo-obstruction. N Engl J Med 341:137–141, 1999.
10. Wilson JAP, Rogers EL: Gastroenterologic disorders. In Cassel CK, Cohen HJ, Larson EB, et al (eds): Geriatric Medicine, 3rd ed. New York, Springer-Verlag, 1997.

50. CARE OF THE ELDERLY CANCER PATIENT

Angela DeMichele, M.D., Richard H. Greenberg, M.D., and David J. Vaughn, M.D.

1. Is loss of immune surveillance the reason cancers are more common in older patients?

The question of how the loss of immune surveillance in the elderly contributes to their higher incidence of cancer is quite complicated. Theories suggest that tumor cells express specific antigens that lead to their recognition and removal by the intact immune system. Support comes from the greater incidence of neoplasia in the AIDS or organ transplant populations. Dissenters argue that the narrow range of tumor types (lymphoma, Kaposi's sarcoma) seen in these latter populations does not support the applicability of immune surveillance as a general mechanism in the control of cancer. With lymphoid and plasma cell dyscrasias, evidence suggests that loss of normal cellular regulation of the growth of these specific cell types has more to do with their malignant transformation than the absence of adequate immune surveillance. The mild loss of cellular immunity seen in the elderly may actually lead to more indolent behavior of tumors due to lower levels of nonspecific growth or angiogenesis factors in the cellular milieu.

2. What are the principal modalities for the treatment of cancer in the elderly? What are the goals?

The three main modalities of cancer treatment—chemotherapy (including biologic, hormonal, and immune therapies), radiotherapy, and surgery—may be used singly or in combination. The underlying intent of treatment can be cure, palliation, or comfort-care/symptom control. The goals of therapy typically dictate the aggressiveness of treatment and the acceptable level of toxicity.

3. Should the physician approach the management of cancer differently in the elderly than in the young?

Elderly men and women have the same right to participate fully in the planning and implementation of their cancer care and to be informed fully of their therapeutic options. Assumptions based solely on age and treatment nihilism have no place in the ethical and compassionate development of the therapeutic relationship. Appropriate clinical judgment should be used in dealing with patients with poor functional status and known limited life expectancy. Treatment options with their respective advantages and disadvantages should be presented, along with an analysis of the expected length and quality of survival compared with the level of risk to the patient. The option of focusing on symptom management in lieu of antitumor treatments also needs to be presented. An important component of the personal database for any patient, particularly the elderly, is the inclusion of the patient's wishes regarding advance directives, living wills, durable power of attorney for health care, and preferences regarding levels of resuscitation and artificial life support. (See also Chapter 26.)

4. What is the role of chemotherapy in the elderly cancer patient?

The approach to the elderly cancer patient frequently includes chemotherapy. Decisions about chemotherapy should not be based solely on chronologic age. Consider also the patient's underlying organ function, performance status, and any impairment in functional or cognitive abilities. Because in the past patients older than 65 years were excluded from clinical trials, there is a need for prospective evaluations of chemotherapy efficacy and toxicity in this unique patient population.

5. How does the hematopoietic reserve of the elderly patient influence management?

Aging reduces the amount of active bone marrow, as the proportion of marrow fat increases. Under steady-state conditions, there is little impact on peripheral blood counts. However, with the toxicity of radiotherapy and chemotherapy, myelosuppression occurs, and the recovery of the bone marrow is delayed and diminished. An increase in severe hematopoietic toxicity observed in phase II clinical cancer therapy trials in patients of age > 65 as compared to their younger counterparts has been demonstrated. Modern blood-banking techniques and the use of recombinant hematopoietic growth factors (e.g., granulocyte–colony-stimulating factor) have made it easier to utilize myelosuppressive chemotherapy at higher doses and on schedule in the elderly with demonstrated decreases in neutropenia. Alternately, dose modification or the selection of less myelosuppressive drugs can avoid much of the bone marrow toxicity.

6. How does renal function influence their care?

Differences in renal function between elderly patients and their younger counterparts are the most significant determinants of alterations in cancer chemotherapy pharmacokinetics (see also Chapter 45). Changes with aging include:
- Reduced renal blood flow
- Reduced glomerular filtration

Renal impairment leads to decreased clearance and therefore the increased risk of toxicity from drugs that are renally eliminated (esp. methotrexate, bleomycin, streptozocin, and the platin-complex agents). Careful determination of renal function (creatinine clearance) as part of treatment planning is more important than assumptions based solely on age. Nephrotoxic supportive agents, such as aminoglycoside antibiotics and amphotericin, must also be approached with care in the setting of renal insufficiency. Although amifostine has been developed to protect renal function in patients receiving cisplatin-based chemotherapy, its role in the treatment of elderly patients remains to be defined.

7. Does hepatic function influence their care?

- Age-related decreases in hepatic mass, hepatic blood flow, and microsomal oxidation and reduction have been noted.
- Metabolism of chemotherapeutic agents occurs principally by hepatic phase I oxidative and reductive modification to active or inactive compounds.
- No accepted biologic marker of hepatic function exists, but appropriate clinical judgment should be exercised in the setting of significant hepatic compromise.
- The conjugating (phase II) functions of the liver do not appear to change significantly in the elderly, because alterations of metabolism at this level are typically seen only in severe hepatic dysfunction.

8. What pharmacologic issues influence the cancer care of the elderly?

Intact hepatic and renal functions are critical to the normal metabolism and excretion of cancer chemotherapeutic agents. Poor drug tolerance in the elderly is largely a product of the narrow therapeutic index of most anticancer drugs superimposed on a tendency of declining organ function reserve. Chronologic age alone should not be used as the determinant of dose modifications in chemotherapy. Adjustments in treatment intensity rather should be made based on the presence of comorbid conditions that could affect the disposition or toxicity of the intended drug. Although allowing avoidable toxicity can lead to treatment delays that compromise dose intensity, undue fear of first-line chemotherapy drugs at optimal doses is likely a major source of the observed worse response to cancer treatment seen in the elderly.

- Elderly cancer patients may have clinically relevant impairment in many pharmacokinetic processes.
- Absorption of oral drugs may be affected by the higher gastric pH, delayed gastric emptying, and altered membrane transport typical of the elderly. (However, these effects have not proved to be of significant clinical relevance.)
- Changes in body composition in the elderly (decreased body water, decreased lean body mass, increased body fat, and decreased plasma-binding proteins) can affect the volume of distribution, elimination half-life, and peak or steady-state concentrations of drugs used in anticancer therapy.

Additionally, persons aged > 65 years take an average of 4 daily medications for preexisting chronic illnesses. Evidence suggests that older adults exhibit some degree of noncompliance when required to take > 4 medications/day, as is often required by the chemotherapeutic regimen. Noncompliance stands to be exacerbated further by the multiple therapeutic and symptom control drugs, as well as their potential interactions, prescribed in the course of cancer care.

9. How does the cardiovascular function of elderly patients influence their care?

- The use of radiotherapy to the left chest or cardiotoxic chemotherapy (anthracyclines such as doxorubicin, high-dose alkylators) may require careful pre-evaluation and treatment planning.
- Cardioprotectant agents, such as dexrazoxane (ICRF-187, Zinecard), are now available that may help in extending the safe use of cardiotoxic chemotherapeutic drugs.
- The aggressive hydration associated with the standard use of many chemotherapeutic agents must be approached with caution to avoid fluid overload.

10. How does pulmonary function influence their care?

The presence of comorbid pulmonary disease is of greater significance than age alone in determining a patient's tolerance of surgical procedures or pulmonary-toxic chemotherapy (e.g., bleomycin). However, in the well-conditioned elderly individual without significant pulmonary disease, surgical and chemotherapeutic management of malignancy should not be precluded.

11. How does mucosal integrity influence care?

- Decreased cellular proliferation, skin/subcutaneous tissue thickness, and collagen production/remodeling in the elderly lead to poorer wound healing that may complicate surgical procedures and increase the likelihood of mucositis from chemotherapy or ionizing radiation.
- Potential for decreased mobility following surgery further increases the risk of skin breakdown/ulceration and infection.
- Enhancing nutrition, increasing mobility, and careful planning of radiation or chemotherapy dosing can help alleviate the potential loss of mucosal integrity.
- Cryotherapy (sucking on ice chips) during treatment with such agents as 5-fluorouracil decreases local perfusion and can significantly reduce the incidence of the associated mucositis.

12. Describe how neurologic function is affected by cancer treatment.

- Sensory and cognitive impairments are more common in the elderly, leading to a much higher incidence of treatment- and disease-related delirium.
- Losses in taste and olfaction can intensify the decreased appetite associated with chemotherapy, head/neck radiotherapy, and malignancy.
- Great care (dose modification, aggressive laxative regimen) must be exercised in the use of agents such as vincristine due to the potentially severe adynamic ileus that can result.
- The cumulative fatigue experienced with the use of cisplatin is enhanced in the elderly.

13. What factors can contribute to delirium in the elderly cancer patient?

Cancer patients are at risk for delirium due to a large number of potentially reversible causes: direct tumor invasion of the central nervous system (CNS), sensory overload or deprivation (e.g., removal of glasses or hearing aid), isolated or unfamiliar environment, sleep deprivation, fluid/electrolyte and nutritional imbalances, organ failure or encephalopathy, disordered bowel function, infection, fever, and hypoxia. Drugs associated with cancer management, such as chemotherapy, corticosteroids, biologic response modifiers, antiemetics, antihistamines, anticholinergics, and antispasmodics, commonly contribute to delirium.

14. How well do the elderly tolerate cancer surgery?

Despite their higher incidence of comorbid medical illness, with appropriate preparation, most elderly cancer patients tolerate surgery well. Endoscopic surgical approaches can be particularly well tolerated. Despite multi-year life expectancies that extends into the 90s, the elderly are far more likely to be denied attempts at curative resections of their tumors than younger persons. Older cancer patients are just as likely to suffer local recurrence of their disease if surgical margins are inadequate. Therefore, in the absence of serious comorbidities, age should not preclude an aggressive surgical approach.

15. How well do the elderly tolerate radiotherapy?

Any patient with poor nutritional, hydration, or functional status is likely to experience increased radiotherapy-induced toxicity. However, studies of elderly cancer patients with good performance status demonstrate that these patients tolerate radiotherapy with significant clinical benefit. One exception was radiation for malignant CNS gliomas, in which the elderly fared poorly. Despite this, radiation for metastases to the brain is tolerated just as well by the elderly as by younger patients. There is a need for disease-specific preoperative evaluation of radiotherapy in the elderly population to determine tolerability and efficacy compared with younger counterparts.

16. Do elderly patients with cancer experience symptoms differently?

Studies comparing cancer patients by age, but controlling for stage of disease and life expectancy, reveal that the elderly report very similar symptoms referable to their illness and treatment. All groups, regardless of age, tend to have progressively more complaints of greater intensity at diagnosis and at recurrence, with the peak occurring as they enter the terminal phases of their disease. Other studies have suggested that increasing age is associated with less sensitivity to pain. At present, it should not be assumed that the elderly are tolerant of pain or that their analgesic program need not be as aggressive. (See also Chapter 27.)

17. Are there special considerations regarding breast cancer in the elderly?

Breast cancer continues to rise in incidence as women age. Controversy surrounds the issue of whether breast cancer is less aggressive in the elderly. Studies demonstrate that healthy elderly women tolerate the same treatment that would be proposed for their younger counterparts including surgery, cytotoxic chemotherapy, and radiotherapy; enjoy equivalent benefits from such therapy; and suffer poorer outcomes if their treatment is compromised. Elderly patients who are candidates for breast conservation (lumpectomy plus radiotherapy as opposed to mastectomy) should be offered this treatment option. In light of the high proportion of estrogen and progesterone receptor-positive breast cancers in the elderly, the appropriate use of tamoxifen and other antiestrogens is important in both the adjuvant and metastatic settings. The selective estrogen receptor modulators (SERMs), a new class of compounds, offer the potential of lowered serum cholesterol, decreased risk of cardiovascular death, and conservation of bone density to postmenopausal women. Education of older women and their physicians is crucial to encourage greater participation in screening and breast self-examination in an attempt to increase the chance of diagnosing earlier-stage disease.

18. Are there special considerations regarding colorectal cancer in the elderly?

In the treatment of colorectal cancer, surgery, radiotherapy, and chemotherapy are considered standard in their appropriate settings. The resultant benefits to the elderly in terms of cure and palliation are comparable to those enjoyed by younger patients. Colorectal surgery in the elderly is well tolerated with appropriate preparation and the control of comorbid medical conditions. Poor outcome is associated with emergent surgeries (e.g., perforation or obstruction), so efforts should be made to react quickly to symptoms and screen for early detection.

The difficult adjustment associated with the creation of a colostomy in the elderly should encourage creation of primary anastamoses and sphincter-sparing procedures whenever possible. Transanal excision with radiotherapy may be considered for early-stage rectal tumors. Adjuvant chemosensitized radiotherapy is beneficial for transmural, node-positive, or locally advanced rectal carcinomas. Adjuvant chemotherapy with a 5-fluorouracil-containing regimen is considered standard for node-positive and some high-risk node-negative colon cancers. Age alone should not preclude the optimal use of chemotherapy.

19. Discuss special considerations for the management of prostate cancer in the elderly.

Prostate cancer is largely a disease of older men. Standard options for treatment of localized tumors include radical prostatectomy, radiotherapy (external beam or brachytherapy), and, in select cases, observation. Radiotherapy for prostate cancer in the elderly has equivalent efficacy and toxicity compared with its use in younger men. For localized disease in patients with estimated survival < 10 years, surgery and radiotherapy are equivalent. Some well-differentiated prostate carcinomas can even be followed without active treatment in some elderly patients. Surgery may be superior for patients with a life expectancy > 10 years. In locally advanced disease, radiotherapy has less morbidity than surgery. Metastatic disease requires hormonal therapy. Surgical castration is fully effective, safe, economical, and ensures compliance but is personally unacceptable in 50% of patients. Gonadotropin-releasing hormone analogs are safe and effective but are costly and require long-term compliance. Cytotoxic chemotherapy continues to be studied in the metastatic setting. Studies have demonstrated that mitoxantrone plus prednisone is more effective than prednisone alone in palliative treatment of painful metastases from hormone-refractory prostate cancer. Strontium-89 also is of some value in the palliation of painful bony disease.

20. Are there special considerations regarding lung cancer in the elderly?

Non–small cell lung cancer in the elderly tends to present more often as localized disease, due in part to the higher proportion of squamous cell histology. Despite more limited disease, the elderly, particularly those with comorbid cardiopulmonary disease, are often denied curative surgical approaches and less frequently receive chemotherapy and radiation. Newer surgical techniques, including thoracoscopic lung resections, could make definitive surgical management more applicable to the elderly. Radiotherapy of non–small cell lung cancer can offer effective palliation. Recent data from the Royal Marsden Hospital demonstrate that the use of palliative chemotherapy in the setting of non–small-cell lung cancer can provide symptom relief and objective tumor responses in the elderly population. Small-cell lung cancer in limited stage is curable in the elderly at the same rates as in younger patients as long as renal and cardiac function allow use of standard treatment. For patients who are elderly and infirm, abbreviated chemotherapy strategies may result in effective palliation.

21. What about gynecologic cancer in the elderly?

Gynecologic cancers, regardless of cell type (cervical, uterine, ovarian), present at later stages of disease in older women. Tolerance of standard surgical and chemotherapeutic treatment approaches is similar irrespective of age when adjusted for comorbid illness. More than 50% of ovarian cancers occur in women over 65 years of age. Elderly women with epithelial ovarian cancer have a worse prognosis than younger women, because they present with more advanced malignancies of higher grade or aneuploid DNA content. Despite the fact that age is not clearly associated with increased surgical morbidity or treatment toxicity, elderly women less often receive definitive surgery and/or chemotherapy.

22. Lymphoma?

The epidemiology of Hodgkin's disease predicts for a bimodal age-related incidence, with the second increase occurring in late adulthood. Age itself represents an independent prognostic variable, with age > 60 years at presentation predicting a more advanced initial stage, lower response rate, decreased survival, and increased toxicity from therapy.

Non-Hodgkin's lymphoma is also highly prevalent in the elderly with 25–35% of patients > 70 years. Low-grade subtypes of non-Hodgkin's lymphoma are more common in the elderly. While not considered curable, these tumors can behave indolently over many years. Survival is not improved by early treatment in most patients. Treatment usually is reserved for patients with symptoms, organ involvement, or transformation into higher-grade histologies. Alternatives to standard cytotoxic chemotherapy include monoclonal antibody therapy. With respect to intermediate and high-grade histologies of non-Hodgkin's lymphoma, the elderly consistently have worse survival independent of death from other causes. Evidence suggests that significantly improved response to treatment and survival could be attained with the use of fuller doses of chemotherapy than those typically used in the elderly. Alternate treatment regimens and improved supportive measures such as growth factors may prove helpful in maximizing treatment tolerance in such individuals.

23. Acute myelogenous leukemia (AML)?

AML occurs with a median age of 60 years. Despite successes in the treatment of younger patients, the elderly have lower rates of response, remission, and cure. Poor prognostic factors occur at a higher rate in the elderly and include unfavorable chromosomal aberrations, greater proportions of less-favorable subtypes, antecedent myelodysplastic syndromes, and comorbid medical conditions. Therapy is based on an anthracycline combined with cytarabine. High-dose chemotherapy approaches are particularly poorly tolerated. Despite the use of optimal regimens, efficacy of treatment in the elderly is substantially worse than that in comparable younger patients. Optimal consolidative approaches are still the subject of investigation. An exception is acute promyelocytic leukemia, in which the use of all-transretinoic acid has resulted in high remission rates with acceptable tolerance. Elderly patients too frail to tolerate standard chemotherapy may benefit from the use of palliative low-dose cytarabine.

24. What are some issues concerning sexuality in the elderly cancer patient?

The diagnosis of cancer brings potential threats to the sexual function of the elderly. Four of the principal issues are loss and grief, distressing symptoms, body image changes, and changes in self-esteem and self-control. Physical and sensory dysfunction may come as a result of drug side effects and sedation, hormonal blockade or ablation, psychogenic impairment/depression, and treatment-related nerve or vascular damage and fibrosis. A disruptive loss of privacy is associated with progressive physical disability, presence of outside caregivers, and the typical nursing-home living environment (semiprivate rooms, single beds, unlocked doors, lack of staff comfort with sexual issues).

The elderly patient or couple needs the assistance of the health care provider to recognize and validate these changes and to assist in the process of re-establishing sexuality and a sense of normalcy. Physical rehabilitation should include attention to sexual issues. A program of exercise gives general benefits in terms of endurance, mobility, self-image, and mood. Nutritional support and counseling improve healing, energy level, and general sense of well-being. The physical approach to sexuality may require alterations to accommodate changes in function or comfort level. Attention to rest and normalcy of sleep patterns aids energy level and concentration. Sedatives should be kept to a minimum. Counseling concerning appearance and grooming can help offset some of the changes in appearance associated with surgeries and the effects of chemotherapy or radiation. Medical interventions, such as lubricants, hormonal supplements, penile implants or injections, and vacuum erection aid devices, may have applicability to specific situations. Psychiatric referral should also be considered, when appropriate. Even in the absence of sexual intercourse, the validation of the patient's concerns and the encouragement of closeness and intimacy can provide security when the outside world threatens with hazards and losses.

25. What social needs are prominent in elderly cancer patients?

Cancer death rates are higher among the socioeconomically disadvantaged. A growing number of elderly find themselves enduring worsening financial constraints as old age advances. Almost one-third of Americans aged > 65 live alone, and approximately 30% of these have no children. Such issues impact directly on the safety and effectiveness of oncologic care, patient compliance, home-based care, and access to medical facilities for evaluation, treatment, and follow-up. A complete and understandable educational process for the elderly is important to dispel potential misconceptions about their disease and treatment. Attention must be paid to potential sensory and cognitive deficits when medical information is communicated. Rehabilitation (physical, occupational, psychological, prosthetics) is an essential component of any cancer treatment plan for the elderly and often benefits from a multidisciplinary approach.

26. How does the caregiver of the elderly cancer patient cope with the illness?

Studies have compared the experience (depression, lifestyle change, change in health, level of care provided to the patient, level of assistance provided to caregiver by friends and family) of the caregiver based on the age of the patient and the stage of the illness. When the patient is younger, the caregivers tend to be more depressed and experience greater impact on their lifestyle. These same caregivers tend to derive more support from their family and friends. As the patient's disease progresses to its terminal phases, all caregivers, regardless of age, experience higher levels of depression, greater health and lifestyle impact, and increased demands to provide care to the patient. Early phases of the patient's illness tend to place largely emotional stresses on the caregivers, while the burden of providing care to the patient dominates the late phases of the disease. Caregiver strain develops as increasing difficulty arises in the fulfillment of the caregiver's perceived responsibilities. Additionally, the level of practical and social support provided by friends and family tends to remain constant or decrease in the late stages of the illness, leaving the patient and caregiver increasingly isolated.

Physicians and social workers can intervene in this situation to provide caregivers with:
- Home care support (home health aids)
- Financial analysis/assessment of eligibility for resources
- Referral to "wellness community" (community-based psychological support groups)
- Treatment-center based support groups

BIBLIOGRAPHY

1. Byrne A, Carney DN: Cancer in the elderly. Curr Probl Cancer 17:147–218, 1993.
2. Feldman EJ: Acute myelogenous leukemia in the older patient. Semin Oncol 22(suppl 1):21–24, 1995.
3. Fleming RA, Capizzi RL: General aspects of cancer chemotherapy in the aged. Adv Exp Med Biol 330:271–286, 1993.
4. Hickish TF, Smith IE, O'Brien ME, et al: Clinical benefit from palliative chemotherapy in non–small-cell lung cancer extends to the elderly and those with poor prognostic factors. Br J Cancer 78:28–33, 1998.
5. McKenna RJ Sr: Clinical aspects of cancer in the elderly: Treatment decisions, treatment choices, and follow-up. Cancer 74:2107–2117, 1994.
6. Tannock IF, Ozoha D, Stockler MR, et al: Chemotherapy with mitoxantrone plus prednisone or prednisone alone for symptomatic hormone resistant prostate cancer: A Canadian randomized trial with palliative endpoints. J Clin Oncol 14:1756–1764, 1996.
7. Weinrich S, Sarna L: Delirium in the older person with cancer. Cancer 74:2079–2091, 1994.

51. DERMATOLOGY

David Margolis, M.D., and Jeffrey Miller, M.D.

1. What happens to the skin as an individual ages?

Skin changes with aging include the formation of skin cancers and precancers, wrinkles and furrows, increased "dryness," easy bruising, and impaired healing response. These changes are due to alterations in the architecture of the epidermis, dermis, and subcutaneous fat layer and in the interactions among the various cells of the skin and the immune system.

The keratinocyte is the major cell type found in the epidermis. These cells are prone to environmental insults that accumulate with age. The most important repetitive insult is from sunlight, and this is believed to be the chief risk factor for premature aging of the skin, such as the formation of wrinkles and all types of skin cancer. Aging and photodamage alter the way the epidermis and dermis interface, resulting in increased cutaneous fragility. Fibroblasts, which are the chief cellular component of the dermis and are responsible for the formation of much of the extracellular matrix of the dermis, enter a period of senescence with biologic aging of the body. Aged fibroblasts are unable to replicate and respond properly to growth factors, thereby leading to degenerative collagen and elastic components. The subcutaneous fat layer degenerates with age, contributing to the lax, inelastic feel of aged skin.

2. Why does the skin of older individuals flake?

The frequency of complaints related to dry skin increases with aging. This increased frequency is probably related to a decrease in the production of sebum and keratinocyte-produced fatty acids, an increase in water vapor permeability across the dermal-epidermal barrier, and harsher methods used to care for the skin. Clinically, these skin problems can be manifested as mild scaling to frank excoriation. Dry skin is often associated with pruritus.

Treatment includes the frequent use of emollients and moisturizers. Since the geriatric population is at increased risk of developing contact dermatitis, care must be exercised to ensure that any topical product used is not a sensitizing agent for that patient. These products may need to be applied as frequently as four times daily. Patients should also be instructed in gentle skin care, which includes the use of a moisturizing soap, infrequent bathing or showering using tepid water, and gentle drying of the skin by patting rather than rubbing.

3. How is pruritus approached in the elderly?

Many older persons present with the chief complaint of pruritus (itching). Pruritus may be due to a primary skin disease, systemic disease, or multifactorial or idiopathic causes. Xerosis, defined as rough, dry, scaling skin, is the most common cause of pruritus in the elderly. This type of pruritus is often called senile pruritus. Xerosis may be related to winter and its low humidity, excessive bathing, medications (e.g., opiates), and atopy (e.g., history of hay fever, eczema, asthma). Other causes of pruritus include psychogenic factors related to stress and depression and manifestations of systemic disease, such as renal, thyroid, hepatic, anemia, diabetes, and malignancy.

Therapy is directed at the underlying cause of the pruritus. Emollient cream and ointment (e.g., Dermasil), decreased bathing, application of nonmedicated soap (e.g., Dove) limited to the axilla and genital areas, moderate strength topical corticosteroids (e.g., fluocinolone or triamcinolone ointment), and systemic antihistamines are used for pruritus related to xerosis. If no skin disease is evident, an underlying systemic disorder needs to be investigated based on history and physical exam.

4. Why do the lower extremities become red and swollen?

Lower extremity swelling can be related to impaired venous or lymphatic flow. These abnormalities can be secondary to congenital disorders, such as lymphedema praecox, or acquired disorders, such as deep venous thromboembolism or congestive heart failure. Edematous limbs frequently become dermatitic and clinically may mimic cellulitis. In patients with venous disease, the chronicity of the edema may lead to sclerosis of the cutaneous structures and a skin finding called **lipodermatosclerosis**. Both dermatitis and lipodermatosclerosis are most likely due to trauma to the cutaneous structures from the edema. In addition, a significant increased incidence of contact dermatitis is noted in edematous limbs.

It is important to understand the cause of the edema before treating it. For example, diuretics work well for edema related to congestive heart failure but poorly for venous-related edema, which responds to external compression. Treatment should include the use of topical emollients. Petrolatum is the least likely to cause a contact dermatitis. The use of topical steroids should be limited. They initially appear to be helpful but are treating only a symptom, dermatitis, and not the problem, limb edema.

5. What is shingles?

Shingles, or herpes zoster, is the reactivation of the latent herpes varicella-zoster virus usually in a dermatomal pattern. Reactivation tends to occur in the elderly population, as well as in patients who are immunosuppressed secondary to collagen vascular disease, malignancy, or medications. Patients often note a prodrome of burning in the involved dermatome. The disorder is then manifested by grouped vesicles or pustules within a dermatome. The most common sites of involvement are the trunk, face, and scalp. The disease may disseminate to involve more than one dermatome, a presentation that is more likely in immunocompromised hosts. The reactivation of varicella-zoster virus is usually self-limited with full resolution within 2 weeks. Antiviral agents such as acyclovir, 800 mg 4 times/day for 5 days, are approved for the treatment of varicella-zoster infections. However, a sizable group of patients will develop chronic discomfort called post-herpetic neuralgia.

6. Define post-herpetic neuralgia.

No consensus exists for defining post-herpetic neuralgia. An acceptable definition is the persistence of skin discomfort in an area of recent varicella-zoster reactivation. However, the definition of persistence ranges from pain after all lesions are healed to pain that is present > 30–90 days after all lesions have been healed. Post-herpetic neuralgia most commonly occurs in the elderly with an increasing prevalence with increasing age. The discomfort can vary from burning to a sharp pain that can be debilitating.

Studies show that early treatment of the initial reactivation of varicella-zoster with oral antiviral agents can avoid the development of post-herpetic neuralgia. Early intervention with these agents is probably indicated for patients at highest risk to develop this sequela, the aged. Past reports examined the use of corticosteroids and antiviral agents. Corticosteroids are probably helpful for pain management but do not ultimately alter the disease. Once post-herpetic neuralgia has occurred, treatments are relatively unsuccessful. Treatments for the chronic pain associated with post-herpetic neuralgia include capsaicin, anticonvulsants, narcotics, antidepressants, electrical stimulation, acupuncture, ketamine, and lidocaine.

7. Describe the different causes of leg ulcers.

Leg ulcers afflict approximately 1% of the population, with at least two thirds of those afflicted being over age 60 years. Causes of chronic leg ulcers include venous disease, arterial insufficiency, insensate ulcers, pressure ulcers, sickle cell ulcers, and vasculitis.

Insensate ulcers or neuropathic ulcers are usually related to diabetes mellitus but can be related to other diseases that cause a sensory neuropathy, such as leprosy, and are usually located on the plantar areas of the foot. The wound may be associated with a Charcot joint. Lower extremity wounds associated with **arterial insufficiency** are usually accompanied by claudication. Claudication is pain that occurs suddenly in the lower extremity after a metabolic challenge and is quickly relieved after resolution of this challenge. The most common chronic leg ulcer is related to **venous disease**. Venous disease occurs because of elevated ambulatory venous pressures.

These pressures can be elevated because of obstruction of the deep venous system of the leg (e.g., clot), loss of valvular competence of the veins communicating between the deep and superficial venous system (e.g., varicose veins), or loss of the muscular tone of the calf. It is also not uncommon for an individual to suffer from more than one cause of leg ulcer (e.g., venous *and* arterial disease) concomitantly.

Treatment of chronic wounds depends on the correct diagnosis. Once the diagnosis is made, treatment should be based on removing the cause of the wound. For example, an individual with venous disease needs to have the ambulatory venous hypertension decreased by augmenting venous return with external compression, while an individual with arterial insufficiency needs improved arterial flow that may require surgical intervention. Good wound care should be provided for the ulcer. This includes the use of moist dressing, removal of necrotic tissue, and gentle cleansing.

8. What is the most common blistering disease in the elderly?

Bullous pemphigoid. Most cases appear in patients over age 60 years. Bullous pemphigoid is characterized by a chronic, nonscarring vesicular bullous eruption in which nongrouped bullae occur on normal or urticarial skin. Lesions are most common on flexural surfaces, with the oral mucosa affected in one-third of patients. Nikolsky's sign (induction of blister with lateral skin pressure) is negative. The blistering results from autoantibodies directed against a 230-kilodalton antigen which anchors the basal cells of the epidermis to the basement membrane. Biopsy of an early small blister reveals a subepidermal blister. Diagnosis is often confirmed through direct and indirect immunofluorescence that identifies the patient's autoantibodies. The disease typically lasts a year with a variable number of flareups.

Bullous pemphigoid is to be distinguished from **pemphigus vulgaris**. Pemphigus vulgaris produces widespread erosions and flaccid bullae with a positive Nikolsky sign. Mucous membranes are commonly affected. Age of onset is frequently in the 4th to 5th decade. The blistering is caused by autoantibodies directed against adhesion molecules between keratinocytes in the epidermis. Direct and indirect immunofluorescence is diagnostic.

9. Do the elderly get acne?

Rosacea, a condition often confused with acne, commonly affects the middle-aged to elderly. Found in 10% of the general population, the disease is characterized by flushing, facial erythema and telangiectases, papules and pustules, and rhinophyma. Most patients present with facial erythema and telangiectases. The absence of comedones and different age prevalence distinguish rosacea from acne. The differential diagnosis of rosacea includes carcinoid syndrome, seborrheic dermatitis, lupus erythematosus, contact dermatitis, and steroid-induced rosacea.

10. What is a reasonable approach to hair loss in the elderly?

At menopause in women and at age 20–40 years in men, thin hair and hair loss may become a severe problem. A good medical and drug history needs to be taken, and simple tests for thyroid function, free testosterone, and dihydroepiandrosterone sulfate levels as well as complete blood count should be conducted in the appropriate setting. Correction of the medical problem may help, especially in nutritional and metabolic deficiency states. For example, replacement of iron in iron-deficiency anemia can restore hair growth. Spironolactone at a dose of 50–200 mg/day may be helpful if an androgen excess is uncovered. If there is no medical abnormality, other approaches include topical minoxidil, oral finasteride, and surgical approaches such as hair transplants and scalp reductions. Minoxidil and finasteride must be used for several months before hair regrowth can be observed. Shedding of hair occurs if the patient uses less than the recommended dose or stops treatment.

11. How common is melanoma?

The incidence of melanoma continues to rise throughout the world. In the United States, its incidence has nearly tripled in the past four decades, growing faster than that of any other cancer. By the year 2000, projections suggest that melanoma will develop in 1 out of 75–90 white

Americans. African-Americans and Asians have decreased rates of melanoma because of greater degrees of pigmentation. It is important to note that the highest age-specific incidence rates occur in the elderly population. Recognizing risk factors for melanoma is important because prognosis is excellent with early detection and treatment of melanoma. Major risk factors for melanoma include:

Higher than average number of benign melanocytic nevi
Atypical nevi (> 6 mm size, irregular border, and variegated color)
Pigmentary characteristics of blue eyes, blond or red hair, and fair complexion
Personal history of melanoma
Family history of melanoma
Immunosuppression
Excessive sun exposure

12. What are the clinical signs of melanoma?

As a visible tumor, cutaneous melanoma can be recognized and detected early. An **ABCDE** rule has been established to help diagnose melanoma in any pigmented lesion.

A—**A**symmetry
B—**B**order irregularity
C—**C**olor variegation
D—**D**iameter > 0.6 cm (size of pencil eraser)
E—**E**levation

Melanoma should also be suspected if a patient reports any change in an existing mole or a new pigmented lesion. Also, itching and burning of a mole should raise suspicion for melanoma, but most patients with melanoma experience no symptoms. A definitive diagnosis requires an excisional biopsy for histologic examination.

13. Which nonmelanoma skin cancers are seen most commonly in the elderly?

Basal cell carcinomas and **squamous cell carcinomas** are common nonmelanoma skin cancers in the elderly. More than one-third of all cancers in the United States are nonmelanoma skin cancers. Basal cell carcinoma commonly presents as a translucent flesh-colored or pink pearly papule with prominent telangiectases. Squamous cell carcinoma typically presents as a firm, erythematous nodule with elevated borders and occasional central ulceration. Both types of cancer commonly occur in sun-exposed areas, such as the head, neck, and arms. Basal cell carcinomas have a low risk of metastases (< 1/400 cases). Squamous cell carcinomas also have a low risk of metastases, except when they appear in the setting of immunosuppression or at sites of chronic inflammation, scar tissue, and radiation.

14. Are sunscreens important for the elderly?

Chronic exposure to the sun's ultraviolet rays, UVB and UVA, is thought to be the primary cause of skin cancer and skin aging. It is estimated that about 75% of the total lifetime dose of UV radiation is accumulated before age 20 years. Sunscreens are important in the battle against skin cancer and skin aging. Regular use of a sunscreen in the elderly population is important because this practice can minimize the risk of sun-induced skin cancer, slow the effect of photoaging, and prevent drug-induced photosensitivity.

15. How does sun protective factor (SPF) work?

The best chemical sunscreens provide UVA and UVB coverage. The effect of a sunscreen's SPF number depends on the patient's minimal erythemal dose (MED), defined as how long it takes the sunlight in a particular place, on a particular day, to turn skin barely pink. Whatever the patient's MED for a particular time and place, a sunscreen's SPF value can be used to estimate how long he or she can safely stay outdoors. Just multiply the MED by the SPF number.

Sensitivity to UVB radiation is determined by the melanin content of skin. This has led to the assignment of skin types I to VI based on sun sensitivity and pigment response. Sun exposure results in sunburn in a shorter period of time with skin type I compared to skin type IV. Therefore, a person's MED increases with higher skin types.

SKIN TYPE	COMPLEXION	MED UVB (mJ/cm²)	RECOMMENDED SPF	SUNBURN/TANNING HISTORY
I	Very fair	15–30	15–30	Always burns; never tans
II	Fair	25–35	15–30	Often burns; tans mildly
III	Light	30–50	15–30	Sometimes burns; tans gradually
IV	Medium	45–60	10–15	Rarely burns; tans easily
V	Dark	60–90	10–15	Never burns; tans easily
VI	Darkly pigmented	90–120	6–10	Never burns; deeply tans

16. Name the most common dermatologic conditions seen in the geriatric population.

Patients who presented to a geriatric clinic and noninstitutionalized volunteers who underwent a full skin examination were evaluated for skin conditions. Although this survey is limited by sample size and bias, the following skin conditions were commonly seen in this geriatric population (age > 65 years old):

Seborrheic keratosis (benign neoplasm of epidermal cells appearing as a pasted-on papule)
Actinic keratosis (precancerous neoplasm of the epidermis caused by sunlight)
Pruritus
Tinea pedis (fungal skin infection characterized by plantar scale)
Seborrheic dermatitis (chronic, superficial, inflammatory process especially affecting the scalp, eyebrows, and face)
Venous stasis dermatitis
Nonmelanoma skin cancers

BIBLIOGRAPHY

1. Bolognia JL: Aging skin. Am J Med 98(1A):99S–103S, 1995.
2. Koh HK: Cutaneous melanoma. N Engl J Med 325:171–182, 1991.
3. Kurban RS, Kurban AK: Common skin disorders of aging: Diagnosis and treatment. Geriatrics 48:30–42, 1993.
4. O'Donoghue MN: Cosmetics for the elderly. Dermatol Clin 9:29–34, 1991.
5. Sunderkotter C, Kalden H, Luger TA: Aging and the skin immune system. Arch Dermatol 133:1256–1262, 1997.
6. West MD: The cellular and molecular biology of skin aging. Arch Dermatol 130:87–95, 1994.

V. Health Systems and Innovations

52. HEALTH CARE SYSTEMS

Christopher L. Vojta, M.D., M.B.A., and Risa Lavizzo-Mourey, M.D., M.B.A.

1. Why is health care for the elderly such an important issue?

In 1999, there were approximately 34 million Americans over the age of 65. This number is expected to double by 2030. In addition, the oldest of the old is the fastest growing segment of the senior population with 11.7 million Americans between 75 and 84 years old and 3.9 million over 85. Fifty-two percent of the elderly live in nine states: California, Florida, New York, Texas, Pennsylvania, Ohio, Illinois, and New Jersey. Although the percentage and number of elderly Americans living in poverty has declined dramatically since the 1960s, one in six older persons continues to live within 125% of the poverty line. Thirty-five percents of households with heads over 65 years old report net income less than $15,000.

Income in Households with Head of Household 65 Years and Over, 1997

Under $5,000	3%
$5,000–9,999	16%
$10,000–14,999	16%
$15,000–24,999	23%
$25,000–34,999	14%
$35,000–49,999	12%
$50,000–74,999	8%
$75,000–99,999	4%
$100,000 and over	4%

Source: U.S. Bureau of the Census: Current Population Reports, P60-200. Money Income in the United States: 1997 (With Separate Data on Valuation of Noncash Benefits). Washington, DC, U.S. Government Printing Office, 1998.

The health status of the elderly is dominated by chronic conditions. In 1995, 37% of seniors reported limitations due to chronic conditions, and 10.5% were unable to carry out a major activity. In addition, 4.4 million elderly Americans report difficulty with at least one activity of daily living, and 6.5 million report difficulty with at least one instrumental activity of daily living. As a result, over 70% of health expenditures in the U.S. are for chronic conditions. In addition, the elderly account for 40% of hospital stays and 49% of hospital days and average 11.1 doctor contacts per year.

Medicare Spending by Type of Benefit—Fiscal Year, 1997

	BENEFIT PAYMENTS (BILLIONS OF DOLLARS)	PERCENT DISTRIBUTION
Total: Part A	116.5	100
Inpatient hospital	86.8	74
Skilled nursing facility	10.7	9
Home health agency	17.5	15
Hospice	2.0	2

Table continued on following page

Medicare Spending by Type of Benefit—Fiscal Year, 1997 (Continued)

	BENEFIT PAYMENTS (BILLIONS OF DOLLARS)	PERCENT DISTRIBUTION
Total: Part B	72.7	100
Physician/other suppliers	42.4	58
Outpatient hospital	17.4	24
Other	12.9	18

Source: Medicare Payment Advisory Commission: Health Care Spending and the Medicare Program: A Data Book. Washington, DC, Health Care Financing Administration, 1998.

2. What is Social Security?

Social Security consists of four trust funds: Old-Age Survivors Insurance (OASI), Disability Insurance (DI), Hospital Insurance Trust Fund (Medicare Part A), and Supplementary Medical Insurance (Part B). OASI is a federally funded program that covers all employed Americans. It is designed to provide income to the elderly after they retire and is funded through payroll taxes. In 1999, over 144 million people worked in Social Security-covered employment, each paying 6.2% of earnings to the OASI and 1.45% of earning to Medicare Part A (to a maximum of $72,600 in 1999). Corporations also pay OASI and Part A taxes of 6.2% and 1.45%, respectively. Self-employed workers, therefore, pay a total of 15.3% in Social Security-related taxes.

The OASI has allowed retirees to maintain income at the level of other Americans; it provides 36% of income for people over 65 years old. Until recently, full benefits began at age 65, but for people born after 1959, benefits begin at age 67. Beneficiaries can choose to begin receiving benefits as early as age 62, but at a lower level. In 1996, 37.7 million retired workers and survivors received total payments of $302.9 billion, or an average monthly payout of $720. Benefit amounts for each person are calculated on the highest average indexed earnings over 35 years. In 1999, OASI is partially prefunded, but this surplus is projected to disappear by 2012; at present rates, assets of the OASI trust fund will be depleted by 2032.

3. What is the Older Americans Act?

Title II of the Social Security Act was passed in 1965 with the goal of fostering community-based services for the elderly. The stated mission was to help older persons achieve adequate retirement income; best possible physical and mental health; suitable and affordable housing; institutional, home, and community-based long-term care; and employment without age discrimination. Initially, it provided small grants to state agencies on aging to fund social services programs, but in the 1970s its budget rose as a national nutrition program (including "meals on wheels") and area agencies on aging were established. The programs generally are not means-tested.

4. What is Medicaid?

Medicaid is a state and federally funded program designed to provide health care for the poor. The federal government mandates that states provide a basic package of services, including hospital, doctor, and nursing home services, but because the states have wide latitude in designing their programs, Medicaid varies widely in different states. Between 1980 and 1990 spending on Medicaid increased 300%. In 1995, total program costs were $152 billion, of which the federal government paid $86 billion and the states paid $66 billion.

In 1996, there were about 37.5 million Medicaid recipients, of whom 4.4 million were elderly. Although the majority of the elderly do not meet Medicaid income requirements, those who enter nursing homes often quickly spend down their assets to pay for care and then look to Medicaid for continuing support. Thus, Medicaid is the largest payor of long-term care for all Americans, covering 68% of nursing home residents and over 50% of nursing home costs.

5. What is meant by dual eligibility for Medicaid and Medicare?

Dually eligible people are covered by both Medicare and Medicaid. Generally they include the poor elderly. Approximately 6 million Americans received both Medicare and Medicaid benefits in 1995, and another 3–4 million were eligible but not receiving benefits. This population tends to be at greater risk than other elderly, accounting for 30% of Medicare and 35% of Medicaid expenditures.

Of the 6 million dually eligible Americans, 5.4 million qualify for the full range of benefits, and 500,000 are Qualified Medicare Beneficiaries or Special Low-Income Medicare Beneficiaries (SLMBs) who receive varying levels of help to cover Medicare out-of-pocket expenses. SLMBs usually are the near poor with incomes at 100–120% of the poverty level.

6. How important is the Veterans Administration (VA) system?

The VA is one of the largest health care systems in the world and the largest integrated health system in the U.S. The VA provides care to over 3.1 million patients with nearly 827,000 inpatient stays and 32 million outpatient visits in 1997. It owns and operates approximately 171 hospitals, 127 nursing homes, and 93 clinics. The VA has an annual health care budget of $15 billion, of which $1 billion goes to research. Although these funds traditionally have come from the federal government, increased emphasis will be placed on cost sharing with third party payors such as Medicare in the future.

In 1995, the VA began a fundamental realignment from specialty-based inpatient care toward outpatient primary care. The system was divided into 22 regional Veteran Integrated Service Networks charged with budgeting and planning functions for all medical care within their respective boundaries. Traditionally, eligibility for VA health benefits has been restricted to veterans with service-connected disabilities and those who are poor. This is a small proportion of the roughly 26 million veterans. Of those eligible, however, approximately 40% receive some care through the VA system. A major component of the VA's new strategic direction is its Special Emphasis Programs.

Veterans Health Administration Special Emphasis Programs

Addictive disorders	Preservation/amputation care
Blind rehabilitation	Prosthetics and rehabilitative medicine
Geriatrics and long-term care	Readjustment counseling
Gulf War veterans	Seriously mentally ill
Homelessness	Spinal cord injury and disorders
Posttraumatic stress disorder	Women veterans

Source: Veterans Health Administration: Annual Report and Strategic Forecast. Washington, DC, Department of Veterans Affairs, 1998, p 43.

7. How did we end up with our current health system?

In the past two centuries, the American health care system has been transformed from one in which the doctor-patient relationship predominated to one dominated by third party payors. Throughout the 1800s, patients generally sought health care on a fee-for-service basis and negotiated payments with their physicians. With the Industrial Revolution, the first significant insurance policies sprouted to protect injured workers. The depression speeded the proliferation of insurance as doctors and hospitals sought to protect steady streams of income by encouraging the formation of insurance plans. After World War II, an era of hospital construction reigned, and the government encouraged workers to accept health care benefits in lieu of higher wages. The 1960s were marked by the creation of the first large safety nets in the form of Medicare and Medicaid. Unexpectedly large increases in costs of financing these programs led to attempts to curb costs, beginning with the Tax Equity and Fiscal Responsibility Act in 1973, which allowed the creation of managed care organizations. Hospitals were subsequently targeted with the introduction of the prospective payment system and diagnosis-related groupings in 1983. The 1990s have brought the increasing ascendency of managed care organizations in various forms, despite the 1996 defeat of the Clinton health plan.

Milestones in the Development of the United States Health Care System

YEAR	MILESTONE	IMPLICATIONS
1800s		Patient-doctor relationship only. Health care provided on fee-for-service basis.
Early 1900s	Industrial Revolution	Industrial policies develop to pay for medical bills and funeral costs of injured workers.
1929	Great Depression	Expansion of traditional insurance plans. Start of Blue Cross movement when Baylor University enrolls 1250 public teachers in insurance plan.
1935	Formation of National Institutes of Health	
1938	Formation of Food and Drug Administration	
1946	Hill-Burton Act	Favors building of hospitals. Exempts health care benefits from wage and price controls by making corporate contributions to health care tax-deductible.
1963	Health Professions Educational Assistance Act	Provides direct federal aid to medical and allied health professional schools.
1965	Medicare/Medicaid and Older Americans Act	Medicare protects elderly from catastrophic health events. Medicaid provides safety net for the poor. Older Americans Act provides for community-based services for the elderly.
1973	Tax Equity and Fiscal Responsibility Act	Encourages growth of managed care through grants and federal demonstration projects.
1983	Prospective Payment System	Replaces Medicare fee-for-service payments to hospitals with prospective payments based on diagnosis-related groupings
1996	Clinton health plan defeated	Attempt at implementing universal health coverage defeated. Managed care continues to gain members.
1998	Medicare + Choices	Medicare members given option of receiving Medicare benefits under managed care plans.

BIBLIOGRAPHY

1. Department of Veterans Affairs–Veterans Health Administration: Journey of Change II. Annual Report and Strategic Forecast. Washington, DC, 1998.
2. Harper-Alport J (ed): 1998 Medicare Explained. Chicago, CCH Incorporated, 1998.
3. Health Care Financing Administration internet website.
4. Health Care Financing Administration, Bureau of Data Management and Strategy: Data from the Division of Health Care Information Services and the Office of the Actuary: Data from the Office of Medicare and Medicaid Cost Estimates, Washington, DC, 1998.
5. Iglehart JK: The American health care system—Medicaid. N Engl J Med 340:403–408, 1999.
6. Iglehart JK: The American health care system—Medicare. N Engl J Med 340:327–332, 1999.
7. Medicare Payment Advisory Commission: Health Care Spending and the Medicare Program: A Data Book. Washington, DC, Health Care Financing Administration, 1998.
8. Schultz HA, Young K: Health Care USA. Understanding Its Organization and Delivery. Gaithersburg, MD, Aspen Press, 1997.
9. Starr P: The Social Transformation of American Medicine. New York, Harper Collins, 1982.

53. THE ABCs OF MEDICARE REIMBURSEMENT

Dennis S. Hsieh, M.D., Madhurika Samakur, and
Risa Lavizzo-Mourey, M.D., M.B.A.

1. What is Medicare? Which patients are covered by Medicare?

Medicare was implemented in 1966 as part of the Social Security Amendments of 1965 and pays for the health care expenses of people over the age of 65. By 1973, people who qualified for Social Security or Railroad Retirement disability benefits for at least 24 months and people with end-stage renal disease became eligible to receive Medicare benefits. Medicare consists of hospital insurance and supplementary insurance. Hospital insurance, also known as Part A, helps to cover the costs of hospital stays, skilled nursing care, home visits, and hospice care. Supplementary insurance, known as Part B, helps to pay for physician services, outpatient hospital services, and various other outpatient health services, studies, and supplies. Medicare beneficiaries are automatically enrolled in Part A. For enrollment in Part B, Medicare beneficiaries must pay a premium that usually is taken out of their monthly Social Security checks. In addition, the enrollee is responsible for deductibles and copayments under both Parts A and B.

2. An elderly woman broke her hip and was hospitalized for 1 week. She then had a 2-week stay in a skilled nursing facility. What is covered? What does she have to pay?

Hospital stays are covered by Medicare Part A. Coverage amounts and limits are determined by the spell of illness. Part A coverage pays for inpatient care for up to 90 days of a spell of illness. Once a deductible is paid ($768 in 1999), Medicare pays for all covered services for the first 60 days. For the next 30 days, the patient is required to pay a coinsurance ($192/day in 1999), after which Medicare pays for all covered services. If more than 90 days are needed in the hospital, the Medicare beneficiary can choose to use any number of her 60 lifetime reserve days, paying a coinsurance ($384/day in 1999) for each reserve day used.

For an approved stay in a skilled nursing facility (some of which are nursing homes), Medicare pays for up to 100 days of nursing care during a spell of illness (in addition to the 90 days of hospital coverage), starting on the day she enters the facility. All skilled nursing care services are covered by Medicare for the first 20 days. The next 80 days require a daily coinsurance ($96.50/day in 1999). If more than 100 days of skilled nursing care are needed, the beneficiary is responsible for all costs.

3. Explain "spell of illness" and "reserve days."

A spell of illness begins the day when the patient enters the hospital and ends when the patient has been out of the hospital for 60 consecutive days. For each hospital spell of illness, the patient is required to pay a separate deductible. For example, if a patient has been in the hospital for 1 week after a hip replacement and is readmitted 3 weeks later because of a stroke, Medicare considers both hospitalizations as part of one spell of illness. Conversely, if a patient is admitted for congestive heart failure and then readmitted for the same illness 61 or more days after discharge, the two hospital admissions are considered separate spells of illness, even though they were for the same diagnosis.

For the 61st to 90th days in a spell of illness, the patient must pay a daily copayment. Medicare stops paying for hospital costs after 90 days for any given spell of illness. However, each Medicare recipient is entitled to 60 lifetime reserve days. These days may be used if a spell of illness lasts longer than 90 days. The patient decides when and how many reserve days to use. Patients should choose wisely, budgeting their use of the 60 days over their lifetime.

4. How does Medicare pay for office visits?

Medicare Part B pays for all physician services (including physician services provided in the inpatient setting), outpatient medical services (such as physical therapy, occupational therapy, speech therapy, and medically required podiatric services), and supplies not covered by Part A. Part B also covers outpatient tests and procedures, even if they are done at a hospital.

Medicare pays for services only by participating providers. Because of the regulations for reimbursement, most providers participate in Medicare. Recipients are responsible for paying an annual deductible of $100. After the deductible, Medicare pays 80% of allowable charges for the rest of the calendar year. Beneficiaries are responsible for the remaining 20% of the allowable charges. The participating provider may not bill the beneficiary for any charges that exceed the maximum allowed by Medicare. The provider may bill beneficiaries for services that Medicare does not cover (for example, a face lift); however, the provider must disclose the charges before the services are rendered.

Beneficiaries, in addition, must pay a premium for Part B coverage ($45.50 per month in 1999). Theoretically, the premium covers one-fourth of the cost of Medicare Part B services; usually, however, collected premiums fall short of this percentage. The premium usually is deducted automatically from monthly Social Security checks.

5. An elderly man needs to see a cardiologist and may need a stress test. He is worried about the cost. Does Medicare pay for consults and tests?

Because the cardiology consult is a physician service and the stress test is an outpatient procedure (even though it may be done at the hospital), all of the services are covered by Medicare Part B. The patient is responsible for the annual $100 deductible and 20% of Medicare-allowed charges. The $100 deductible applies to the first $100 of allowed charges in any given calendar year. Thus, if the patient receives services from multiple providers, payment of the $100 may be split among different providers. Once the $100 deductible is met, there are no more deductibles until the next calendar year.

6. An elderly man cannot afford prescribed medicines, whereas other patients get their medicines at little cost. Why do only some patients get prescription coverage?

Part A of traditional Medicare covers medicines given as part of the hospital stay. Part B, however, does not provide prescription coverage for the outpatient setting. Medicare-eligible patients who have prescription coverage either are enrolled in Medicare Part C or receive prescription coverage from other sources. Common options include private insurance (such as Medigap) and state-administered health programs (such as Medicaid and prescription assistance programs for the elderly).

7. An elderly man may have depression and should see a psychiatrist. He is concerned about the cost of the services. What will Medicare pay?

Inpatient mental health services provided at Medicare-participating psychiatric hospitals are covered by Part A. Patient deductibles and copayments are similar to those for general inpatient care except for the lifetime maximum of 190 inpatient days. However, there is no specific limit to the number of days of psychiatric care that a patient receives in a general hospital. The beneficiary is responsible for the costs of all inpatient psychiatric care after the 190 days are used. Outpatient services from psychiatrists, psychologists, and clinical social workers are covered under Part B. However, outpatient care for psychiatric diagnoses is covered at 62.5%. Thus, the patient is responsible for a copayment of 37.5% of allowable charges for psychiatric services.

8. An elderly woman suffered a stroke and needs skilled nursing services and physical therapy at home. Will Medicare pay?

Home health care services are offered by agencies that provide skilled nursing care, physical therapy, and other therapeutic services. Depending on the circumstances, these services are covered under either Part A or Part B, as long as they are provided by a Medicare-approved agency and as long as the care is acute rather than chronic or supportive. To qualify for this coverage, the patient must need intermittent skilled nursing care, physical therapy, or speech therapy. In addition, the beneficiary must be confined to the home and be under a doctor's care.

In addition to part-time or intermittent skilled nursing care, other covered services include part-time home health aide services, occupational therapy, physical therapy, and medical equipment. Services are covered in full, but beneficiaries are responsible for 20% of Medicare-approved charges for durable medical equipment, plus any amount in excess of the approved amount on unassigned claims. Medicare does not cover full-time nursing care, meals delivered to the home, or homemaker services intended primarily to assist in meeting personal care or housekeeping needs.

9. An elderly woman needs to move into a nursing home. How much will Medicare pay?

Medicare does not cover custodial care. Patients who require short-term, acute skilled nursing care after a hospital stay often go to a nursing facility before discharge home. If the nursing home is a certified skilled nursing facility, acute care is covered by Medicare. The patient is responsible for paying for custodial care (long-term care) in the nursing home. If the patient is financially unable to pay, state Medicaid programs may help. To qualify for Medicaid, patients must "spend down" their assets and reach poverty levels.

It is estimated that one-half of all Americans turning 65 will be in nursing homes at least once; of those, one-fifth will stay for at least 1 year. Long-term care (LTC) insurance has been advocated as a method to finance nursing home care. Despite certain tax incentives for purchasing LTC insurance, it is prohibitively expensive for most older people. In addition, LTC insurance covers part, but not all, of the expenses associated with nursing home care. Analysis of whether and when to purchase LTC insurance is somewhat complicated. A person may pay significant premiums over many years and never use the insurance. Crude estimates place the optimal age to start purchasing LTC insurance in the 50s.

Across the board, over one-half of nursing home reimbursement comes from state Medicaid programs. One-third of the payments come directly from patients and their families. Less than 10% comes from Medicare, and only 2% comes from private insurance.

10. An elderly patient has terminal lung cancer. Will Medicare pay for hospice care?

Hospice care, which provides care for terminally ill people, is paid by Medicare Part A if the care is provided by a Medicare-certified hospice and if the beneficiary has a life expectancy of 6 months or less. Hospice services covered under Medicare include:

- Physician services
- Nursing care
- Medical equipment
- Short-term inpatient care
- Medical social services
- Physical and occupational therapy
- Speech and language pathology services
- Nutritional counseling
- Home health aide and homemaker services

A Medicare recipient can receive up to 5 days of inpatient care. There are no deductibles for this coverage. Prescriptions directly related to hospice care (such as pain medicines) also are covered. However, there is a copayment of 5% of the reasonable cost of drugs, not to exceed $5 per prescription. For respite care, copayment is $5/day. If Medicare benefits are used for the treatment of an illness unrelated to the terminal illness, the patient is responsible for paying any applicable deductibles and coinsurance.

11. Give examples of services that Medicare does not cover.

- Outpatient medications
- Custodial services, such as custodial care, routine maintenance services, and nonmedical therapeutic services (as determined by Medicare regulations; not based on physician approval or approval by the Food and Drug Administration)
- Traditional nursing home care (although Medicare covers acute care in skilled nursing facilities, it does not cover long-term home nursing care for chronic and stable illnesses)
- Any service that is not necessary or reasonable (as determined by Medicare regulations; not based on physician approval or approval by the Food and Drug Administration)
- Personal care items

- Cosmetic surgery
- Telephone, television, and other such personal items
- Routine foot care and related services
- Private room and private nursing

Depending on the plan, patients may receive coverage for some of the above services if they are enrolled in Medicare Part C or have Medigap (private supplemental) insurance.

Medicare Cost Summary

	BENEFICIARY PAYS (IN 1999)	MEDICARE PAYS
Part A services		
Inpatient hospital stays	$768 deductible for days 1–60 $192/day for days 61–90 $384/day for days 91–150 (if lifetime reserve days are used) All costs after day 150	All approved costs after deductible and copayments
Skilled nursing care	Nothing for days 1–20 $96/day for days 21–100 All costs after day 100	Approved costs after copayments
Home health care	Nothing for services 20% of approved amount for medical equipment	100% of services 80% of approved amount for medical equipment
Hospice care	5% of prescription drugs $5/day for respite care	All costs except limited cost for drugs and respite care
Inpatient psychiatric services	Same as general inpatient care, except for lifetime maximum of 190 inpatient psychiatric days	Same as general inpatient care, except for lifetime maximum of 190 inpatient psychiatric days
Part B services		
Physician services	$100 deductible (paid once a year) 20% of approved amount	80% of approved charges after $100 deductible
Home health care	Nothing for services 20% for durable medical equipment	All costs for services 80% for medical equipment
Outpatient hospital services	$100 deductible (same as above) 20% of hospital charges	80% of hospital charges
Laboratory services	Nothing	100% of approved amount
Outpatient psychiatric services	$100 deductible (same as above) 37.5% of approved charges	62.5% of approved charges

12. What are Medigap policies?

Medicare pays many of the health care costs of the elderly, but it is not a comprehensive plan. Beneficiaries must pay coinsurance and deductibles. Medigap is private insurance regulated by federal and state laws that helps to pay these costs. Medigap policies pay for most or all of Medicare coinsurance amounts, and some also provide coverage for Medicare deductibles. Each Medigap plan has a different combination of benefits. Some plans pay for services not covered by Medicare, such as outpatient prescription drugs, preventive screening, and care outside the United States. However, Medigap policies with comprehensive benefits have high premiums that many people cannot afford.

13. With traditional Medicare (Parts A and B), how much freedom do beneficiaries have to choose doctors and hospitals?

Traditional Medicare allows beneficiaries to pick any doctor or hospital without restriction to access. It is still the most prevalent option. However, this option tends to be costly for the government because there tend to be few limitations on the total amount of care provided. Traditional Medicare is also costly for patients because total deductible, copayment, and prescription costs often are significant. As a result, many patients purchase private supplemental insurance (Medigap) or choose a Medicare Part C plan.

14. Various advertisements on television advise patients to switch from traditional Medicare to a private insurance program. What should patients know when picking a plan?

Currently, $180 billion (11% of the federal budget) is spent on Medicare. Nonetheless, because of high deductibles and copayments, the Medicare package offers less than 80% of what the average the employer-based plans offer. Out-of-pocket health care costs consume a big portion of the income of the elderly. As a result, increasing emphasis has been placed on managed care techniques to bring down Medicare costs and improve quality.

The Balanced Budget Act of 1997 created Medicare Part C, more popularly known as Medicare + Choice. On January 1, 1999, Medicare patients became eligible to receive health care coverage from private insurance companies. Under Medicare + Choice, the government pays a private organization a set amount for each beneficiary that it enrolls. The beneficiary continues to be responsible for paying Part B premiums. The plan (and no longer the government) is responsible for paying for services that member beneficiaries require. At a minimum, Part C plans must provide all services that traditional Medicare covers. Before the Balanced Budget Act of 1997, managed care plans were the only insurance option available to beneficiaries. These plans restrict care to participating providers and limit care through various managed care techniques. Medicare + Choice introduced additional options. Although Medicare + Choice plans are still in flux, the major types are summarized in the table below.

Major Types of Medicare + Choice Plans

PLAN TYPE	ADVANTAGES OVER TRADITIONAL MEDICARE	DISADVANTAGES OVER TRADITIONAL MEDICARE	PLAN COSTS
Health maintenance organizations (HMOs) Health insurer (HMO) receives capitated sum from government and becomes responsible for all of patient's care	Significantly lower or no deductibles and low copayments Often include limited prescription plan Some cover services not covered by traditional Medicare (e.g., eyeglasses, hearing aids, dental benefits, alternative medicine)	Restricted choice of doctors and hospitals Must go through primary provider for approval and referral to specialists Use of medical services is "managed" by plan	Typically, beneficiaries continue to pay Part B premiums, without additional premiums
Provider-sponsored organizations (PSOs) Health care providers (PSO) receive capitated sum from government and become responsible for all of patient's care	Similar to HMOs	Similar to HMOs Significant concern that some PSOs will become insolvent Because PSOs initially are exempt from state regulations, patients may receive poor quality of care	Similar to HMOs, but because no HMO takes portion of money, patients theoretically pay less
Preferred provider organizations (PPOs) Patients are able to choose providers but save extra money if they use in-network providers	Similar to HMOs and PSOs; patients save money if they use network providers Unlike HMOs and PSOs, no gatekeeper restricts services and patients may go out of network	If patient uses providers out of network, final costs may be higher than in traditional Medicare	Total costs to patient probably will be higher than with HMOs or PSOs, but less than with traditional Medicare Parts A and B Patients may need to pay additional insurance premiums

Table continued on following page

Major Types of Medicare + Choice Plans (Continued)

PLAN TYPE	ADVANTAGES OVER TRADITIONAL MEDICARE	DISADVANTAGES OVER TRADITIONAL MEDICARE	PLAN COSTS
Medical savings-accounts (MSAs) Government deposits money into patient's MSA. Patient purchases high deductible major medical policy and pays for medical services out of MSA	Patients control utilization of services; they can negotiate type of service and price Unused money (surpluses) can be applied to future years for services such as long-term care	Plans have high deductibles If patient becomes significantly ill, total costs can be much higher than with other plans If patients make poor investment decisions, they can "lose" significant portion of MSA	If patient uses more services than what Medicare deposits into MSA, patient is responsible for difference
Private contracting	Patients are able to use any provider Because of better reimbursement, patients will be sought after by providers Theoretically, quality of services will be best	Insurance premiums for private contracting plans will be very expensive; only richest people will be able to afford these plans	Of all Medicare Part C plans, private contracting is likely to cost beneficiaries the most In addition to higher out-of-pocket costs, patients probably will need to pay additional insurance premiums

15. How does a patient enroll in Medicare?

People sign up for Medicare at the Social Security office. The enrollment period of seven months begins three months before the 65th birthday and ends three months after. After this enrollment period, people may enroll during the general enrollment period from January 1 through March 31. Medicare coverage begins on the first July 1 after enrollment. For people who delay enrollment beyond the initial enrollment period at age 65, any Part A or B charge that they subsequently pay will be higher.

16. Medicare rules seem to be complex and constantly changing. Where can I get more information?

Information is available through brochures published by the Social Security Administration. You also may call the Social Security Administration at 1-800-772-1213 or the Medicare Hotline at 1-800-MEDICARE (1-800-633-4227). The Health Care Financing Administration (HCFA) also publishes several leaflets of interest to Medicare beneficiaries. They can be requested by writing to HCFA at 7500 Security Blvd., Baltimore, MD 21244-1850 or viewed on the HCFA Web site at www.hcfa.gov and www.medicare.gov.

BIBLIOGRAPHY

1. Getzen T: Health Economics: Fundamentals and Flow of Funds. New York, John Wiley & Sons, 1997.
2. Health Care Financing Administration: 1998 Guide to Health Insurance for People with Medicare. Baltimore, Health Care Financing Administration, 1998.
3. Institute on Aging: Improving the Medicare Market. Bethesda, MD, Institute on Aging, 1996.
Additional Web site:
www.hiv.hcfa.gov/medicare/ormedmed.htm#medicare

54. HOME CARE

Hollis Day, M.D., M.S., *Bruce Kinosian*, M.D., *and Jean Yudin*, M.S.N., R.N., C.S.

Mrs. W.

Mrs. W. is a patient introduced in the first chapter of this book. She is a 68-year-old female with complications of diabetes mellitus that included peripheral neuropathy and autonomic nervous system dysfunction. Mrs. W. is the beneficiary of the interdisciplinary team approach that includes physicians, nursing staff, social workers, and family members to coordinate the patient's care, improve her quality of life, and decrease her need for hospitalizations for hypo- and hyperglycemia. As Mrs. W.'s diabetes progresses, she will be one of many patients who benefit from home health care services that allow her to remain at home, in the community and not in a nursing home, while still receiving excellent medical and social support.

1. What is home health care?

Home care is a subset of the broad range of health and social services that are provided to an individual living in the community. Care provided to the patient in the home environment could be either health-related in the sense that a patient is receiving therapy (e.g., speech or physical therapy, wound care, medication monitoring), or social, as in assistance with activities of daily living (e.g., meals-on-wheels, household chores, paying bills).

2. What is the purpose of home care?

The purposes of home care vary in accordance with the perspectives of society, providers, payors, and consumers. Traditional (Medicare-funded) home care is designed to be post-acute care, intended to restore individuals to their pre-illness level of functioning. Historical (pre-Medicare) home care had a substantial public health function, with a focus on infants, children and communicable diseases. Care at home can enable individuals to live with their families, instead of in institutions (e.g., patients on home ventilators). Long-term care (LTC) services in the community range from highly technical medical supports, such as chronic parenteral infusions, to meeting nonmedical needs such as cooking, shopping, and cleaning. Consequently, maximizing a patient's functional status and allowing him or her to live in the least restrictive environment possible becomes an important goal of long-term home care.

3. Why should physicians consider home care as an option for patients?

Patient preferences are very important when instituting a plan of care. If a patient is more invested in his or her care, the plan is more likely to be thoroughly implemented. Patients prefer to remain in their homes as long as possible. Therefore, if feasible, everything possible should be done to manage a patient at home, because he or she will be happier and more likely to comply with treatment in a familiar environment.

4. Does home care improve survival?

Studies have demonstrated that home care improves survival and morbidity. Although past data failed to demonstrate that home care reduces nursing home placement, more recent data support the belief that home care is cost-effective for discharge planning and preventing re-hospitalization.

5. Who is eligible for home care?

The most common consumers of home care are the geriatric population. Patients appropriate for home care may be recovering from an acute illness that required hospitalization, patients with a disability that prevents them from coming into the office, patients with a terminal illness, and patients with an acute exacerbation of a chronic illness.

Generally, home care is reserved for patients who are considered homebound. The current definition of a homebound individual according to the Health Care Finance Administration (HCFA) is one for whom the "ability to leave home creates a considerable/taxing effort and when [the patient] leaves home it is for infrequent or short time periods (e.g., to receive medical treatment)." Proposals have been made to more quantitatively define the term *homebound* but to date have not been adopted. However, managed care plans have taken a more restrictive view of medical home care, restricting skilled services to those specifically required for post-acute recovery and disallowing provision of nonskilled services that individuals need to remain in the community. Other programs provide aides and nonskilled services to individuals residing in the community in order to maintain them independently at home.

Eligibility does not equal need. Individuals with a chronic, relapsing condition, such as class IV congestive heart failure, may need a daily home health aide to maintain function. However, Medicare and most HMOs will not pay for assistance in maintaining function but only for assistance with progression toward a "goal of therapy." Once the goal has been met, these types of insurance no longer will pay for assistance.

6. Who provides care for homebound patients?

In the ideal setting, an interdisciplinary group provides medical and social care for a patient. They often are linked to providers of durable medical equipment. A patient's primary care physician is considered part of a "team" of home health agency (HHA) personnel, the physician, the family, and the patient, because the physician is required by HCFA to authorize all care provided by the HHA.

The core team provided by HHAs consists of physicians, nurses, nurse practitioners, social workers, home health aides, physical and occupational therapists, and sometimes speech therapists as well. In settings with strong community based long-term care programs, such interdisciplinary groups may include members from the local community agencies (i.e., the local area agency on aging), which provides much of the nonskilled services for a care plan. The importance of communication is never lessened; however, in settings with less interdisciplinary structure, communication burdens, particularly upon the primary physician, primary nurse, and primary aide, are heightened.

The implementation of a successful home care plan depends on frequent, clear, well-documented communication among the members of the team. Equally, the success of a home care plan depends not only on the team members but on the ability of the patient and informal caregivers (family, friends) to execute the plan.

7. What is the role of the physician in providing home care?

Historically, the physician routinely made house calls and provided primary care in the patient's home. Over the past few decades, this practice has declined as the emphasis on either acute hospital care or outpatient office practice increased. More recently, however, there has been a resurgence of interest in physicians seeing patients at home, and some physicians have made this a full time profession. Home visits are highly rewarding for the physician: a special bond develops when patients realize that the physician has made an effort to see them in their natural setting. Similarly, the physician can enjoy getting to know the patient in a more social context, learning about the family and seeing what the patient truly values. Still, in general, the office-based physician's role is to be actively involved in the interdisciplinary plan of care that has been jointly developed with the nursing provider in charge of the case, the patient, and the patient's caregivers; to participate in team meetings; and to facilitate changes in the care plan as circumstances demand.

8. What new or different information can be gained through a home assessment that may not be achieved through a routine history and physical in the office?

An assessment of the patient in his or her home environment can be highly educational. A patient's functional status depends on the interaction between his or her physical and cognitive capacities and the environment in which he or she lives. In the office the physician can test physical and cognitive ability, but he or she cannot fully appreciate the patient's functional capacity until the demands that the patient's environment make upon these abilities (and vice versa) are seen. For example, the physician can see what medications the patient actually is taking including any over-the-counter, outdated, or duplicate medications. New light may be shed on a patient's complaint of incontinence when you see that the bathroom is unable to be reached easily. Equally important, a home visit provides a thorough comprehension of the caregiver's burdens and a clearer understanding of why a particular care plan is difficult to implement.

9. **List services that can be provided in the home.**
   - A complete geriatric assessment with an emphasis on physical/basic and instrumental activities of daily living
   - Physical (PT), speech, and occupational therapy (OT)
   - Phlebotomy and home monitoring of specific measures such as INRs
   - X-rays, including ultrasound, echocardiography, sleep studies, nerve conduction/electromyography (EMG), Doppler's, pulmonary function testing
   - Nutrition support services, such as total parenteral nutrition or enteral feeding using g-tubes, jejunostomy tubes
   - Home infusion services, such as parenteral antibiotics, transfusions, chemotherapy, and hydration
   - More advanced therapies, such as home dobutamine infusions and home ventilators
   - Social services, including evaluation of abuse or neglect, need for home-delivered meals
   - Home safety evaluations
   - Assessment of caregiver's burden

10. **What are some conditions that can be treated as safely in the home as in the hospital?**
    - Deep venous thrombosis (DVT)
    - Uncomplicated community-acquired pneumonia
    - Cellulitis
    - Uncomplicated urinary tract infection

These conditions have been extensively studied and offer relatively easy medication administration, do not require intensive monitoring of laboratory values (e.g., with low–molecular-weight heparin in DVT you do not have to monitor prothrombin times), and do not require close monitoring of vital signs. Families and patients are instructed how to administer many of the treatments, and nurses are sent to the home to administer intravenous medications and monitor a patient's progress. Treatment of these conditions at home is both cost-effective and more comfortable for the patient.

11. **Describe the elements of a home safety evaluation.**
    A home safety evaluation is designed to evaluate a patient's ability to function safely in the home both in the routine setting and in the event of an emergency. Often individuals are more stable in a familiar home setting than they appear to be when evaluated in an unfamiliar hospital or office site.
    One portion of a home safety evaluation includes the search for potential environmental factors that contribute to falls. Environmental factors that may precipitate falls include:
    - Throw rugs or carpeting that may not be tacked down
    - Uneven steps or flooring that may cause a person to trip
    - Shaky or absent handrails that do not extend far enough at the ends of the stairs
    - Poor lighting
    - Beds and toilets from which it is difficult to arise
    - Bathtubs and showers that are difficult to enter and exit and do not have non-skid surfaces
    - An extremely cluttered environment that provides no access to an immediate exit in the case of an emergency

Other elements of the home safety evaluation:
- Check the temperature setting on the water heater to prevent scalding
- Assess safety features on doors and windows to prevent forced entry
- Survey the kitchen for potential fire hazards
- Test fire alarms to ensure their proper functioning
- Guarantee easy access to a telephone

12. Why is the assessment of caregiver burden important?

Informal caregivers, usually a spouse or other family member, provide the bulk of care for most homebound patients. When they become stressed, the patient is affected, often leading to hospitalizations or ultimately to placement in a long-term care facility. An assessment of the caregiver in the home can reveal how many hours a day the caregiver is attending to the needs of the patient, what type of tasks they are performing, and the obstacles (physical, mental, and social) that may prevent adequate implementation of the care plan. It also may reveal who the actual caregivers are.

13. How do patients gain access to home care?

In the traditional model, patients commonly enter the home care system at the time of discharge from the hospital. In this situation, case managers develop a plan of care with the help of the physician and make referrals to home care agencies that then follow a patient's progress. They are followed for a brief period of time and services are subsequently discontinued after all goals have been met.

More commonly, however, home care services are being used to provide long-term care in the community. Patients often are referred from the physician's office when they frequently fail to arrive for their appointments or are known to have significant difficulty in leaving the house. One recent study demonstrated that 78% of home care visits occurred more than one month after a patient had been discharged from the hospital and that 61% of visits were to patients who received home care for 6 or more months. These often are patients who gain access to nonmedical home services through their area agency on aging or other community sources.

14. What are the different levels of care that are available at home?

The highest level of care available is skilled nursing care, often designated as home *health* care. Skilled professional or nursing services focus on assessment and management of medical problems and provide family education and recommendations for additional support services (e.g., social work, physical therapy). Other professional services include physical, occupational, and speech therapy.

An additional level of home care is that provided by paraprofessionals known as home health aides, or personal care assistants. These assistants help patients with activities of daily living (ADLs), taking medication at the appropriate time, and maintaining a safe environment. Homemakers provide chore services, such as cooking, cleaning, and shopping. They are provided by payors for community-based LTC services, but not (officially) by HCFA. However, many HHAs will provide homemaker services for clients who require such assistance.

15. Who pays for these services?

Medicare will pay for home care if a patient has a skilled nursing need. Payment is dependent on constant reassessment and ongoing improvement in the patient's condition. Medicare will not pay for daily skilled services unless they are of finite duration. Medicare may not pay for a patient's medications. For example, if a patient is receiving antibiotic therapy at home, he or she must pay for it privately or have another type of insurance that will cover the medication. A physician must supervise the patient's progress and adequately document the patient's need for ongoing care so that all parties involved can receive payment. Medicare will pay for a limited amount of paraprofessional services (maximum of 20 hours/week) and again, only if the patient has a skilled nursing need. These home care services are therefore generally paid for by the individual or family and can lead to substantial expense.

For individuals who require assistance with ADLs for chronic conditions, the short "post-acute" period may often leave them without needed services after their skilled need ends. Through the use of allowed services—that is, skilled nursing to monitor changes in therapies, new diagnoses, to teach families about aspects of care, manage a complex care plan, or through subsequently requiring PT for mobility or OT to help with ADL performance, aide services can be maintained for individuals with chronic conditions for extended periods. However, annual caps on total home health services require that such services be viewed as stop-gap measures until waiting lists for community-based services can be negotiated and community based LTC services can begin.

No standardized system is in place for long-term care of the frail patient in the community. Thus, it is important that every physician be aware of local resources through which services—both medical and nonmedical—can be obtained to allow as many patients as possible to function safely and at maximum capacity outside of an institution. Further, as a patient advocate, it is important for the primary care physician to challenge agency assertions of "Medicare doesn't allow . . ." or "Medicare requires. . . ." Often local agency policy is portrayed to ordering physicians as federal regulation, an inaccuracy that does disservice to needy, frail elders.

16. What is the difference between home care, palliative care, and hospice?

Hospice is care of the terminal patient whose life expectancy is 6 months or less. Although hospice care can be provided in the home, it also can be provided in more institutional settings. Hospice care has traditionally been associated with oncology, although recently criteria have been promulgated for individuals with a number of other terminal conditions, such as congestive heart failure, chronic obstructive pulmonary disease, renal failure, and dementia. In addition to the services that HHAs provide, hospices often provide augmented volunteer support services and pastoral and social work counseling services. Providers from HHAs and hospices, however, may apply principles of **palliative care**. These principles are generically focused on relief of symptoms and attention to individual patient's spiritual, emotional, and physical concerns, rather than resolving specific illness episodes. Some hospices have affiliated HHAs for individuals not yet willing to accept all the restrictions of hospice (e.g., many hospices require that individuals renounce treatment of infections or hospitalizations, no matter how transitory).

Home care, however, is for any patient who meets the criteria previously mentioned, not just for someone who is terminally ill.

17. Where can I go for more information about home care?

More information can be found through the American Academy of Home Care Physicians at www.aahcp.org/aahcp/ or by calling 410-676-7966.

BIBLIOGRAPHY

1. American Medical Association Home Care Advisory Panel: Guidelines for the medical management of the home-care patient. Arch Fam Med 2:194–206, 1993.
2. Boling PA: Home care physicians in the interdisciplinary team. In The Physician's Role in Home Health Care. New York, Springer, 1997, pp 42–69.
3. Health Care Financing Administration: The Home Health Agency Manual, publication number 11. Revised. Washington, D.C., Department of Health and Human Services, 1996.
4. Ramsdell JW, Swart JA, Jackson JE, Renvall M: The yield of a home visit in the assessment of geriatric patients. J Am Geriatr Soc 37:17–24, 1989.
5. Repetto L, Granetto C, Venturino A: Home care in the older person. Clin Geriatr Med 13:403–413, 1997.
6. Van Gerpen BS, Scott CB: Home care: What is it? J Med Assoc Ga 86:119–120, 1997.
7. Vladeck BC, Miller NA: The Medicare home health initiative. Health Care Financing Rev 16:7–16, 1994.
8. Welch HG, Wennberg DE, Welch WP: The use of Medicare home health care services. N Engl J Med 335:324–329, 1996.

55. NURSING HOMES

Joan Weinryb, M.D., C.M.D.

1. What is a nursing home? What is its place in the continuum of long-term care?

A nursing home or facility is a long-term care institution that maintains at least three inpatient beds. It offers around-the-clock nursing care as well as medical, social, and personal services to persons in need of restorative care or long-term maintenance. Nursing homes are part of the continuum of health services outside acute care hospitals, ranging from home-bound through community-based to institutional settings. Nursing homes in the United States have their origin in the following:

- Nineteenth-century British workhouse infirmaries
- County poor houses
- State mental hospitals
- Voluntary homes for the aged
- Proprietary boarding homes
- Hospital-affiliated nursing homes

2. What are the types of nursing homes in the U.S.?

Nursing homes may be freestanding, associated with hospitals, part of chains of similar facilities, or linked with other facilities in a continuum of care.

- 68% are certified for provision of Medicare services.
- 56% of nursing home income comes from Medicaid payments.
- 73% of nursing homes are for-profit.
- 22% of nursing homes are not-for-profit or have religious affiliation.
- 4% are government-run.

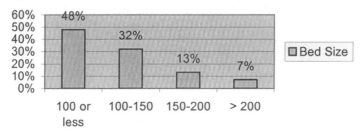

Breakdown of U.S. nursing homes by number of beds (bed size).

3. How are the demographics of the United States population and changes in social structure affecting nursing home care?

The frail geriatric population is the most rapidly growing segment of U.S. society. By the year 2030, the number of Americans over age 85 is expected to double. Almost half of these have some degree of dementia. Of Americans 75 years or older, 20% of men and 50% of women live alone. One-third have no children. Elderly Americans with families have fewer children and tend to be more geographically separated from their children than previous generations. Much formal and informal care is arranged by daughters. More women now work outside the home, making caregiving for frail, elderly relatives more stressful and difficult. Institutional care thus becomes a more needed alternative.

It has been predicted that 52% of women and 33% of men turning 65 in 1990 will reside in a nursing home at some time before they die. Twenty-five percent will stay at least 1 year, and 9% will reside in a nursing home for 5 years or longer.

4. What are the characteristics of elderly adults most often found in nursing homes?

Current rates of nursing home usage vary with age, sex, race, and bed availability, which differ from state to state. Chronically mentally ill, developmentally disabled, and physically disabled Americans of all ages are residents in nursing homes. The proportion of an age group in nursing homes increases with advancing age, with a greater proportion of caucasian women than caucasian men in each age group. Unavailability of community caregivers and decreased functional status are independent risk factors for nursing home admission.

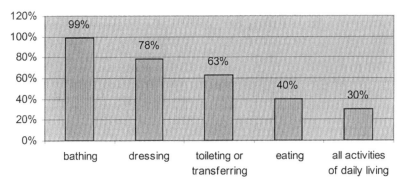

Number of patients residing in nursing homes who require assistance with activities of daily living.

5. Of whom is the population of U.S. nursing homes composed?

Nursing homes contain short-term (< 6 months) and long-term (> 6 months) residents. Short-term residents are divided almost evenly between those who are admitted for terminal care and those admitted for rehabilitation or convalescence. Long-term residents may have physical and/or cognitive impairment, which precludes their continued management in the community. Most nursing home residents have a combination of physical and cognitive impairment. The prevalence of mental disorders, including dementia, delirium, and psychiatric illness, among nursing home residents is said to be about 90%.

Noninstitutional long-term care services are becoming more accessible but are not practical or appropriate for a substantial portion of the frail, dependent geriatric population. Need and demand for nursing home care are likely to continue to grow over the next several decades as the elderly population lives into extreme old age in increasing numbers.

6. How has the nursing home population changed in recent years?

The nursing home population has grown more dependent and more medically ill. Dramatic shortening of hospital stays has created a demand for subacute care. Managed care utilizes the nursing home setting as a more cost-effective alternative to hospital care. Capitated systems have a strong financial incentive to treat acutely ill patients in less expensive settings such as nursing homes.

7. What factors put elderly people at risk for nursing home admission?

Increasing age and frailty combined with:
1. Mental, behavioral, or physical conditions that make management by a community caregiver difficult
2. Functional disabilities that preclude independent living
3. Lack of a social support system
4. Shortage and expense of available, accessible community-based long-term care services

8. How expensive is nursing home care?

Generally, cost can be estimated at $30,000–$45,000 per year per patient. Expenditures for nursing home care exceed $50 billion. Medicare pays less than 3% of nursing home cost; 68% is reimbursed by Medicaid; and 42% comes out of pocket. Twelve percent of elderly people live below the poverty line before nursing home admission and are already eligible for Medicaid grants. Others are forced to "spend down" their assets until they become impoverished and qualify for Medicaid.

9. How is medical care regulated and reimbursed in nursing homes?

Nursing home care is highly regulated by state and federal governments. Reimbursement for care depends on compliance with regulations as demonstrated during nursing home surveys and other oversight. The intent of nursing home regulations is to improve quality of care by requiring periodic comprehensive assessment of each resident, providing standards for training nurses' aides, and reducing the use of physical and pharmacologic restraint. The Omnibus Budget Reconciliation Act of 1987 (OBRA '87) mandates that each resident be assisted to "attain or maintain the highest practicable physical, or mental and psychosocial well being." Nursing home oversight focuses on the process of care.

Formerly, nursing facilities billed Medicare, Medicaid, or private sources for services rendered to each resident. As of July 1998, nursing facilities are reimbursed under the prospective payment system (PPS) mandated by Congress. Patient acuity is classified according to resource utilization groups (RUGs), which are subdivided into 44 categories. Each RUG category is reimbursed at a specific level based on utilization of nursing and therapy staff time. Reimbursement depends on the computer transmission of the minimum data sheet (MDS), which describes the resident's problems through objective behavioral observations rather than diagnoses. Analysis of patient care needs is based on the following factors:
- Rehabilitation requirements
- Cognitive function
- Distressed mood
- Special care needs
- Ability to perform activities of daily living
- Behavioral symptoms

A per-diem rate based on (1) acuity of the residents, (2) local employment costs, and (3) rural versus urban location is paid to the nursing home to cover the cost of all services expected as part of the patient's care plan.

PPS was designed to cut $9.5 billion per year from the long-term care budget as part of the effort to reduce Medicare expenditures by $115 billion. Nursing home surveys for quality of care are henceforth to be based on electronically transmitted MDS data. Such data will identify the percentage of residents within a facility with conditions targeted as issues for care. Examples of such conditions include:
- Decubitus ulcers
- Dehydration
- Involuntary weight loss
- Untreated depression
- Use of medications possibly or probably contraindicated in elderly persons

The same data trigger the survey process.

10. How are nursing homes staffed?

Nursing homes are staffed by registered nurses (RNs) with supervisory responsibilities, licensed practical nurses (LPNs) who administer medications and treatments, and nurses' aides. Nursing home staffing does not resemble that of the acute care hospital. RN coverage may include only one person with supervisory responsibilities. Nurses' aides, often undereducated and poorly paid, administer the bulk of personal care. In a single year, staff turnover rates may be as high as follows:
- Aides: 90%
- LPNs and RNs: 50%
- Directors of nursing and administrators: 30%

The U.S. has a shortage of physicians willing to provide care in nursing homes. As the elderly population most at risk for needing nursing care increases, a large proportion of physicians attending nursing home patients is approaching retirement.

11. How are the diagnosis and treatment of medical problems affected by nursing home residence?

Making an accurate diagnosis tends to be more difficult because of the effects of multiple chronic illnesses, multiple medications and their side effects and interactions, and the uncommon presentations of common illnesses in elderly patients. History-taking is complicated by the cognitive disability of the patient and the failure of communication between different nursing staffs and ancillary staff about the onset of pathologic signs and symptoms. Assessing all symptoms in search of a unifying diagnosis is often unsuccessful and confounds identification of the acute problem embedded in the matrix of chronic symptoms. Atypical presentations (e.g, confusion or falls in urinary tract infection without dysuria) and nonspecific presentations (e.g., shortness of breath in pneumonia or myocardial infarction without cough or chest pain) may complicate decision-making. Delay in examination by a physician or in diagnostic testing may occur because of (1) the facility's location, (2) the facility's access to laboratories and radiologists, and (3) practitioners' other commitments. Delay also may occur because nonspecific symptoms are overlooked by staff who have become accustomed to cognitive dysfunction and dependency in daily activities, whose scheduling constraints cause time pressure, or who are unfamiliar with a particular resident because of the facility's policy of "floating" staff assignments.

12. Are falls a problem in nursing homes?

Unintentional injury is the sixth leading cause of death in people 65 years or older. Falls are a frequent and serious problem in nursing homes. More than two-thirds of nursing home patients fall at least once a year. Falls may result in injury or in postfall fear syndrome. Risk factors for falls, including sedative drugs, antidepressasnts, antipsychotic medications, absolute number of medications taken, balance problems, hip weakness, poor functional status, and intermittent use of restraints, have been identified and ameliorative strategies proposed. Nursing home financial constraints, leading to minimal staffing, suboptimal physical features (e.g., slippery, hard floors, dim lighting, high beds), and increased utilization of the most highly trained staff to complete required paperwork, are contributing factors. Customized seating, alarm devices, floor pads, and pharmacologic modifications can be utilized in mitigation. Physical therapy to increase strength and balance may be efficacious. Aggressive treatment for osteoporosis in nursing home patients is just beginning to be implemented.

13. Is urinary incontinence a problem in nursing homes?

Over 50% of nursing home patients are incontinent of bladder and/or bowel. Often incontinence is the deciding factor leading to nursing home admission. Medical consequences of urinary incontinence include skin breakdown and use of urethral catheters, which may act as conduits for infection. Normal aging leads to decreased bladder capacity, increased detrusor irritability, and decreased urethral length and closing pressure. Additive factors of immobility, cognitive impairment, medication effects, inaccessibility of toilet facilities, and chronic illnesses such as diabetes mellitus increase incontinence problems. The work-up for reversible conditions includes history, physical examination, urinary studies, determination of postvoid residual, and cytometric evaluation. Pharmacologic treatment depends on the cause of the incontinence. Toileting schedules, treatment of impaired mobility, and removal of impediments to mobility such as bedrails and other restraints often are helpful to nursing home patients.

14. Is nutrition an issue in nursing homes?

Poor nutritional status alters tissue regeneration, inflammatory reaction, and immune function, placing nursing home residents at higher risk for death, sepsis, and infections. Loss of $\geq 5\%$ weight in 1 month or $> 10\%$ in 6 months is considered significant. Nutritional assessment identifies residents at risk. Body weight and laboratory indices (e.g., albumin, plasma transferrin, he-moglobulin) can be monitored.

Risk Factors for Malnutrition

Conditions that can cause wasting (e.g., cancer, pulmonary disease, cardiac disease, abnormalities of the esophagus, liver and biliary tract disease)

Cognitive disturbances (e.g., depression, anxiety, dementia, psychosis)

Infectious diseases (e.g., tuberculosis, AIDS)

Movement disorders (e.g., Parkinson's, essential tremor, tardive dyskinesia)

Metabolic disorders (e.g., hypo- and hyperthyroidism, hyperparathyroidism, adrenal insufficiency)

Mechanical problems (e.g., arthritides, dental abnormalities, oral lesions)

Increased metabolism, anorexia, swallowing difficulties, and absorption problems contribute to protein energy malnutrition. Functional difficulties with eating, medication effects, and unpalatable diets (texture, low salt, low cholesterol) can be corrected. Regulatory guidelines suggest use of enteral feeding tubes for patients with dysphagia or aspiration, decreased alertness, and malnutrition not attributable to a single cause that can be reversed. Tube feeding can be complicated by aspiration, diarrhea, electrolyte and fluid imbalance, gastric bleeding, and skin irritation at the tube site. Some nursing home residents or their families may consider enteral feeding as aggressive therapy not in keeping with the patient's wishes. This information must be carefully documented in the nursing home record. Studies of enteral feeding in nursing homes residents have failed to demonstrate benefits in terms of weight gain or albumin normalization.

15. Given the level of cognitive impairment of nursing home patients, are people commonly restrained?

Formerly, restraint was common, but the past decade has shown tremendous change in this area. Federal regulation has contributed to the impetus to reduce both physical and chemical restraints. Before the passage of OBRA '87, use of restraints ranged from 25% to 85%. Despite widespread use, no studies demonstrated reduction of falls or injuries. Numerous complications (e.g., pressure sores, pneumonias, urinary tract infections, contractures, agitation, delirium) were documented. Nursing home residents now have the legal right to be free of physical restraints or psychoactive drug administration not required for treatment of their medical symptoms. Before restraints are used, the nursing facility must demonstrate that less restrictive measures were tried but proved ineffective. Restraints are to be used for the shortest time possible, and documentation must be provided to verify that the restraint enables the resident "to maintain the highest practicable physical, mental and psychosocial function." Psychoactive drugs, used to control mood, mental status, or behavior, are permitted only for specific conditions. Gradual dose reductions and behavioral interventions, unless clinically contraindicated, must be implemented, and the absence of negative side effects must be documented. Since institution of OBRA '87 regulations, use of physical restraints has declined by 50% and use of psychoactive drugs unrelated to a psychiatric diagnosis has declined by 25–36%.

16. Is infection common in nursing facilities?

Infection and infection control are important issues in nursing homes. Fifteen percent of nursing home residents suffer the effects at any one time. Clinical clues to acute infection include:
- Increase in temperature of 2.4°F above baseline
- Acute confusion
- Unexplained changes in behavior or functional status
- Loss of appetite
- Weight loss
- Weakness
- Lethargy

• Urinary incontinence
• Falls
• Orthostatic hypotension
• Tachypnea

17. Which infections are of particular concern in nursing homes?

Pneumonia, caused mainly by pneumococci, gram-negative bacilli, staphylococci, influenza, and anaerobes. Complications include respiratory failure, bacteremia, and empyema. The mortality rate is 12–35% and increases with bacteremia, severity of underlying disorders, pulmonary involvement, and virulence of pathogens (especially gram-negative bacilli). Prophylactic immunization against influenza and pneumococcal infection should be undertaken because it has been shown to decrease infection significantly.

Urinary tract infection is common. The nursing home population has rates of asymptomatic bacteriuria as high as 50%. Research has indicated no beneficial effect from treatment of asymptomatic bacteriuria. Symptomatic nursing home patients require treatment but often do not manifest fever, dysuria, frequency, or hesitancy; they may present instead with confusion, hypotension, nausea, or anorexia from reactive ileus of the intestine or worsened cognitive impairment.

Infected pressure sores and lower extremity cellulitis pose another frequent problem. About 10–15% of pressure sores can become locally infected, some developing contiguous osteomyelitis and some progressing to systemic infection.

Cellulitis related to peripheral vascular disease, chronic venous insufficiency, edema, and trauma occurs commonly. Appropriate preventive strategies and treatment decrease morbidity and mortality.

Elderly persons have the highest risk for developing **tuberculosis** of any population group in the U.S. except patients with AIDS. The case rate in nursing facilities is 4 times that of elderly community dwellers and 14 times that of the general population. Sixty percent of all tuberculosis deaths in the U.S. occur in nursing homes. Tuberculosis screening by admission and annual purified protein derivative (PPD) tests and prophylactic treatment of recent converters with isoniazid limit morbidity and mortality.

Increasing numbers of nursing home residents return from the hospital colonized with **methicillin-resistant** *Staphylococcus aureus* (MRSA) or **vancomycin-resistant enterococci** (VRE). Rates increase with increased acuity of the residents. Some nursing homes have the facilities to group such patients. Others ensure that they do not share rooms with patients who have enteral feeding tubes, indwelling urethral catheters, or tracheotomies and thus are at higher risk of infection. Universal precautions, if exercised assiduously by the staff, limit spread of these organisms.

18. Is medication use different in nursing homes?

Nursing home residents use more medication than community elders—on average, over eight concurrent prescriptions. This reflects the frailty of the population as well as possibly inappropriate prescribing practices. Consensus about what constitutes appropriate medication is poor in many areas. Medications such as sedative-hypnotics, antidepressants, antihypertensives, nonsteroidal anti-inflammatory drugs, oral hypoglycemics, analgesics, dementia treatments, platelet inhibitors, histamine-2 blockers, decongestants, iron supplements, muscle relaxants, gastrointestinal antispasmodics, and antiemetics have come under scrutiny. Medications should be related to particular diagnoses. Appropriateness of prescribing should be based on risk-benefit ratios. Important issues include scrutiny for medications that generally should be avoided in the elderly and doses, frequencies, or durations that should not be exceeded. Diagnoses, disease severity, symptoms, and signs must be included in the analysis of medication appropriateness. Nursing home regulations require avoidance of long-acting benzodiazepines in people over 65 years old, unless short-acting medications cannot be substituted. Anxiolytic/sedative drugs must be prescribed for particular indications in specified doses. Proof of symptoms, attempt to reduce or discontinue the medication, and efficacy of treatment must be documented. Antipsychotic medications must be used for specific psychotic symptoms. Patients must be followed for onset of abnormal involuntary movements, dyskinesia, and therapeutic effect.

Because of its narrow therapeutic range and considerable toxicity, the use of digoxin has been questioned in nursing home patients with congestive heart failure.

Antibiotics often are prescribed for unclear indications, leading to increased levels of resistant organisms.

As many as 50% of residents entering nursing homes from the community have not been taking their medications as prescribed. Diligent dispensing of every medication that the resident was supposedly taking may lead to toxicity.

Knowledge of differences in geriatric pharmacokinetics and pharmacodynamics, combined with educated assessment by the nursing staff and review by the consultant pharmacist, as mitigated by financial constraints, guides drug usage in nursing homes. Treatment of pain, depression, psychosis, agitation, infection, bowel problems, and other diseases can be managed appropriately.

19. Are pressure sores a consequence of nursing home residence?

Pressure sores, localized areas of tissue necrosis, are a serious consequence of immobility and debilitation. About 60% of pressure sores develop in the hospital, 18% in nursing homes, and 18% at home. Most occur in elderly patients. The longer the nursing home stay, the more likely the patient is to develop a pressure sore. The four key factors involved in causing skin breakdown are pressure, shearing force, friction, and moisture; thus, immobility, malnutrition, fecal and urinary incontinence, and altered level of consciousness are risk factors common among nursing home patients. Efforts to limit pressure sore development in nursing homes include risk assessment with standardized instruments (e.g., Norton scale) and nutrition evaluation by following body weights and laboratory tests (e.g., cholesterol, albumin, total lymphocyte count). Repositioning schedules and assistance devices (including cushions, mattresses, splinting devices) to counteract immobility and pressure effects are useful. Strategies for prevention have been formalized into clinical guidelines published by the U.S. Department of Health and Human Services. An estimated 29–79 minutes of nursing time per day is needed to implement the guidelines. Traditionally, little reimbursement is available for preventive strategies, even though development of pressure sores causes much suffering and may lead to complications of cellulitis, osteomyelitis, infection of adjacent structures such as joints, sepsis, and death. Capitated systems have a financial incentive to prevent pressure sores, because prevention is much less expensive than healing.

20. How are pressure sores characterized and treated?

Pressure sores are characterized by a standardized staging system:

Stage I   Nonblanching erythema
Stage II   Partial-thickness skin loss
Stage III   Full-thickness skin loss with necrosis of subcutaneous tissue
Stage IV   Extensive destruction involving muscle, bone, or supporting structures; large area involved; presence of exudate

Treatment involves positioning devices to relieve pressure, dressings that create an optimal environment for healing, debridement of nonviable tissue, improvement of nutritional status, and management of complications.

21. How is dignity jeopardized by nursing home life?

The nursing home resident has the legal right to dignity, self-determination, and communication with and access to persons and services outside the nursing home. Areas to be protected include:

- Privacy and respect
- Medical care and treatment
- Right to refuse treatment
- Freedom from abuse and restraint

• Freedom of association and communication in privacy, activities, work, personal possessions, grievances and complaints, and financial affairs
• Transfer and dismissal from the nursing home

Facilitating personal autonomy for physically and mentally impaired nursing home patients involves problems of identifying what is appropriate and eliminating barriers. Living in a nursing home often means living in a shared room. Space is reduced to a few feet around the bed. Only personal possessions that can fit into the available storage space may be kept. Confused and lucid patients are often housed together. Life is defined by routines for baths, meals, getting up, and going to bed. Entertainment is often geared to the lowest common denominator. There are often long, empty spaces of time. Rules designed to protect often circumscribe the activities of less impaired residents. Nursing homes must work to reconcile the need to provide medical and nursing care to a diverse population with the ideal of providing a home-like setting.

22. How can the dignity of nursing home residents be protected at the end of life?

Many cognitively impaired patients have lost the capacity for medical decision-making. The physician must judge whether the patient, in the context of each individual decision, understands the consequences of his or her decision. When the patient appears to be unable to make an informed decision, a hierarchy of decision-making should be followed. Advance directives, made when patients were competent, should prevail. Advance directives often include a durable power of attorney for health matters, which empowers a surrogate decision-maker to make decisions when the patient is no longer able. If no advance directive exists, physicians may seek advice from family or friends, often according to a hierarchy decided by state law. A court may be asked to appoint a guardian to act for the incapacitated patient.

Conflict may exist between family members or between family and physician about what treatment is in the patient's best interest. Areas in which problems may occur include resuscitation decisions and decisions related to feeding and hydration. Physicians and other nursing home staff can decrease the stress of decision-making at crisis times by discussion in advance of crucial decisions about resuscitation, invasive interventions, and enteral nutrition.

BIBLIOGRAPHY

1. Avorn J, Gurwtiz JH: Drug use in the nursing home. Ann Intern Med 123:195–204, 1995.
2. Beers MH, Ouslander JG, Rollingher I, et al: Explicit criteria for determining inappropriate medication use in nursing home residents. Arch Intern Med 151:1825–1832, 1991.
3. Drew J: Changing a legacy: The Eden Alternative in the nursing home. Ann Long-term Care 7:115–121, 1999.
4. Evans J: Medical care of nursing home residents. Mayo Clin Proc 70:694–702, 1995.
5. Evans JM, Andrews KL, Chutka DS, et al: Pressure ulcers: Prevention and management. Mayo Clin Proc 70:789–799, 1995.
6. Gillick M, Berkman S, Cullen L: A patient-centered approach to advance medical planning in the nursing home. J Am Geriatr Soc 47:227–230, 1999.
7. Kane R: Everyday Ethics: Resolving Dilemmas in Nursing Home Life. New York, Springer, 1990.
8. Levenson S: Medical Direction in Long Term Care. Durham, NC, Carolina Academic Press, 1993.
9. Norton D, et al: An Investigation of Geriatric Nursing Problems in Hospital. Edinburgh, Churchill Livingstone, 1975, pp 193–236.
10. Ouslander J: Medical Care in the Nursing Home. New York, McGraw-Hill, 1997.
11. Panel for the Prediction and Prevention of Pressure Ulcers in Adults: Clinical Practice Guidelines, No. 3. Rockville, MD, Agency for Health Care Policy and Research, 1992 (Pub. No. AHCPR 92-0047).
12. Smith D: Pressure ulcers in the nursing home. Ann Intern Med 123:433–442, 1995.
13. Thomas D: Nutritional deficiencies in long-term care. Ann Long-term Care III 6:325–332, 1998; 6:250–258, 1998.
14. Schrier RW: Geriatric Medicine. Philadelphia, W.B. Saunders, 1990.

56. ALTERNATIVE LONG-TERM CARE

Thomas Lawrence, M.D.

1. What is alternative long-term care?

In past years, the term *long-term care* most often referred to care provided in the nursing home setting. Nursing homes had two designated levels of care: skilled nursing and intermediate care. Skilled nursing referred to caring for the most frail nursing home residents who often were completely dependent in activities of daily living (ADLs), were unable to ambulate, and had medical needs that required a registered nurse. Included in the skilled care group of nursing home residents are patients with needs such as wound care, use of gastrostomy tubes, and intensive treatment of medical conditions such as diabetes. Intermediate care encompassed higher-functioning residents who did not have major nursing needs and were able to ambulate and self-feed.

Nontraditional long-term care, also called alternative long-term care, includes a wide variety of programs, most of which have developed and become widely available in the past 15–20 years in the United States. Like traditional long-term care services, alternative long-term care refers to longitudinal supportive services and health care designed to meet the care needs of frail, dependent people, the majority of whom are elderly and often would be eligible for nursing home placement.

2. What are the most commonly used institutional sites of alternative long-term care?

1. Assisted-living facilities (known as personal care facilities in some states) and senior housing with services
2. Retirement communities, which include continuing care retirement communities (also known as life-care communities)
3. Adult day-care programs, often augmented with in-home support services
4. Home-based community care (services in this area are growing at a rapid rate)

Less commonly used sites of care include long-term care hospitals and community-based continuing care programs. Day hospitals, which provide multidisciplinary patient assessment and rehabilitation services, are common in England and elsewhere but are not widely available in the United States.

3. Explain continuum of care.

As a wide variety of alternative institutional and community-based long-term care options have become available, continuous care with minimal disruption during times of health transitions has become a reality. Complete continuum of care refers to a spectrum of services designed to provide all of the social and health care needs of people as they age. This spectrum ranges from independent living to acute hospital-based care and nursing home-based long-term care. Many community facilities in the U.S. currently house the two most commonly used long-term alternatives, assisted living and nursing care, within one facility. Within this model, an important goal is to accomplish transitions from one setting to another with a minimum of disruption in care.

A broader definition of continuum of care includes caregiver continuity and continuity within an individual's health domains. This concept promotes the continuance of a patient's caregiving team, medical care, and physician services, including primary care physicians and consultants, as the patient moves from office-based care to home care services, assisted living, and nursing home care. Continuity of health domains involves creating links among issues relating to health promotion, disease prevention, treatment of acute disease, and management of chronic diseases and conditions. Creating linkages in care between physical health domains and spiritual and psychosocial health also is receiving increasing attention.

The continuing care retirement community (see question 5) is an example of a long-term care continuum that covers the full spectrum of individual needs. The challenge in the future will be for health care providers to develop fully functioning continuums of care in community settings that are accessible and affordable to those in greatest need.

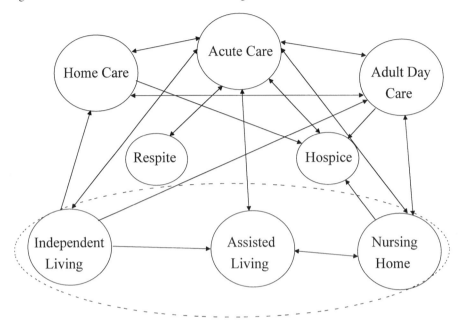

The long-term care continuum. Arrows indicate transitions in care. Dotted lines indicate continuing care retirement community.

4. What are assisted-living facilities?

Assisted-living facilities provide a combination of housing, personalized support services, and health care services. They are among the fastest growing markets in senior housing. Currently an estimated 30,000 assisted-living residences in the U.S. house more than a million Americans. The typical assisted-living resident is age 83 or older, widowed or single, and most often female. These facilities range in size from a few beds to several hundred; typical facilities have between 25 and 120 beds. They may be freestanding or part of a retirement community or nursing home. The term *assisted living* encompasses the older designations of personal care home, residential care home, domiciliary care home, and group home.

Typical services provided in assisted living include support with the instrumental activities of daily living (IADLs) of meal preparation, transportation, shopping, housekeeping, laundry, and activities. Support with ADLs, such as bathing, dressing, eating, toileting, and ambulation, is more variable and depends on the specific facility and population. The number of services usually reflects increasing charges to residents.

Assisted-living facilities are extremely heterogeneous; of this form of senior housing it has been said, "When you've seen one assisted-living facility, you've seen one assisted-living facility." Nonetheless, one common finding is that resident acuity (level of infirmity) is continuing to climb as residents from intermediate care nursing home units are placed in assisted-living sites. Some assisted living or personal care facilities provide on-site nursing care for all or part of the day, but, unlike nursing homes, they are not required to provide this service according to state licensure. Health care services generally are supervised by most assisted-living facilities, including medication assistance and emergency call systems. Many provide on-site physician care, especially those that are part of a retirement community or nursing home. Some facilities are specialty-based; the most common type serves residents with Alzheimer's disease and other dementias. Assisted-living dementia units frequently provide care with greater attention to resident dignity, autonomy, safety, and quality of life than is ordinarily available in a nursing home dementia unit.

5. What is a continuing care retirement community?

Continuing care retirement communities (CCRCs) are retirement communities that provide a spectrum of services ranging from independent living to assisted living or nursing facility care. These programs also are called life care communities because the long-term contract provides for housing, community services, nursing care, and other health care programs for the duration of the recipient's life. There are three common types of CCRC contracts. The first may offer nursing care with little or no increase in monthly payments. The second may place a cap on the amount of nursing care that is covered; beyond the cap additional payments are made. The third type of contract may require full per-diem rates for all nursing care. CCRCs generally require a one-time entrance fee that may or may not be partially refundable. Monthly fees generally depend on the size and amenities of the resident's housing.

The average age at entry of CCRC residents is about 77, younger than with assisted living. About 23% of CCRC residents are married couples, whereas most assisted-living residents are single or widowed. Many CCRCs contract with primary care physicians who then manage the care and health care services provided in all settings. Most CCRCs have on-campus assisted living and nursing care, but some have one or both levels available off site, although they still are covered by contract.

6. What is adult day care?

Adult day care offers various supportive and social services and health care in a community-based environment during daytime hours. Services may be used part-day or full-day, usually 1–5 days weekly. The clients of adult day programs typically have a mix of physical and cognitive impairments for which they need assistance. Most but not all clients live with caregivers who are unable to provide full daytime care because of work schedules or the need for daytime respite care. Typically one meal and a schedule of activities are the focus of the program. Some programs offer specialized services, including dementia programs, incontinence management, and pain management. Some offer more extensive services, including rehabilitation therapies and physician services. Transportation often is coordinated by the center, and some centers offer transportation services directly for a fee.

7. What other community-based alternative long-term care programs are available?

The most commonly used alternative to nursing home care for frail elders in need of assistance with daily functioning is informal caregiver services in the home setting. Most older Americans prefer to live independently in their own homes for as long as possible, and although this is not possible for all dependent elders, most are able to remain in the community, often living with family or other caregivers, while receiving community-based services. For every older person being cared for in an institutional long-term care setting, at least three or four with equal impairment are cared for in the community.

8. What is respite care?

Respite care provides relief for usual caregivers. Most often it involves a short admission, ranging from a few days to a few weeks, to a nursing home or assisted-living facility. Respite care has become widely available in recent years at most community long-term care facilities and is financed on a per-diem rate paid by the patient. The cost of this service may be less than half the cost of nursing home care; however, most insurance plans, including Medicare and Medicaid, do not cover the costs of respite care. Respite care may be needed to provide caregiver relief for vacation, provision of personal health needs, or periodic relief to prevent caregiver stress and exhaustion. It generally is believed that the availability of respite care delays or prevents the need for institutionalization for many functionally impaired elders living in community settings.

9. What is PACE?

One unique community-based program covered by Medicare is the Program for All-inclusive Care for the Elderly (PACE). PACE is an optional benefit under both Medicare and Medicaid that provides comprehensive community-based care for people who qualify for nursing home care according to state standards. The PACE program uses a case-management approach to provide medical, rehabilitation, social, and personal services to its enrollees. Services are available 7 days per week; usually an adult day health center serves as the base of operations. PACE care may include care at the day center as well as in-home care. Primary care physicians and nurses provide continuous care, including treatment of acute illness. The PACE program currently operates nationally in 24 centers with plans for annual expansion. Since its beginning in 1986, the PACE program has proved to be successful in providing high-quality community-based long-term care as well as preventing nursing home placement and reducing hospitalization. At the same time, most programs have demonstrated cost savings in caring for extremely frail and chronically ill elderly patients compared with usual options.

10. What factors determine which level of care an individual requires?

The two most important factors that determine level of care are functional status and medical needs. **Functional assessment** is the process through which an individual's ability to perform basic and instrumental activities of daily living is evaluated. The pattern of functional deficits predicts what services the person will need. For example, unmanaged bowel incontinence, complete feeding dependency, and requirement of two persons for transfers are functional problems that frequently predict the need for nursing home care rather than alternative types of long-term care. Assisted-living facilities often will not accept residents with unmanaged urinary incontinence, any degree of feeding dependency, or inability to transfer independently and ambulate with minimal assistance. The two IADLs indicating that an independent elder with basic ADLs may be safely left alone for brief periods in a community setting are the ability to provide meals and hydration and the ability to use a telephone to call for emergency assistance.

Medical needs that may predict nursing home care rather than alternatives include extensive wound care needs in bed-bound patients and management of complex comorbid active diseases (e.g., diabetes, congestive heart failure, chronic obstructive pulmonary disease, coronary heart disease) that require close monitoring and adjustment of treatment regimens.

11. What principles of preventive health care apply to alternative long-term care?

Typical health promotion and disease prevention activities that are appropriate for independent, high-functioning elderly people may not be effective or desired by frail older populations in need of long-term care. Examples include cancer screening and cardiovascular risk reduction in people without known cardiovascular disease. There are, however, several areas in which prevention is quite important. Depression is extremely prevalent in long-term care populations (50–60% of nursing home residents have symptoms of depression). Periodic screening for depression can be accomplished with such tests as the 15-item Geriatric Depression Scale. Frail, functionally impaired elders also are at high risk for weight loss with subsequent malnutrition. Monitoring monthly weights and checking baseline serum albumin levels are effective measures for early diagnosis of protein malnutrition. Prevention of infectious disease by maintaining vaccination with pneumococcal, influenza, and tetanus vaccines is recommended for elders in all long-term care settings. Residents in long-term care programs generally are at high risk for falls and fall-related injuries, including hip fracture. Prevention of falls is best achieved by implementing a formal program to identify risk factors and to design specific interventions that reduce or eliminate those risks.

12. What role do physicians play in the care of patients in alternative long-term care settings?

Physicians have a central role in the care of nursing home residents, in part due to extensive state and federal regulations that mandate regular visits by physicians to nursing home residents. Although regular on-site physician visits are not required by regulations in other settings, the role of physicians and mid-level practitioners is vital to the delivery of high-quality care in alternative long-term care settings. Physicians see residents in assisted-living facilities at a growing rate, partly because reimbursement recently has been improved and partly because the boom in the development of larger assisted-living facilities makes them an efficient site for physician practice. The physician's role in home care visits to chronically ill elderly people is also a growing trend nationally. On-site physician services usually are an integral part of continuing care retirement communities. Most adult day programs do not incorporate on-site physician services.

13. What factors indicate the need for hospitalization to manage acute illness among individuals in long-term care programs?

Hospitalization for long-term care residents usually is indicated by the need for medical services that are not available in the current setting or by the development of barriers to services, such as poor coordination of care or financing problems. Common medical conditions that lead to hospitalization include inadequate oral intake, dehydration, infections, acute respiratory failure, unstable angina, gastrointestinal bleeding, and fractures of the lower extremity. Inadequate intake of food and fluid causing dehydration, due to either acute illness or progressive dysphagia, may result in the need for hospitalization for intravenous fluid or to establish access for enteral nutrition. Infections that require intravenous antibiotics are a common cause for hospitalization. However, many currently available broad-spectrum antibiotics have good oral bioavailability and have reduced the need for hospitalization to treat infection. Hospitalization for more intensive treatment or closer monitoring often is needed in patients with acute respiratory failure, unstable angina, and gastrointestinal bleeding. In addition, people who have multiple chronic comorbid conditions, such as chronic obstructive pulmonary disease, coronary heart disease, and diabetes, may have acute problems that require hospitalization.

Barriers to the management of acute illness in long-term care settings may involve lack of diagnostic or therapeutic services or delays in accessing these services; examples include laboratory, radiology, and pharmacy services. Long-term care settings may have nursing staffs that are less experienced or are not as highly trained in the management of acute illness as hospital nursing staffs. Lack of physician availability for diagnosis and treatment of acute illness may result in hospitalization of long-term care residents. In addition, there is the financial incentive of higher reimbursement for physicians for hospital-based care. Poor information transfer from prior health care settings in the long-term care continuum or between consultants and primary care physician may result in unnecessary hospitalization due to incomplete medical information upon which to make treatment decisions.

BIBLIOGRAPHY

1. Eng C, Pedulla J, Eleaser GP, et al: Program of All-inclusive Care for the Elderly (PACE): An innovative model of integrated geriatric care and financing. J Am Geriatr Soc 45:223–232, 1997.
2. Goldberg TH, Chavin SI: Preventive medicine and screening in older adults. J Am Geriatr Soc 45:344–354, 1997.
3. Gordon M: On-site acute care for residents of long-term care facilities. J Am Geriatr Soc 44:606–607, 1996.
4. Kane RA: Expanding the home care concept: Blurring distinctions among home care, institutional care, and other long-term-care services. Millbank Q 73:161–185, 1995.
5. Krothe JS: Giving voice to elderly people: Community-based long-term care. Public Health Nurs 14:217–226, 1997.
6. Phillips-Harris C, Fanale JE: The acute and long-term care interface: Integrating the continuum. Clin Geriatr Med 11:481–501, 1995.
7. White M: Eligibility in the ever-changing continuum of care. Ann Long-Term Care 7:112–114, 1999.

57. COMPLEMENTARY AND ALTERNATIVE MEDICINE

Elizabeth R. Mackenzie, Ph.D.

1. What is complementary and alternative medicine?

The National Center for Complementary and Alternative Medicine (NCCAM) at the National Institutes of Health (NIH) defines complementary and alternative medicine (CAM) as "those treatments and health care practices not taught widely in medical schools, not generally used in hospitals, and not usually reimbursed by medical insurance companies." This definition covers a wide array of modalities, from chiropractic manipulation, therapeutic massage, and reflexology to homeopathy, herbal medicines, traditional Chinese medicine (including acupuncture, tai chi, qigong), Ayurvedic medicine (including yoga and meditation), spiritual healing, and shamanism. These examples are only a small fraction of the kinds of unconventional healing practices available in the U.S. However, most have some underlying assumptions or perspectives in common. CAM purports to be holistic; that is, it treats the whole person, including physical, mental, emotional, and spiritual dimensions.

Biomedicine has been the dominant form of health care in the U.S. since the mid-nineteenth century. It relies largely on sophisticated surgical techniques, vaccines, antitoxins, and other pharmaceutical preparations. Biomedicine rose to dominance in large part because of its many impressive successes (e.g., vaccines to reduce childhood diseases, antibiotics to treat infection). Despite growing interest in biopsychosocial approaches to health among providers and health researchers, conventional medicine typically has compartmentalized the practice and study of medicine into separate specialties and subspecialties. Although allowing greater intellectual precision, this compartmentalization has resulted in a somewhat fragmented approach to understanding health and disease. Generally speaking, "holism" is one way to differentiate CAM from conventional biomedicine. A corollary is that CAM seeks to heal the person rather than to cure the disease.

CAM systems focus on prevention and health promotion (or wellness) rather than on treating symptoms after they have arisen. Because conventional health care has a growing interest in health promotion and because consumer demand for access to holistic forms of medicine has increased, certain facets of CAM are gradually finding their way into the mainstream, often making it difficult to distinguish among systems that are alternative, complementary, integrated, integrative, or conventional. For example, the use of vitamin E for Alzheimer's disease began as a CAM intervention but has been largely adopted by mainstream medicine. Acupuncture used to be viewed askance by the medical community and is now practiced in many large hospitals nationwide. Many health systems are adding CAM clinics or holistic programming. This pattern of inclusion of CAM modalities into conventional medicine, shown to be effective, is part of the process of creating "integrated medicine," a health care system that uses the perspectives and techniques of both biomedicine and CAM.

Ambiguities surrounding the categorization of particular modalities and systems probably will become even more pronounced as managed care organizations and insurers begin to cover CAM modalities and as medical schools offer courses in CAM or integrated medicine, according to their own definitions of the category.

An often overlooked characteristic of CAM modalities is that many originated in the healing traditions of specific cultural or ethnic groups, typically from non-Western societies. In fact, these healing traditions (or ethnomedicine) have engendered a vast array of CAM systems. Traditional Chinese medicine or traditional Oriental medicine, the Indian Ayurvedic tradition, and herbal and shamanic healing from tribes across North and South America, Africa, Australia, and Eurasia have contributed much to our knowledge of nonbiomedical healing systems. Only a few modalities have their roots in Western Europe (e.g., chiropractic manipulation, homeopathy, naturopathic medicine, European folk medicine, and certain religious healing traditions). Various modalities developed in the past few decades do not have explicitly ethnomedical roots, such as numerous body work techniques designed to help people achieve enhanced structural balance (e.g., Rolfing, Alexander, and Feldenkrais techniques, cranial-sacral therapy), treatments that require special technology (e.g., biofeedback, transcutaneous electrical nerve stimulation), and the use of various nutritional supplements (e.g., glucosamine sulfate to treat arthritis). Nonetheless, there is a significant overlap between CAM and ethnomedicine.

2. Do older adults use CAM?

Over one-third of older adults (aged 50+) in the U.S. use CAM. In a survey of 101 primary care physicians treating persons diagnosed with probable Alzheimer's disease, Coleman et al. found that over one-half administered at least one CAM therapy. Among the most popular CAM therapies for Alzheimer's disease are vitamins, health foods, herbal medicine (especially ginkgo biloba), music therapy, and home remedies. Patients with osteoarthritis also appear to be frequent users of CAM modalities; both acupuncture and glucosamine sulfate are popular CAM treatments for arthritis. Because so many of the chronic conditions most likely to be treated with CAM modalities are prevalent in older adults, and because the highest reported use nationally is in the 35–49-year-old group, CAM use among older adults can be expected to increase over the next several years.

3. How can the physician discuss CAM use with patients?

Despite the de facto integration of CAM into the health care landscape, a 1990 survey found that approximately 70% of persons who use CAM modalities do not discuss the topic with their physicians. Given the high probability that CAM use will affect conventional treatment plans and health outcomes, clinicians should include questions about CAM use. Eisenberg recommends the following approach: "Patients with [chief complaint] frequently use other kinds of therapy for relief. For example, some patients use chiropractic, massage, herbs, vitamins, etc. Have you used or thought about using any of these or other therapies for your [chief complaint] or for any other reason?" It is extremely important that the question be asked in a nonjudgmental and nonthreatening manner. Patients who sense that their medical provider disapproves of, ridicules, or disparages attempts to explore the potential benefits of CAM usually conceal their interest. Concealment may have seriously adverse consequences for the physician–patient relationship, possibly leading to lower quality of care. Clinicians should keep in mind that it is possible to acknowledge patients' beliefs about CAM without sharing them. Creating a psychological environment that supports forthright, respectful dialogue is the first step toward better understanding of CAM by both patients and providers.

4. To integrate or not to integrate?

Given the current trends in use of CAM, most clinicians probably will have to face the question of how comfortable they are with discussing and perhaps integrating aspects of CAM into their practice. There are three salient dimensions to this question: (1) Does it work? (2) Can it harm? (3) By whom should it be delivered?

5. Are CAM modalities efficacious?

Perhaps the most important piece of information about CAM from the point of view of the practicing clinician is, "Does it work?" The past decade or so has seen numerous U.S. studies of the efficacy of CAM modalities for particular conditions, many funded by the NIH. Although many studies have been inconclusive and some modalities have been shown to have dubious therapeutic value, investigations into a wide array of therapies indicate some promise. CAM modalities previously suggested to be efficacious for conditions common within the population of older adults are summarized in the following tables.

CONDITION	CAM TREATMENT	STUDY
Cognitive decline	Ginkgo biloba (herb)	Kanowski et al: Proof of efficacy of the ginkgo biloba special extract Egb 761 in outpatients suffering from primary degenerative dementia of the Alzheimer type and multi-infarct dementia. Pharmacopsychiatry 4:149–158, 1995.
Frailty, poor balance, falls	Tai chi	Wolf et al: Reducing frailty and falls in older persons. J Am Geriatr Soc 44:489–497, 1996.
Depression	Exercise	Moore, Blumenthal: Exercise training as an alternative treatment for depression among older adults. Alt Ther Health Med 4:48–56, 1998.
Osteoarthritis	Acupuncture	Bareta: Evidence presented to consensus panel on acupuncture's efficacy. Alt Ther Health Med 4: 22–30, 102, 1998.
Coronary artery stenosis	Support groups/ lifestyle changes	Ornish et al: Can lifestyle changes reverse coronary heart disease? The Lifestyle Heart Trial. Lancet 336:129–133, 1999.
Fibromyalgia	Acupuncture	Berman et al: Is acupuncture effective in the treatment of fibromyalgia? J Fam Pract 48:213-238, 1999.

CAM Modalities Currently under Investigation via NIH-NCCAM Grants

CONDITION	TREATMENT	STUDY
Sleep disorders (Parkinson's disease)	Melatonin	University of California at San Francisco (Dowling)
Agitation	Music and message	University of Massachusetts (Remington)
Knee osteoarthritis	Acupuncture	University of Maryland (Berman)
Depression	Hypericum (St. John's wort)	Duke University (Davidson)
Alcoholism	Acupuncture	Minneapolis Medical Research Foundation (Bullock)
Depression	Acupuncture	University of Arizona (Allen)

6. Can CAM modalities harm the patient?

For providers interested in integrating some CAM modalities into their practice, it is important to be aware of contraindications, herb-drug interactions, and other potential harmful effects of CAM use. Of greatest concern, especially in terms of toxicity, is herbal medicine or phytomedicine. Although herbal preparations often have fewer side effects than synthetically produced drugs and many are so benign that they can be used in large quantities under most circumstances (e.g., chamomile, red clover), some have the potential to harm when used improperly. For example, licorice root is known to raise blood pressure and should not be used by hypertensive patients. St. John's wort must be stopped 1 week before anesthesia/surgery. Echinacea, an herb used as an immune system booster, is contraindicated for persons with autoimmune disorders. Ginkgo biloba inhibits platelet-activating factor and therefore can interact adversely with antithrombotic drugs. Many herbs can induce menstruation (e.g., pennyroyal, feverfew), and pregnant women are well advised to use herbal teas, tinctures, and extracts with caution. Essential oils used in aromatherapy, although plant-derived and therefore a type of phytomedicine, are the extremely concentrated volatile oils of a plant (the "essence" of the plant) and should rarely if ever be taken internally.

Patients also may stop taking their prescribed medication, replacing it with a CAM treatment without their physician's knowledge. Although the hypertensive patient whose blood pressure becomes significantly lowered as a result of biofeedback or meditation may actually no longer require antihypertensive medication, it is best for this transition to occur gradually and under a physician's supervision.

7. By whom should CAM be delivered?

Because CAM covers such a broad array of modalities, philosophies, and cultural traditions, it is not always clear how to judge a practitioner's competence. Some modalities have rigorous licensing and training requirements (e.g., traditional Chinese medicine, massage, naturopathy), and licensed practitioners can be assumed to have reached a certain level of competence. National and state level associations usually publish lists of licensed and certified practitioners. However, some modalities have no such oversight, and many of the most skilled practitioners may be self-taught or educated under an informal apprenticeship (e.g., herbal medicine and various forms of ethnomedicine, such as curanderismo, santeria, Native American healing). Knowing who to trust is often best determined by the practitioner's local reputation among patients and health professionals alike. Another method for choosing a CAM practitioner is to seek out physicians or nurses who have undergone training in a specific modality. Numerous physicians now practice as acupuncturists, homeopaths, herbalists, or other CAM specialists.

8. What reliable resources are available for accurate information about CAM?

1. The NIH's National Center for Complementary and Alternative Medicine (NCCAM) offers information about use of CAM, including current and past research into efficacy and definitions. Their clearinghouse for information can be reached at 1-888-644-6226; their Web address is http://altmed.od.nih.gov/nccam/.

2. The American Holistic Health Association (AHHA) serves as a national association for CAM practitioners and a clearinghouse for information about CAM for the public. Web site: http://ahha.org; telephone: 714-779-6152.

3. Fleming T (ed): PDR for Herbal Medicines. Montvale, NJ, Medical Economics Company, 1998.

4. Blumenthal M (ed): The Complete German Commission E Monographs: Therapeutic Guide to Herbal Medicines. Newton, MA, Integrative Medicine Publishers/American Botanical Council, 1998.

5. Dossey L (ed): Alternative Therapies in Health and Medicine: Aliso Viejo, CA, Innovision Communications. Telephone: 1-800-899-1712.

6. Gordon J: Manifesto for a New Medicine: Your Guide to Healing Partnerships and the Wise Use of Alternative Medicine. Reading, MA, Perseus Books, 1996.

7. Eisenberg D: Advising patients who seek alternative medical therapies. Ann Intern Med 127:61–69, 1999 [includes an appendix listing information resources].

8. NIH, Office of Alternative Medicine: Alternative Medicine: Expanding Medical Horizons [Workshop on Alternative Medicine's Report to the NIH, Chantilly, VA]. Washington, DC, U.S. Government Printing Office, 1992.

BIBLIOGRAPHY

1. Astin JA: Why patients use alternative medicine: Results of a national study. JAMA 279:1548–1553, 1998.
2. Coleman LM, Fowler LI, Williams ME: The use of unproven therapies by people with Alzheimer's disease. J Am Geriatr Soc 43:829–830, 1995.
3. Eisenberg DM: Advising patients who seek alternative medical therapies. Ann Intern Med 127:61–69, 1997.
4. Eisenberg DM, Davis RB, Ettner SL, et al: Trends in alternative medicine use in the United States, 1990–1997: Results of a follow-up national survey. JAMA 280:1569–1575, 1998.
5. O'Connor BB: Implications for the health professions. In Healing Traditions: Alternative Medicine and the Health Professions. Philadelphia, University of Pennsylvania Press, 1995, pp 161–195.

INDEX

Page numbers in **boldface type** indicate complete chapters.

Terminally ill patients. *See also* Advance directives;
Palliative care
in nursing homes, 331
terminal sedation for, 145
Tests
false-positive/false-negative results of, 56, 57
sensitivity and specificity of, 56
Tetanus immunization, 66, 335
Thalamotomy, 177
Thalassemia, 203, 206
Thallium testing, preoperative, 131–132
Theophylline
drug interactions of, 96, 113
as insomnia cause, 46
Thromboembolism
postoperative, 130
preoperative prophylaxis for, 132–133
relationship to hormone replacement therapy,
159, 160
Thrombolytic therapy, 70, 912, 210, 218
Thrombosis
deep venous, 210
home health care for, 321
lower-extremity swelling associated with,
303–304
prophylaxis for, 134, 253
stroke-related, 193
as myocardial infarction cause, 210
as stroke cause, 187, 189, 210
Thrush, oral, 107
Thyroid, examination of, for involuntary weight loss
evaluation, 32
Thyroid cancer, 232
Thyroid disorders, **227–232**. *See also* Goiter;
Hyperthyroidism; Hypothyroidism
Thyroid function, evaluation of, 227–228
Thyroid hormones. *See also specific thyroid
hormones*
overdose of, 230
Thyroiditis, 230
autoimmune, 228
Thyroid nodules, 230
"cold," 231–232
Thyroid-stimulating hormone, 227, 228, 229–230,
231, 232
as heart failure indicator, 222
Thyroid storm, 231
Thyroid supplementation, as osteoporosis risk
factor, 256
Thyrotropin-releasing hormone, 227
Thyroxine, 227, 230–231, 232
as heart failure indicator, 222
as hypothyroidism therapy, 228–229
Ticlopidine
antiplatelet activity of, 210, 211
as stroke prophylaxis, 194–195, 214
Tinea cruris, 276
Tinea pedis, 307
Tissue plasminogen activator, 192, 218
Tobacco. *See also* Smoking
smokeless, 94
Tolcapone, as Parkinson's disease therapy, 174

Total knee replacement patients, anticoagulant
prophylaxis in, 133
Toxicosis, triiodothyronine, 230
Toxins, environmental
as Parkinson's disease cause, 173
role in aging, 7, 8
Trachea cancer, smoking-related, 95
Tramadol
as osteoarthritis therapy, 246
use in palliative therapy, 142
Transcutaneous electrical nerve stimulation
(TENS), 141, 246
Transdermal fentanyl system, 144
Transient ischemic attacks, 187
constipation-related, 40
diagnostic work-up of, 193
mimicking conditions of, 189–190
as stroke risk factor, 192, 194, 195
Transportation Department, mandated reporting of
impaired drivers to, 119
Travelers, immunization of, 68
Tremor, essential, 172
Tricyclic antidepressants, 167
as delirium cause, 17
as fatigue cause, 21, 22
as insomnia therapy, 48
as pain medication, 142, 144
as risk factor for falls, 198–199
Trigger point injections, 141
Triiodothyronine, 227, 228
Triiodothyronine resin uptake, 227–228, 230, 232
Trimethobenzamide, adverse effects of, 111
Trimethoprim, as acute renal failure cause, 264
Trimethoprim-sulfamethoxazole, as folate
deficiency cause, 205
Tritec triple therapy, for *Helicobacter pylori*
infections, 290
Troglitazone, as diabetes mellitus therapy, 236
Tuberculosis, 31, 329
Tumor necrosis factor, 31

Ulcers
diabetic, 236, 304
of the leg, 304–305
Marjolin's, 276
pressure. *See* Pressure ulcers
Ultrasound, of urinary bladder, 281
Undernutrition. *See* Malnutrition
Urea breath test, for *Helicobacter pylori* infection
diagnosis, 289
Urinalysis
for urinary incontinence evaluation, 282
use in heart failure diagnosis, 222
Urinary incontinence. *See* Incontinence, urinary
Urinary retention, as nortriptyline contraindication,
144
Urinary tract
aging-related changes in, 280
evaluation of, 280–282
in parkinsonism, 173
Urinary tract infections, 321, 329
Urine osmolarity, as dehydration indicator, 270

Uropathy, obstructive, 263, 264, 270
Uterine cancer, 161, 300

Vacuum tumescent devices, 36
Vaginal bleeding, 152, 153, 161–162
Vaginal discharge, 152, 156
Vaginal pessaries, 154–155
Vaginitis, atrophic, 156
Valproic acid, adverse effects of, 113
Values history, 135
Valvular heart disease, 210, 221
Vancomycin
    drug interactions of, 112
    enterococcal resistance to, 329
Vascular disease, 286
    peripheral, diabetes mellitus–related, 236
    smoking-related, 94
Vascular dysfunction, as erectile dysfunction cause, 34, 35
Vasodilators
    direct, as heart failure therapy, 224
    as fatigue cause, 22
Vasopressin, aging-related decrease of, 268–269
Venlafaxine, 167
Venous disease, as leg ulcer cause, 304–305
Venous insufficiency, as urinary incontinence cause, 277
Vertigo, **24–28**
    benign paroxysmal positional, 26, 27, 198
    differentiated from dizziness, 24
    differentiated from lightheadedness and dysequilibrium, 25
    as falls risk factor, 198
    stroke-related, 188
Vestibular dysfunction, as dizziness cause, 26
Vestibular rehabilitation, 26, 27
Vestibular suppressants, as vertigo therapy, 27
Veterans Administration system, 310–311
Vibratory sense, loss of, 54
Vigilance, 12
Viral infections. *See also* specific viral infections
    as septic arthritis cause, 248
Visceral pain, 140, 141, 142
Vision impairment
    aging-related, 50–51
    diabetes mellitus–related, 237
    effect on driving ability, 118, 119
    giant cell arteritis–related, 239–240
    parkinsonism-related, 173
Visuospatial tests, 184
Vitamin A, as pressure ulcer therapy, 275
Vitamin B$_{12}$ deficiency, 203, 205
Vitamin C
    as osteoarthritis therapy, 247
    as pressure ulcer therapy, 275
Vitamin D, as osteoporosis prophylaxis, 259
Vitamin D deficiency, as osteoporosis risk factor, 256
Vitamin E
    as Alzheimer's disease therapy, 184, 186
    antiplatelet activity of, 210
    as osteoarthritis therapy, 247

Vitamin K, effect on warfarin kinetics, 214
Voiding records, 282
Volume depletion, 269
    as acute renal failure cause, 264
Volume repletion, in hospitalized hypernatremic patients, 269–270
Volvulus, 40
Vulva, disorders of, 162

Walking, as exercise, 78, 235
Warfarin
    age-related sensitivity to, 110
    as atrial fibrillation therapy, 212
    drug interactions of, 113, 213, 214
    interaction with alcohol, 93
    as osteoporosis risk factor, 256
    pharmacokinetics and pharmacodynamics of, 211, 214
    preoperative use of, 132, 133
    as secondary stroke prophylaxis, 212
    as stroke prophylaxis, 193, 195
Weakness, differentiated from fatigue, 20
Wear and tear theories, of aging, 7, 8
Weber-Rinne test, 26
Weight gain, hormone replacement therapy–related, 160
Weight loss
    as diabetes mellitus therapy, 235
    as hypertension therapy, 101
    involuntary, **30–33**
        cancer-related, 30, 31
        diabetes mellitus–related, 233, 234
        infection-related, 328–329
        in long-term care residents, 326, 327, 328–329, 335
        malnutrition-related, 275
        significant, 81
    for osteoarthritis management, 245
Wheelchairs, 125–126, 201–202
    pressure ulcer-preventive seating systems for, 272–273
"Widower's syndrome," 34, 35
Wilson's disease, 173
Withdrawal
    from aclohol, 92
    as delirium cause, 17
    as insomnia cause, 46
    naloxone-related, 145
    from smoking, 96
Women's health issues, **152–163**
    menopause, 155–162
        definition of, 155
        hormone replacement therapy for, 156–162
        symptoms of, 156
    pelvic relaxation, 152–155
Wrinkles, 303

Xerosis, 303
Xerostomia, 30, 31, 107–108
X-rays
    of chest, for heart failure diagnosis, 222
    of osteoarthritis, 245